Treatment and Therapy of Addictions

Treatment and Therapy of Addictions

Edited by **Don Boles**

FOSTER
ACADEMICS

New Jersey

Published by Foster Academics,
61 Van Reypen Street,
Jersey City, NJ 07306, USA
www.fosteracademics.com

Treatment and Therapy of Addictions
Edited by Don Boles

International Standard Book Number: 978-1-63242-409-9 (Hardback)

This book contains information obtained from authentic and highly regarded sources. Copyright for all individual chapters remain with the respective authors as indicated. A wide variety of references are listed. Permission and sources are indicated; for detailed attributions, please refer to the permissions page. Reasonable efforts have been made to publish reliable data and information, but the authors, editors and publisher cannot assume any responsibility for the validity of all materials or the consequences of their use.

The publisher's policy is to use permanent paper from mills that operate a sustainable forestry policy. Furthermore, the publisher ensures that the text paper and cover boards used have met acceptable environmental accreditation standards.

Trademark Notice: Registered trademark of products or corporate names are used only for explanation and identification without intent to infringe.

Printed in the United States of America.

Contents

Permissions

List of Contributors

Preface

The researches compiled throughout the book are authentic and of high quality, combining several disciplines and from very diverse regions from around the world. Drawing on the contributions of many researchers from diverse countries, the book's objective is to provide the readers with the latest achievements in the area of research. This book will surely be a source of knowledge to all interested and researching the field.

Addiction, increasingly recognized as a heterogeneous brain disorder, is one of the most distinct psychiatric pathologies in that its management includes miscellaneous, often non-overlapping, resources from the biological, psychological, medical, economic, social, and legal realms. Despite various researches, till now there are no dependably effective treatments of addiction. This may result from a lack of acknowledgement of the etiology and pathophysiology of this disease and also from the lack of concern into the potential differences among patients in the way they interact compulsively with their drug. This book presents an outlook of the psychobiology of addiction and its therapeutic strategies from pharmacological, social, behavioural, and psychiatric approaches. This book would serve as a valuable guide for those involved in the field of addiction control.

In the end, I would like to express my deep sense of gratitude to all the authors for meeting the set deadlines in completing and submitting their research chapters. I would also like to thank the publisher for the support offered to us throughout the course of the book. Finally, I extend my sincere thanks to my family for being a constant source of inspiration and encouragement.

Editor

Addiction Treatment – Pharmacology

1

N-Acetylcysteine as a Treatment for Addiction

Jennifer E. Murray[1,2,*], Jérôme Lacoste[3] and David Belin[2,4]
[1]Department of Experimental Psychology, University of Cambridge, Cambridge,
[2]INSERM European Associated Laboratory, Psychobiology of Compulsive Habits,
[3]Unité de Recherche Clinique Intersectorielle,
Centre Hospitalier Henri-Laborit, Poitiers,
[4]INSERM U1084 - LNEC & Université de Poitiers,
AVENIR Team Psychobiology of Compulsive Disorders, Poitiers,
[1,2]UK
[2,3,4]France

1. Introduction

Drug addiction is a chronic relapsing disorder characterized by compulsive use despite negative consequences and relapses even after years of abstinence (Leshner, 1997). Criteria put forth by the American Psychiatric Association (2000) for diagnosing drug addiction require at least three of the following symptoms associated with drug use: tolerance; withdrawal; a loss of control over drug intake; unsuccessful attempts to reduce intake; a significant amount of time spent acquiring, using, or recovering from the substance; reduced interest in social or work activities; and continued use despite awareness of adverse physical and psychological consequences (American Psychiatric Association, 2000). In the United States, 22.5 million people, or 8.9% of the population meets the criteria for substance dependence or abuse (Substance Abuse and Mental Health Services Administration, 2010), and in Europe, drug, and especially cocaine, use has been increasing over the last ten years in the general population, with a more pronounced trend in young individuals (EMCDDA, 2009), suggesting that cocaine addiction may continue to spread in western countries. Worldwide estimates suggest more than 8% of the population have an alcohol use disorder and more than 2% have an illicit drug use disorder (World Health Organization, 2010).

The prevalence of drug use despite obvious health and financial consequences is a testament to the tenacity of addiction as a brain disease affecting cognition, motivation and memory (Leshner, 1997). At the psychobiological level, addiction has been hypothesised to reflect the development of loss of executive control over aberrant incentive habits (Belin et al., 2009a, Belin & Everitt, 2010), resulting from drug-induced neuroplasticity processes in vulnerable subjects. These plasticity processes have been suggested to stem from the impact of drug action on the mesolimbic dopamine system, through which drug use can induce a host of changes in the brain resulting in significant neural reorganization (see Lüscher & Malenka, 2011, Russo et al., 2010). Much of this reorganization is due to long term potentiation, or strengthening, of excitatory synapses as a result of drug use. As recently reviewed, the

---

* Corresponding Author

dopamine signals from neurons originating in the ventral tegmental area (VTA) targeting the nucleus accumbens (NAc) in the ventral striatum modulate glutamate synaptic plasticity and are believed to be critically involved in the pathophysiology of addiction (Chen et al., 2010).

In animal models using passive drug exposure, these neurons show an N-methyl-$_D$-aspartate (NMDA) receptor-dependent strengthening of excitatory synapses (long term potentiation) 24 hrs following an acute experimenter-administered injection of cocaine, amphetamine, nicotine, ethanol, and morphine (Saal et al., 2003; Ungless et al., 2001). Interestingly, this strengthening was not found with the non-abused psychoactive drugs, fluoxetine or carbamazepine, suggesting the role this plasticity may play in determining whether a drug is abused or not.

Although of interest, these data capture neither the volitional aspect of drug use nor the instrumental nature of drug seeking and taking, thereby greatly limiting their translation to the pathophysiology of addiction (Belin et al., 2009b, Belin & Dalley, 2012). Therefore, in preclinical models, a more valid approach to the human drug administration situation is the self-administration paradigm in which – akin to the human experience – an animal, rather than the experimenter, voluntarily administers the drug through instrumental conditioning (see later).

Following two weeks of cocaine self-administration, long term potentiation of glutamate function in DAergic VTA neurons is maintained even after 90 days of abstinence – an effect not found in a yoked, non-contingent control group receiving the same cocaine exposure (Chen et al., 2008). Similarly, measurements in the core of the NAc (NAcC) – where VTA projections are now known to co-release glutamate along with DA (Stuber et al., 2010) – following at least two weeks of cocaine self-administration, showed long-lasting resistance to the induction of long-term synaptic depression compared to yoked controls or controls lever pressing for food reinforcement. Finally, cocaine self-administration followed by either a 3-week abstinence period or 3 weeks of extinction training induced a state of long-term potentiation of glutamate synapses that was resistant to further potentiation (Moussawi et al., 2009). The resistance to further potentiation has been attributed to the prolonged expression of AMPA receptors that had been trafficked to the cell membranes during the drug exposure (Chen et al., 2010) and is indicative of long-lasting neural reorganization brought about by drug abuse. Combined, these data indicate that volitional administration of cocaine results in prolonged changes in NMDA receptor-dependent synaptic plasticity within the nucleus accumbens (Martin et al., 2006).

This long-term strengthening of glutamatergic synapses within the brain reward circuitry as a result of chronic voluntary drug use is also related to dysregulation of glutamate homeostasis (for a review see Kalivas, 2009). Glutamate homeostasis refers to the balance between synaptic glutamate levels and extracellular, extrasynaptic glutamate levels that regulate stable neurotransmission (see Figure 1). If synaptic glutamate release is the key component of glutamate-induced excitatory synaptic transmission, extrasynaptic glutamate is vital for the negative feedback of glutamatergic transmission. This negative feedback is necessary for modulating and inhibiting further excitatory stimulation. Such feedback is supported by activation of extrasynaptically-localized Group II metabotropic glutamate autoreceptors (mGluR2/3 receptors) which results in a regulated reduction of vesicular neurotransmitter release whereby synaptic glutamate concentration is greatly decreased (Dietrich et al, 2002; Manzoni et al., 1997).

Extrasynaptic glutamate availability is primarily provided by the cystine/glutamate exchanger antiporter (system xc-) found on brain glial cell membranes (Baker et al., 2002). System xc- transports the extracellular cystine dimer into the astrocytes and intracellular glutamate out of the astrocytes and into the extracellular space in a 1:1 ratio, thereby enhancing extrasynaptic glutamate levels (Bannai, 1986). Glutamate availability inside the astrocytes is provided by the primary glial glutamate transporter, GLT-1 (Haugeto et al., 1996), and these two systems work in concert to maintain homeostatic glutamate levels. Seven days of cocaine exposure (experimenter administered 15-30 mg/kg daily) followed by three weeks of abstinence, or self-administration (0.25 mg/kg in 2-hr sessions until responding stabilized to <10% variation) followed by extinction (until active lever pressing declined to at least 10% of self-administration levels) decrease basal levels of extracellular glutamate by ~50% within the NAcC. Extracellular glutamate levels are then elevated again into a range between about 160-600% of the withdrawal baseline following cocaine re-exposure (e.g., Baker et al., 2003a; Baker et al., 2003b; McFarland et al., 2003; Pierce et al., 1996). This dysregulation of glutamate homeostasis as a result of drug withdrawal has been suggested to be caused by an overall downregulation of system xc- and is in fact mimicked by blocking system xc- in the NAc (Baker et al., 2003b). Indeed, following chronic cocaine or nicotine self-administration, there is reduced NAc expression of both xCT, the light chain and catalytic subunit of the system xc- antiporter heterodimers, and GLT-1 (Knackstedt et al., 2009; 2010a), indicating these mechanisms are involved in the dysregulation of glutamate homeostasis and may impact the development and trajectory of addiction.

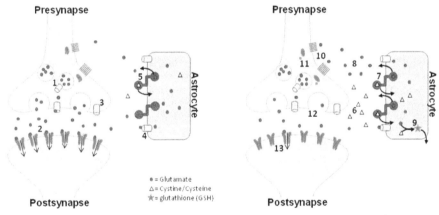

Fig. 1. Actions of N-acetylcysteine on the cystine/glutamate exchanger (system xc-). Glutamate is packaged into presynaptic vesicles by vesicular glutamate transporters (vGluTs) [1]. Following release of glutamate into the synaptic cleft, glutamate binds to postsynaptic localized ionotropic receptors (iGluRs) such as the α-amino-3-hydroxy-5-methylisoxazole-4 propionic acid (AMPA), N-methyl-D-aspartate (NMDA), and kainate receptors [2]. Excitatory amino acid transporters (EAATs) clear extracellular glutamate by taking it back up into cells. These transporters are localized on the presynaptic terminal [3] protecting extrasynaptic receptors from synaptic glutamate and synaptic receptors from extrasynaptic glutamate, and allow for re-packaging glutamate into vesicles. These transporters are also localized on astrocytes [4]. Once in the glial cell, glutamate can be transported into the extrasynaptic

environment by the cystine/glutamate exchanger (system xc-) in a 1:1 ratio [5]. Administration of NAC provides extra synaptic cysteine that is oxidized extracellularly into the cystine [6] required to enhance activation of the cystine/glutamate exchanger [7]. The enhanced xc-activation results in increased glutamate concentration in the extracellular space [8]. Intracellular cystine is rapidly reduced to cysteine where it is combined with intracellular glutamate (and glycine) in the synthesis of glutathione (GSH) which is then released from the astrocyte [9]. Extrasynaptic glutamate binds to and activates mGluR2/3 receptors [10] which negatively regulate adenylyl cyclase [11] thereby suppressing presynaptic glutamate release [12] and reducing postsynaptic iGluR activation [13].

2. Mechanisms of N-acetylcysteine action

The cysteine prodrug and antioxidant precursor, N-acetylcysteine (NAC), has been in use in humans for many years, primarily as a treatment for acetaminophen/paracetamol overdose (Prescott et al., 1977; Scalley & Conner, 1978) and more recently as a mucolytic agent effective in chronic obstructive pulmonary disease (Decramer & Janssens, 2010; Kory et al., 1968) and cystic fibrosis (Dauletbaev et al., 2009; Stamm & Docter, 1965). Further, an evaluation of the potential therapeutic use of NAC in a variety of psychiatric disorders has been recently reviewed (Dean et al., 2011). The aforementioned nature of the neurophysiological changes induced by drug use has also indicated a potential use for NAC treatment in addictions, prompting the initiation of thorough research into NAC as a treatment for addiction in both preclincal models of addiction and drug addicts

In preclinical models of addiction, NAC appears to regulate the systems involved in glutamate homeostasis in the brain. Following 7 days of cocaine exposure and 21 subsequent days of withdrawal, decreased basal extracellular glutamate levels in the NAc are recovered following an IP injection of NAC in rats (Baker et al., 2003a). Notably, inhibition of system xc- prevented the NAC-induced recovery of extracellular glutamate levels in this region, implicating the xc- system in the neurobiological mechanisms whereby NAC normalises cocaine-induced extracellular glutamate dysregulation (Baker et al., 2003a). Thus, NAC may induce a recovery of the downregulated xCT and GLT-1 function (Knackstedt et al., 2009; 2010a). Indeed, the recovery of an altered GLT-1 function allows for increased transport of glutamate into the astrocyte while the recovery of altered system xc-function by xCT recovery allows for increased export of glutamate back into the extrasynaptic space (see Figure 1). The resulting increase in extracellular glutamate then facilitates activation of extrasynaptic mGluR2/3 autoreceptors, ultimately reducing evoked synaptic glutamate release (Moran et al., 2005). This decrease in synaptic glutamate release as a downstream result of NAC administration is the mechanism by which NAC also restores the capacity to induce further long-term potentiation, since blockade of mGluR2/3 receptors prevented this restoration (Moussawi et al., 2009).

NAC is also a known precursor of the endogenous antioxidant, glutathione (GSH), the synthesis of which depends upon the rate-limiting activity of the xc- system. GSH is primarily produced within astrocytes using glutamate and cystine as substrates to generate γ-glutamylcysteine, which is then combined with glycine to create GSH (see Dringen & Hirrlinger, 2003). GSH is released from astrocytes into the extracellular space, where it is broken down by γ-glutamyltranspeptidase into glutamate and a cysteine-glycine dipeptide that is further hydrolyzed into the individual peptides. This reaction is the mechanism by which astrocytes provide the precursors necessary for neuronal GSH production (Dringen & Hirrlinger, 2003). In addition to protecting brain cells from the oxidative stress, GSH has been shown to enhance responsivity of NMDA receptors to glutamatergic stimulation (see Janáky et al., 1999), suggesting some direct modulation of glutamatergic signalling as a result of NAC administration. The role of GSH in addiction has yet to be determined, and thus far, the effects of NAC as a pharmacotherapy for drug dependence appear to be primarily mediated via its actions on system xc- and GLT 1 (Knackstedt et al., 2009; Knackstedt et al., 2010a).

3. N-acetylcysteine in animal models of self-administration, reinstatement, and relapse

The study of the addictive properties of drugs in animals is largely based on variations of the self-administration procedure developed in rats by Weeks (1962; see Belin & Dalley 2012; Panlilio & Goldberg, 2007). Although now conducted with many species, in its simplest and most common form, rats (or mice) are prepared with indwelling intravenous catheters that exit through a backmount to be attached to a tether hanging within a conditioning chamber. Tubing connecting the catheter to a syringe outside the chamber runs through the tether and provides the route by which drugs can be administered directly into the blood stream (see Figure 2).

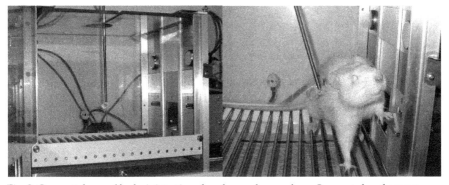

Fig. 2. Operant drug self-administration chamber and procedure. Operant chambers are typically equipped with two retractable levers (assigned as either 'active' or 'inactive') with a cue light above each. When a rat presses the active lever under an FR1 schedule, the resulting drug infusion is accompanied by the onset of the cue light associated with the active lever.

When in the self-administration chamber, two levers are typically available – an 'active' and an 'inactive' lever. Under the most basic Fixed Ratio 1 (FR1) schedule of reinforcement, also called continuous reinforcement, a single press on the active lever results in a drug infusion often paired with a non-drug stimulus, such as a brief presentation of a light. The drug delivery reinforces the behavior, making it more likely the rat will press the active lever again (cf. Hall, 2002). Presses on the inactive lever have no consequence and are used as an index of general activity. This self-administration procedure is particularly useful in determining the abuse liability of psychoactive substances (for a review see O'Connor et al.,

2011). The ability to self administer drugs for short periods of time daily (1-2 hrs per session) results in a stable drug intake over time, a so-called titration process that is suggested to reflect individual control of intake responding to optimal dosing (Wilson et al., 1971; Zimmer et al., 2011) around which blood levels fluctuate in the course of the self-administration session.

Pharmacological challenges during ongoing self-administration, following extinction or abstinence, or before relapse or reinstatement of self-administration (see later) have been useful in identifying potential targets for the development of pharmacotherapies for various forms of addictions (e.g., Schindler et al., 2011; Steensland et al., 2007). Such an approach is based on the common psychodynamic view of the addiction process of which the stages, namely development, maintenance, and relapse/reinstatement, are modelled in Figure 3.

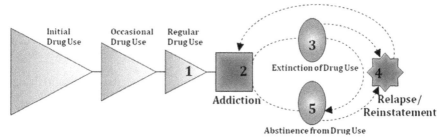

Fig. 3. Stages of the development and maintenance of addiction in humans and animal models. Stages of the addiction cycle that have been targeted with NAC treatment are regular drug use before the development of addiction as defined by the DSM-IV [1], thereby aiming at preventing the transition from controlled to compulsive drug use, the addiction stage (in animal models, when intake has escalated or become habitual) [2], following behavioral extinction of drug seeking predominately seen in animal models – human addicts rarely engage in extinction [3], at the time drug or a drug-associated cue is re-introduced causing reinstatement [4], following short- or long-term abstinence from drug more typical for human addicts and increasingly modelled in animals [5], and at the return to the drug-seeking/taking context, resulting in relapse [4].

A reasonable time point for targeting addiction is when the individual is still regularly engaged in drug use with the intended outcome of reducing intake and eventually stopping use altogether. Therefore, it is of interest to assess potential pharmacotherapies during the self-administration phase. In a standard self-administration task, that is thought to model the stage in which humans engage in regular use but are not necessarily addicted (Figure 3, Stage 1), rats that had access to cocaine for 2 hrs under an FR1 schedule of reinforcement, and administered 60 mg/kg NAC before each daily training session displayed no differential intake as compared with vehicle-treated controls (Amen et al., 2011; Madayag et al., 2007).

The efficacy of NAC on ongoing cocaine intake changes however, with increasing access to cocaine. Indeed, with long (e.g., ≥6 hrs) rather than short (e.g., 2 hrs) daily access to cocaine self-administration, rats no longer titrate intake, but instead tend to increase, or escalate, their intake across days (cf. Ahmed & Koob, 1998). This escalation of drug intake over time, associated with dysregulation of neural networks governing reward (for a review see Koob

& Kreek, 2007), has been suggested to reflect the loss of control over intake that characterises human drug addicts (Figure 3, Stage 2). In an experiment assessing the effects of NAC on cocaine escalation (Madayag et al., 2007), rats initially acquired cocaine (0.5 mg/kg) self-administration in 2-hr sessions under an FR1 schedule of reinforcement until intake stabilized (<10% variation across ≥3 sessions). They were then shifted to 6-hr daily sessions for 11 days in which they were able to self-administer a higher dose of cocaine (1.0 mg/kg) and subsequently given either 60 mg/kg NAC or vehicle pre-treatment. Whereas saline-pre-treated rats displayed typical escalation of their cocaine intake across sessions, NAC-pretreated rats maintained a stable drug intake across days (Madayag et al., 2007). In a similar study, daily pretreatment with the higher dose of 90 mg/kg NAC appeared to reduce cocaine intake across the 12 sessions of long-access cocaine self-administration compared to saline pretreatment (Kau et al., 2008). Combined, the findings that NAC impacts escalation without affecting typical short-access drug self-administration suggests that loss of control over drug intake may be better reflective of dysregulated glutamate homeostasis.

3.1 Treatment during reinstatement of drug seeking

The ultimate goal of any addiction therapy is to achieve and maintain drug abstinence. This therapeutic goal is especially challenging due to the strong associations formed between the interoceptive drug experience and surrounding cues. Re-experiencing a drug or drug cue following a successful quit attempt can evoke and enhance drug craving (e.g., Niaura et al., 1988; O'Brien et al., 1992), thus increasing the likelihood of reinstatement of drug use, often resulting in relapse. As such, finding effective techniques that target the motivational impact of a 'lapse' in drug use (drug-induced reinstatement) or drug-related paraphernalia (cue-induced reinstatement) is of high therapeutic value for maintaining drug abstinence.

From an experimental standpoint, when operant behavior no longer results in the delivery of the reinforcing outcome, extinction occurs, so that instrumental performance declines (Figure 3, Stage 3). Extinction of a behavior is a new learning process that exists alongside the old, previously learned, association (for a review see Bouton, 2002). This new learning is largely dependent on continued absence of the primary reinforcer while the manipulanda (i.e., levers) are still available to press. In humans, these sort of explicit extinction sessions are generally only provided within the context of cue-exposure therapy which aims at presenting inpatients with drug use paraphernalia in the absence of the drug (see Monti & MacKillop, 2007; Siegel & Ramos, 2002). Reinstatement of the previously extinguished behavior can therefore be evoked by presentation of the reinforcer (i.e., drug-induced reinstatement) or a conditioned stimulus (CS) associated with the reinforcer that had not presented during the extinction phase (i.e., cue-induced reinstatement; Figure 3, Stage 4; de Wit & Stewart, 1981).

When an addict 'lapses', or uses once, following abstinence, he is at a much higher risk for re-engaging in regular use. Attenuating the effects of this drug-induced reinstatement may help prevent a 'lapse' in drug abstinence from turning into a full-blown relapse of addiction (e.g., Shadel et al., 2011; Witkiewitz & Masyn, 2008). In rats, cocaine exposure following extinction of self-administration is associated with a glutamate release from prefrontal projections into the NAcC (McFarland et al., 2003), and this release may provide the mechanism that triggers reinstatement of drug seeking. Acute treatment with NAC has been shown to attenuate drug-induced reinstatement. In some of these experiments, rats were trained to self-administer cocaine in 2-hr or 6-hr daily sessions. During the subsequent extinction phase, instrumental responses were reinforced only with contingent presentations of the drug-associated light, and no cocaine was infused, so lever pressing progressively declined. For the drug-induced reinstatement test, rats were injected with a priming dose of cocaine, this pharmacological challenge resulted in a marked increased in the previously extinguished instrumental response, i.e., lever pressing. Pretreatment with 30, 60, or 600 mg/kg NAC before cocaine re-exposure prevented reinstatement of cocaine-seeking behavior (Baker et al., 2003a; Baker et al., 2003b; Kau et al., 2008; Moran et al., 2005). Concurrent blockade of system xc- using (S)-4-carboxyphenylglycine (CPG) during the reinstatement test blocked the reinstatement-attenuating effects of NAC (Kau et al., 2008), thereby suggesting that NAC effects on cocaine-induced reinstatement are mediated through system xc-. Additionally, as measured by in vivo microdialysis during the reinstatement test, NAC administration restored the reduced extracellular glutamate levels that resulted from cocaine self-administration and withdrawal (Baker et al., 2003b). Further, concurrent blockade of mGluR2/3 autoreceptors also prevented the attenuating effects of NAC on cocaine-induced reinstatement (Moran et al., 2005) demonstrating that the effect of NAC restoration of extracellular glutamate on reinstatement may depend upon activation of the mGluR2/3 autoreceptors.

The effects of NAC on drug-induced reinstatement have also been shown when NAC is administered prior to, but not explicitly during, the reinstatement test. In one such experiment, rats were trained to self-administer cocaine under short-access conditions and then underwent extinction followed by cocaine-primed reinstatement (Amen et al., 2011). Following the first test in which cocaine seeking was reinstated, rats were treated with 60 mg/kg NAC for 7 days. The day following the seventh NAC treatment, rats were subjected to a second cocaine-primed reinstatement test. Rats that had received NAC treatment showed significantly reduced cocaine seeking compared to the rats that had received saline treatment during those 7 days (Amen et al., 2011). Although daily treatment with 60 mg/kg NAC before 2-hr cocaine self-administration sessions (see above) had no effect on amount of cocaine taken or subsequent extinction (without NAC pretreatment), cocaine-primed reinstatement was significantly reduced, even though it had been 2-3 weeks since last NAC treatment (Madayag et al., 2007). Similarly, 90 mg/kg NAC pretreatment throughout long-access cocaine self-administration resulted in attenuated cocaine-primed reinstatement that was reversed by inhibition of system xc- following an extinction phase without NAC (Kau et al., 2008). These effects are indicative of the long-lasting protection of glutamate homeostasis as a result of NAC treatment. Indeed, concurrent microdialysis in the NAc immediately prior to the reinstatement test showed that there were lower extracellular basal glutamate levels in rats that had been pretreated with saline during the self-administration stage than in those that had been pretreated with NAC (Madayag et al., 2007). Once cocaine had been administered to induce reinstatement, the saline-pretreated group reached the level of extracellular glutamate that was shown at baseline by the NAC-pretreated group. These findings suggest that NAC administration during self-administration provided protection against the withdrawal-induced downregulation of extracellular glutamate in the NAc and subsequent cocaine-induced reinstatement.

3.2 Treatment during extinction and reinstatement

The effect of chronic NAC treatment during both extinction and subsequent reinstatement tests has also been evaluated (Figure 3, Stages 3 and 4). In one such study (Reichel et al., 2011), rats were trained to self-administer cocaine (50 µg/infusion) under an FR1 schedule until they reached >10 infusions in two hours for twelve consecutive sessions. During the following twelve sessions, lever presses had no programmed consequences (i.e., extinction), and rats were given daily injections of 0, 60 or 100 mg/kg NAC. There was no effect of the lower 60 mg/kg dose of NAC on extinction responding. However, there was a significant enhancement of extinction (i.e., less active lever pressing) when rats were treated daily with 100 mg/kg NAC (Moussawi et al., 2011; Reichel et al., 2011). This effect was also found during extinction of heroin self-administration for which daily administration of 100 mg/kg NAC resulted in enhanced extinction rate (Zhou & Kalivas, 2008). Although NAC treatment was ineffective when applied during acquisition of self-administration, it enhanced extinction learning.

In each of these studies, two tests of reinstatement were then conducted: cue-induced reinstatement and cue+drug- or drug-induced reinstatement. Human addicts are particularly sensitive to cues that had previously been associated with drug use, and exposure to these cues following drug abstinence can reinstate drug seeking and taking behavior, resulting in relapse (see O'Brien et al., 1992; Taylor et al., 2009). Similarly, rats are also quite sensitive to the effects of re-presentation of these drug-associated CSs. As such, the impact of NAC treatment on cue-induced reinstatement of instrumental responding has recently begun to be assessed. For the cocaine self-administration group treated with the lower, 60 mg/kg, dose of NAC, there was a significant reduction in cue-induced reinstatement compared to saline controls, but no effect on cue+drug-induced reinstatement (Reichel et al., 2011). However, when NAC (100 mg/kg) was administered during extinction following either cocaine or heroin self administration, there was a significant reduction in both cue- and cue+drug- or drug-induced reinstatement. These results suggest that, compared to a conditioned stimulus, a higher treatment dose was necessary to disrupt the ability of an unconditioned drug stimulus+drug-associated CS compound to reinstate drug-taking behavior (Moussawi et al., 2011; Reichel et al., 2011; Zhou & Kalivas, 2008). Notably, these effects on reinstatement lasted from two weeks (Moussawi et al., 2011; Reichel et al., 2011) to 40 days (Zhou & Kalivas, 2008) following the last 100 mg/kg NAC treatment, indicating a long-term restoration of glutamate homeostasis in the NAcC brought about by the re-regulation induced by chronic NAC exposure (Moussawi et al., 2011). At the neurophysiological level, rats trained to self-administer cocaine that received saline (rather than NAC) during extinction showed reduced extrasynaptic glutamate levels in the NAcC compared to saline-yoked controls. In rats that received NAC during extinction, there was full recovery of the extrasynaptic glutamate levels two weeks following the last NAC injection – a time period corresponding to the behavioral effect on cue- and cue+drug-induced reinstatement (Moussawi et al., 2011). Furthermore, administration of the mGluR2/3 antagonist, LY341495, into the NAcC prevented the attenuating effects of NAC on cue- and cue+drug-induced reinstatement of cocaine-seeking, again indicating the importance of presynaptic autoreceptors in maintaining glutamate homeostasis (Moussawi et al., 2011).

3.3 Treatment during abstinence

A key concern with the translational potential of the extinction-reinstatement model of drug dependence is that human users are not typically subjected to extinction of responding during presentation of drug-related cues unless they are patients in an explicit cue-exposure therapy session (cf. Monti & MacKillop, 2007). Rather, addicts undergo abstinence – a period in which they either voluntarily (i.e., independently, or by checking into a rehabilitation clinic) or forcibly (e.g., incarceration) abstain from drug use outside the drug-taking environment (Figure 3, Stage 5; Reichel & Bevins, 2009). Following the abstinence period, a person returns home where the associative strength of all the drug-associated cues is still fully intact, and no behavior has been extinguished, and 'relapse' of the addictive behavior often resumes.

A rat model of 'forced abstinence' operationally uses the same drug self-administration protocols as the extinction-reinstatement model, but rather than undergoing an extinction phase in which responding diminishes with repeated non-reinforced lever pressing, the animal is typically left in its home cage for a specified period of time (e.g., 2 weeks) where it can undergo a treatment protocol before returning to the drug-associated conditioning chamber. Notably, extinction and abstinence following cocaine self-administration produce different patterns of protein expression in the NAc (Knackstedt et al., 2010b), warranting further investigation into the efficacy of potential pharmacotherapies in each model of addiction.

The abstinence model has recently been used to assess the efficacy of NAC treatment following cocaine self-administration (Reichel et al., 2011). Rats were trained to self-administer cocaine under an FR1 schedule until they reached >10 infusions in two hours for twelve consecutive sessions. During the subsequent two-week abstinence period, rats were given daily injections of 60 or 100 mg/kg NAC or saline. They were then tested for relapse to cocaine seeking by returning them to the self-administration environment and recording non-reinforced lever presses. Treatment with the lower, 60 mg/kg, dose of NAC during abstinence had no effect on relapse compared to saline, however, treatment with the higher 100 mg/kg dose of NAC during abstinence significantly reduced cocaine-seeking during the relapse test (Reichel et al, 2011). During subsequent tests in which the drug-paired cue, and then the drug+cue, was presented, 100 mg/kg NAC treatment during abstinence maintained a significant effect on drug seeking. Finally, following a second phase of abstinence in which no NAC was administered, there was still a significant attenuation of drug seeking when rats were presented with the drug+cue in the self-administration chamber, again indicative of the long-term re-regulation of glutamate homeostasis provided by NAC administration.

3.4 Treatment during habitual drug seeking

Regular daily drug use is not limited to the taking of the drug. Rather, addicted individuals can invest countless hours 'foraging' for their next high. This foraging takes a person through multiple exposures to stimuli that are predictive of the impending drug experience. As such, not only can these drug-associated CSs reinstate drug-seeking behavior when presented following behavioral extinction but they can also serve as powerful conditioned reinforcers that drive and maintain continued drug foraging over long periods of time when presented contingently. This foraging can continue to persist even after the explicit drug-taking behavior has been extinguished (Olmstead et al., 2001; Zapata et al., 2010), indicating a habitization of the drug-seeking behavior which may be a key characteristic in the transition from casual drug use to addiction (e.g., O'Brien et al., 1998, Everitt & Robbins 2005, Belin et al., 2009a).

Cocaine seeking (see Chapter 2) as opposed to mere cocaine taking, or self-administration, has been operationalized in primates (Goldberg, 1973) and then in rats (Arroyo et al., 1998) and humans (Panlilio et al., 2005) in the so-called second-order schedule of reinforcement. In this specialized model of self-administration, drug seeking is separated from the unconditioned effects of the drug. Cues associated with drug reinforcement function as conditioned reinforcers that maintain persistent, habitual, seeking responses across protracted periods of time without primary drug reinforcement (Everitt & Robbins, 2000; Schindler et al., 2002).

In this procedure, rats are initially trained to self-administer drug under the FR1 schedule of reinforcement with a single lever press resulting in a drug infusion associated contingently with a 20-second cue light presentation. Following stabilization of responding, the response requirement is shifted across days to gradually move the behavior of the rat to what is known as a second-order schedule of reinforcement. There are several ways of increasing the response requirement (cf. Economidou et al., 2011; Vanderschuren et al., 2005, Belin & Everitt 2008), either by introducing ratio / ratio increments or fixed interval schedules with increasing interval durations across days. In the experiment in which NAC effect was measured on early and well-established cue-controlled cocaine seeking (Murray et al., 2012), rats were moved up through the following schedules: FR3; FR5(FR2:S); FR10(FR2:S); FR10(FR4:S); FR10(FR6:S); FR10(FR10:S); FI15(FR10:S). Under each of these schedules of cocaine reinforcement, completion of each unit schedule (given within the parentheses) resulted in a 1-second cue light presentation; cocaine infusions were delivered only upon completion of the first unit schedule according to the schedule outside the parentheses. Therefore, during the final second-order training schedule [i.e., FI15(FR10:S)], cocaine and the 20-second cue light were given on completion of the first FR10:S unit after the Fixed Interval 15-minute period had timed out. In these conditions instrumental responding is no longer under the control of the goal, from which it is now temporally distal, but instead becomes highly dependent upon contingent presentations of conditioned CSs, acting as conditioned reinforcers (cf. Arroyo et al., 1998). As shown in Figure 4, following acquisition of the second-order schedule, removal of CSs (i.e., 1-second light presentations provided under a FR10 schedule of reinforcement are removed, returning the animal to a strict FI15 schedule of reinforcement) results in a decline in lever pressing across sessions in the first 15-minute interval that is reversed when the unit schedule is returned (i.e., 1-second light presentations under FR10). By the time behavior has reached this stage of training, drug seeking during the first 15-min drug-free interval is maintained at very high rates and is thought to reflect cue-controlled habitual cocaine seeking which, at the neurobiological level, has been hypothesised to result of a gradual recruitment of dorsolateral striatal dopamine circuitry (Belin & Everitt, 2008; Ito et al., 2002; Murray et al., in press; Vanderschuren et al., 2005).

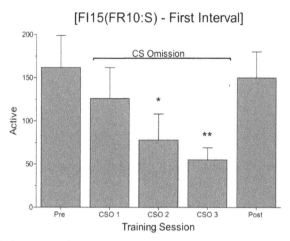

Fig. 4. Control of cocaine seeking by contingent presentations of conditioned reinforcers. Three consecutive days of conditioned reinforcer (1-s cocaine-associated light presentations) omission (CSO 1-3) are compared with performance on the session before conditioned reinforcer omission (Pre) and performance on the session when the reinforcer is returned (Post). * indicates significant difference from Pre, p<.05, **p<.01. Adapted from Arroyo et al (1998) with permission from Springer.

Assessment of drug seeking before actual drug reinforcement can be conducted at both an early stage of acquisition and at a later, well-established stage. To assess drug seeking in the early stage when the behavior had only ever been reinforced under an FR1 schedule of reinforcement by the unconditioned drug stimulus with concurrent CS presentations, a switch in the contingency was instituted for a 15-min test session. This testing procedure allowed for measurement of drug seeking now reinforced by 1-sec cue light presentations. Cocaine was delivered only on the first lever press following the 15-min interval, and each test was immediately followed by an FR1 training session. The effects of acute NAC treatment on cocaine seeking during the early-stage tests are shown in Figure 5A. Drug seeking before the experience of unconditioned cocaine effects was reduced with 60 and 90 mg/kg NAC treatment.

After increasing the response requirements and at least 15 sessions of FI15(FR10:S) training, so that cocaine seeking maintained by regular contingent presentations of the drug-associated conditioned reinforcer was well-established, conditions known to be associated with a shift in the locus of control over behavior from the ventral to the dorsolateral striatum (Vanderschuren et al., 2005; Belin & Everitt, 2008), the effect of NAC pre-treatment on cocaine seeking was measured once again (Figure 5B). At this stage, drug seeking was more sensitive to NAC treatment, with 30, 60, and 90 mg/kg disrupting the conditioned reinforcing effects of the cocaine-associated stimulus. The results of this experiment demonstrate that acute NAC treatment dose-dependently reduced cocaine seeking maintained by conditioned reinforcers both at an early stage of acquisition when drug seeking is considered to be goal-directed and following extensive training on the second-order schedule, when drug seeking is considered to be habitual (Murray et al., 2012). These findings demonstrate that NAC pretreatment may be an aid to establish abstinence by reducing cocaine seeking in individuals that actively seek cocaine on a daily basis, rather than only during relapse following an extinction or abstinence period.

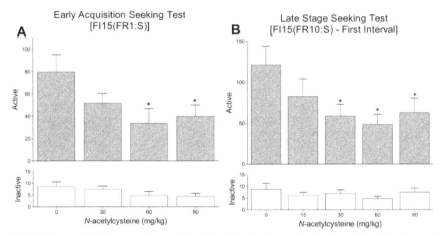

Fig. 5. Effects of NAC on cocaine seeking. Panel A depicts active (top) and inactive (bottom) lever presses during acute NAC treatment in the 15-min cocaine seeking test with contingent conditioned reinforcer presentations (FR1) at an early stage of self-administration. Panel B depicts active (top) and inactive (bottom) lever presses during acute NAC treatment in the first 15-min cocaine seeking interval with contingent conditioned reinforcer presentations (FR10) during the late stage of cocaine self-administration. For both panels, * indicates significant difference from 0 mg/kg NAC, p<.05. Adapted from Murray et al. (2012) with permission from Wiley.

4. N-acetylcysteine in humans: From acetaminophen overdose antidote to addictive and impulsive-compulsive spectrum disorders

NAC, as an antioxidant and gluthatione precursor, has been used for more than 30 years in intravenous or oral protocols as an acetaminophen poisoning antidote. Within this framework, NAC has been shown to have low rates of adverse reactions which nevertheless include nausea, vomiting, as well as cutaneous and systemic anaphylactoid reactions. ECG abnormalities, status epilepticus and fatal reaction due to NAC overdose are rare, the latter having been observed only at doses 10 times greater than the recommended antidote dose (for review see Sandilands & Bateman, 2009). Atopy and asthma are major risk factors for developing adverse and anaphylactoid reactions to NAC (Schmidt & Dalhoff, 2001).

Thanks to its antioxidant effect, NAC has dose dependent protective effects against contrast-induced nephrotoxicity (Briguori et al., 2011). NAC can also be used as both a chelating agent for methylmercury (for review see Dodd et al., 2008) and a mucolytic and anti-inflammatory agent, with controversial efficacy in patients with exacerbations of chronic obstructive pulmonary disease (Decramer et al., 2005). Unlike orally-administered gluthatione and L-cysteine, NAC successfully crosses the blood-brain barrier, and permits restoration of glial and neuronal gluthatione levels, playing a role in the oxidative homeostasis in the brain, protecting neurons against oxidative stress. In addition, NAC treatment reduces levels of some pro-inflammatory cytokines (IL-6, IL-1β, and TNF-α) shown to be implicated in several psychiatric disorders, notably in depressive and bipolar disorders as well as in schizophrenia. NAC has been used to target the prefrontal glutamatergic dysfunction implicated in schizophrenia and impulsive-compulsive behaviors (for reviews see Dean et al., 2011; Sansone & Sansone, 2011). One of the first uses of NAC in psychiatry was a case-report of the amelioration of self-injurious behaviors and craving in a female patient suffering from Post-traumatic Stress Disorder and borderline personality disorder (Pittenger et al., 2005). There are to date very few rigorous studies assessing the efficacy of NAC in the treatment of addiction and impulsive-compulsive spectrum disorders (including behavioral addictions, impulse-control disorders and obsessive-compulsive and related disorders). Those available, despite limited statistical evidence (randomized studies with small size samples, non-randomized cohorts, or case reports), have provided consistent results, in that NAC was always reported to reduce drug use, craving or withdrawal symptoms during the treatment period, sometimes even resulting in a persistent effect on relapse after the end of the trials (Olive et al., 2012).

4.1 NAC and cocaine dependence

NAC treatment for addiction has been primarily studied in cocaine dependent patients, alongside the aforementioned publication of preclinical studies initiated by Kalivas' team (Baker et al., 2003a; Baker et al., 2003b). In one such study, the safety and tolerability of NAC have been assessed in 13 otherwise-healthy, non-treatment-seeking, cocaine-dependent patients with a mean age of 37.1 ± 7.6. During the first hospitalization of the experiment, patients received either four treatments of NAC (600 mg per treatment; 2400 mg total) or placebo spaced 12 h apart. In a cross-over design, the opposite treatment (i.e., NAC or placebo) was given during a hospitalization during the second week. NAC treatment resulted in a significant reduction of withdrawal symptoms (assessed with the Cocaine Selective Severity Assessment, CSSA, a measure of cocaine abstinence signs and symptoms; Kampman et al., 1998) while placebo had no effect. The effect of NAC treatment was not restricted to withdrawal symptoms since it was also accompanied by an overall reduction in self-reported craving (five items, including desire to use, level of craving and other similar constructs, rated on ten-point Likert scales). In this study NAC was well tolerated during the treatment periods, with neither significant adverse effects nor with effects on primary biological parameters (renal and liver functions, complete blood count) between groups. In addition, at completion of the two-week follow-up period patients displayed a marked decrease both in days of cocaine use from 41% ± 7 (in the ninety days before study) to 27% ± 7, and average daily dollar expenditure for cocaine from $30.31 ± 3.44 (in the ninety days before study) to $8.77 ± 2.52, suggesting that a brief NAC treatment, perhaps through promotion of reduced withdrawal symptoms and subjective craving, may have a prolonged efficacy even weeks after the end of the treatment (LaRowe et al., 2006).

In addition to this clinical evaluation, at the end of the treatment period, the same patients were exposed to a cue-reactivity procedure to assess cocaine desire. During two sessions, patients were semi-randomly presented cocaine-related, neutral, and affective (pleasant and unpleasant) slides. Cocaine-related slides produced greater skin conductance than either neutral or pleasant slides. NAC treatment did not modify physiological reactions to any of the slides viewed (i.e., skin conductance and heart rate measures). Cocaine slides evoked higher ratings of craving for, desire to use, and interest in, cocaine, as well as longer viewing times relative to neutral slides. NAC treatment resulted in lower motivation to use cocaine in comparison with placebo when viewing cocaine slides, characterized by a reduced desire to use, a reduced interest in cocaine, and less time viewing cocaine slides. Craving for cocaine was also reported to be lower in NAC- than in placebo-treated participants even though this difference did not reach statistical significance (LaRowe et al., 2007).

In an independent laboratory study in 6 cocaine-dependent patients, with a mean age of 41.8 ± 7.4 and a mean age of drug-use onset of 18.3 ± 4.0, subjective 'high', 'rush', and craving for cocaine were assessed using a computerized version of a ten-point Likert scale. The patient had to use a joystick and move a tab along a horizontal bar with the anchors 'Least Ever' and 'Most Ever' at each extreme end, then push a button at the desired rating after viewing either a neutral or a cocaine video and after a 20 mg/kg IV cocaine infusion. This assessment was conducted the day before and after 3 days of NAC treatment (1200 mg or 2400 mg daily, TID). NAC treatment significantly reduced subjective craving induced by cocaine infusion, as measured before and after treatment. By contrast, NAC affected none of the subjective measures induced by cocaine videos, nor did it affect subjective feelings of high and rush induced by the cocaine infusion (Amen et al., 2011).

Finally, in an open-label study, 23 cocaine-dependent patients, with a mean age of 40 ± 1.4 and a mean lifetime of cocaine use of 13.3 ± 1.5 years, were treated for 4 weeks with three different doses of NAC (1200, 2400 or 3600 mg/day). In a subjective evaluation, the three doses of NAC decreased the mean number of days of use (from 8.3 ± 1.3 to 1.1 ± 1.4) and the dollar amount spent (from $1292.8 ± 508.6 to $52.2 ± 25.9) across the 28 days of treatment. This was in agreement with an objective evaluation revealing that urine drug screens were negative in two-thirds of the sample during treatment (without comparison with baseline due to a lack of significant sampling during this period). Cocaine abstinence symptoms (assessed with the CSSA) decreased during the treatment period. Retention in treatment was significantly better in the 2400 mg and the 3600 mg groups than in the 1200 mg group (88.9% and 83% respectively, vs. 37.5%). Adverse events were mild to moderate, including headache, pruritus and elevated blood pressure, but did not significantly differ among the treatment groups (Mardikian et al., 2007).

These results indicate that administration of NAC (at daily doses of 2400 and 3600 mg) can be an effective treatment for relapse prevention in cocaine-dependent patients, due to its ability to decrease withdrawal symptoms and craving severity. The severity of the cocaine withdrawal symptomatology at treatment entry is negatively correlated with the treatment outcome and the duration of continuous abstinence from cocaine (Kampman et al., 2002). Furthermore, subjective and objective feelings of craving, even during experimental cue-induced and cocaine-infusion procedures, which are predictors of early drug-use outcomes and rapid treatment attrition (Rohsenow et al., 2007), are reduced by NAC, a treatment that results in few mild-to-moderate side effects. Further studies with high-level evidence (i.e., randomized, double-blind, placebo-controlled, long-term studies) must be conducted in cocaine-dependent patients to determine the effective dosing ranges, the optimal duration of treatment, and the indications of NAC as a treatment for cocaine withdrawal or as an anti-addiction drug (used as an adjunct to psychotherapy to help patients in maintain abstinence).

4.2 NAC and marijuana dependence

In an open-label study, 24 cannabis-dependent subjects aged 18-21 were treated for 4 weeks with 1200 mg NAC twice daily (Gray et al., 2010). During the trial, the medication adherence was good (82.6% of scheduled doses), and adverse events were mild-to-moderate – none leading to discontinuation of the treatment. In a subjective evaluation at the fourth week of treatment, NAC significantly decreased the number of days per week cannabis was used, and showed a tendency to reduce the quantity of self-reported marijuana used per day (15.9 ± 2.4 vs. 11.9 ± 2.1 potency-adjusted 'hits'). In an objective evaluation, the cannabinoid content of urine samples was not affected, but craving for marijuana, measured by the Marijuana Craving Questionnaire, was significantly reduced. These results show the potential promise for NAC treatment of cannabis abuse and dependence, especially provided that no effective treatments are available for this particularly vulnerable population. A double-blind placebo-controlled study evaluating the efficacy of NAC (1200 mg twice daily for 8 weeks) combined with Contingency Management on marijuana use in a younger population (ages 13-21) is currently recruiting (NCT01005810).

4.3 NAC and methamphetamine dependence

In a small double-blind placebo-controlled study (Grant et al., 2010), 31 methamphetamine-dependent patients, with a mean age of 36.8 ± 7.12 and a mean age of onset of drug use of 24.3, were treated during 8 weeks with NAC (increased dose from 600 mg daily to 2400 mg daily every 2 weeks) and naltrexone (increased dose from 50 mg daily to 200 mg daily every 2 weeks) or placebo. In a subjective evaluation, at the end of the study, NAC+naltrexone treatment decreased the mean number of days of use every two weeks from 8.1 ± 4.9 to 1.9 ± 1.8 days in comparison with placebo (from 6.3 ± 4.6 to 2.3 ± 3.5 days). In an objective evaluation given at the end of the study however, positive urine drug screens did not differ between groups (46.2% vs. 35.3%). Concerning methamphetamine craving (assessed with the Penn Craving Scale: a self-report measure of frequency, intensity, and duration of craving, ability to resist taking drug, and an overall rating of craving for methamphetamine), NAC+naltrexone treatment did not result in significant improvement since there was no difference between the two groups in their decrease in total score at the end of the study (-43.6% vs. -37.7% for treated and placebo patients, respectively). Rates of adverse events (including nausea and lethargy) did not significantly differ between groups (57.1% vs. 41.2%). This preliminary 8-week study suggested that NAC+naltrexone treatment effectively reduced reported frequency of methamphetamine use even without affecting overall craving for the drug.

4.4 NAC and nicotine dependence

In a double-blind placebo-controlled study, 26 nicotine-dependent patients, with a mean age of 50, who had been smoking for an average of 33 years, were treated for 4 weeks with NAC (2400 mg daily) or placebo (Knackstedt et al., 2009). NAC treatment did not affect the objective measures related to nicotine dependence including carbon monoxide levels, or craving for cigarettes (assesssed with the Questionnaire for Smoking Urges-Brief), nor did it affect withdrawal symptoms (assessed with the Minnesota Nicotine Withdrawal Scale). In a subjective evaluation, there was a trend towards an overall reduction in cigarette use during the study (main effect of time), but no group effect, indicating a lack of efficacy of that dose of NAC on tobacco use. In a separate double-blind placebo-controlled study, 22 students at least twenty years old smoking for an average of 6 years, received NAC (1800 mg twice daily) or placebo for 4 days (Schmaal et al., 2011). None of the subjects reported smoking during the 4 days of treatment. At the end of the experiment, NAC did not affect craving for cigarettes (assessed with the Questionnaire for Smoking Urges-Brief) or withdrawal symptoms (assessed with the Minnesota Nicotine Withdrawal Scale). However, compared to placebo, NAC reduced the subjective rewarding effect of a cigarette smoked at the end of the experiment, suggesting a potential preventative impact of the treatment on relapse.

4.5 NAC and alcohol dependence

NAC has just been evaluated for an 8-week treatment of alcohol dependence, but the results are not yet published (NCT00568087). NAC has only been fully assessed in humans for its antioxidant properties, with some results in combination with corticosteroids and enteral nutrition in the treatment of severe acute alcoholic hepatitis (for review see Reep and Soloway, 2011), while a recent study shows minimal benefits of the combination therapy by prednisolone plus NAC in terms of survival among patients with this indication (Nguyen-Khac et al., 2011). Finally, preliminary findings in rats suggest NAC may also be helpful in the prevention of alcohol-induced heart disease (Seiva et al., 2009). Clearly, further work regarding the potential of NAC treatment for alcohol dependence needs to be conducted.

4.6 NAC and opiates dependence

To our knowledge, NAC has not yet been evaluated in the treatment of opiate dependence in humans.

4.7 NAC and pathological gambling

NAC treatment has been shown to reduce pathological gambling. In an open-label study (Grant et al., 2007), 27 subjects who engaged in pathological gambling, with a mean age of 50.8 ± 12.1 and a mean age of onset of problem gambling of 37.1 ± 12.8, were treated for 8 weeks with NAC (increased dose from 600 mg daily to 1800 mg daily every 2 weeks). Twenty-three patients (85.2%) completed the study for which the primary outcome was the effect of NAC treatment on the pathological gambling score, an adaptation of the Yale-Brown Obsessive-Compulsive Scale (PG-YBOCS), measuring the severity and change in severity of pathological gambling symptoms (Pallanti et al., 2005). Of those that completed the study, 16 patients (69.6%) were responders on the PG-YBOCS, showing a 30% or greater reduction in total score at end-point compared with baseline. Ten patients reported total abstinence from gambling. The total score on the PG-YBOCS decreased during the treatment phase from 20.3 ± 4.1 to 11.8 ± 9.8. On the overall severity and change in clinical symptoms (assessed by the Clinical Global Impression-Improvement scale, a 7 point scale that requires the clinician to assess how much the patient's illness has improved or worsened relative to a baseline state at the beginning of the intervention), 59.3% of patients were 'much' or 'very much' improved at the end of the study. Urge, thought, and self-reported gambling symptoms were improved after NAC treatment. In a second phase, 13 of the patients who completed the open-label study and were considered responders were included in a double-blind placebo-controlled study with NAC treatment at the highest dose or placebo for another 6 weeks. At the end of the 6 weeks, 83.3% of active treatment patients vs. 28.6% of placebo patients still met responder criteria on the PG-YBOCS.

4.8 NAC and impulsive-compulsive spectrum disorders

Finally, NAC has been assessed in several impulsive-compulsive spectrum disorders other than addictions, including trichotillomania, obsessive-compulsive disorder (OCD), and nail-biting in patients suffering from bipolar disorder. In a double-blind placebo-controlled study (Grant et al., 2009), 50 patients with trichotillomania (compulsive hair-pulling), with a mean age of 34.3 ± 12.1 and a mean age of onset of 12.1 ± 5.0 years, were treated for 12 weeks with NAC (1200 mg daily for 6 weeks, then 2400 mg daily) or placebo. Eighty-eight percent of all patients completed the study regardless the group assignment. In a subjective evaluation, NAC-treated patients, as compared to those treated with placebo, displayed significant reductions in the severity of trichotillomania symptoms according to the patient self-rating (using the Massachusetts General Hospital Hair Pulling Scale) and the physician-assessment (with the Psychiatric Institute Trichotillomania Scale), associated with a significant improvement of the severity and the resistance and control dimensions of the disorder. On the severity and change in global clinical symptoms (assessed by the CGI-improvement scale), 56% of NAC patients were 'much' or 'very much' improved at the end of the study compared with 16% of those taking placebo. In a report series, NAC used as an add-on therapy in the treatment of bipolar disorder was associated with a dramatic reduction in nail-biting behavior in three cases (Berk et al., 2009). NAC efficacy on this behavior may be due either to an anti-impulsive action of NAC or to an effect on anxiety or stress. In a case report, NAC has been used in conjunction with fluvoxamine (a serotonin-reuptake inhibitor agent) treatment in a refractory OCD patient. During a total period of 12 weeks, including 7 weeks at the total daily dose of 3000 mg, Y-BOCS scores decreased dramatically and the patient was able to resist her compulsive symptoms during the treatment period (Lafleur et al., 2006).

These findings attest to the promise NAC treatment has for treating the behavioral symptoms of impulsive/compulsive disorders. Three double-blind placebo-controlled studies are currently being carried out, demonstrating the recent interest for NAC in the treatment of impulsive-compulsive spectrum disorders. The first one is evaluating the efficacy of NAC (3000 mg twice daily for 12 weeks) in adult Serotonin Reuptake Inhibitor-refractory obsessive-compulsive disorder and depression (NCT00539513). The second one is evaluating the efficacy of NAC (1600 mg twice daily for 2 weeks then 2600 mg capsules twice daily for the remaining 10 weeks) for the treatment of pediatric obsessive-compulsive disorder (NCT01172275), and the third one is assessing the efficacy of NAC (from 1200 mg daily to 3000 mg daily, during 12 weeks) in pathologic skin picking (repetitive, ritualistic, or impulsive picking of otherwise normal skin leading to tissue damage, personal distress, and impaired functioning; NCT01063348). Moreover, NAC is currently being evaluated in a double-blind placebo-controlled study for children with Tourette syndrome (childhood-onset neuropsychiatric disorder characterised by multiple and chronic motor and vocal tics; NCT01172288).

5. Conclusion

In laboratory studies, NAC has been shown to prevent escalation of cocaine use during long access (6h/day) to the drug (an animal model of loss of control over drug intake, a hallmark feature of addiction) without affecting drug use during short access (1h and 2h/day). NAC also prevents relapse behaviors, reducing drug-associated cues-, cocaine-, and heroin-priming-induced reinstatement after extinction and abstinence protocols (animal models of relapse, when a drug-addicted individual is exposed to different triggers of drug craving and relapse after a period of abstinence). Finally, NAC reduces cocaine seeking, when drug seeking has become habitual (an animal model of the daily behavior of drug foraging, as it can be seen in individuals who spend great deal of time in activities necessary to obtain and prepare the substance, rather than only during relapse following an extinction or abstinence period). These preclinical data resonate well with the human literature which shows overall promising results from clinical trials on drug addiction and impulsive-compulsive spectrum disorders. More specifically, the efficacy of NAC treatment for cocaine addiction appears relevant, with improvement of withdrawal symptoms, attenuation of subjective and objective craving for the drug (during laboratory experiments, NAC attenuates environmental and cocaine-induced urges to use), and persistent reduction in cocaine use even after the end of the treatment. Results in cannabis addiction are less marked but also hold promise, notably due to the absence of available treatment for addicted young adults, who are particularly vulnerable to the development of other, stronger, addictions and psychotic comorbid disorders (Gray et al., 2010). Promising but mitigated results in methamphetamine and nicotine addiction should make us remember that the pathology of addiction may be quite different across drugs of abuse and that a single pharmacotherapy may not be sufficient for all drugs (cf. Badiani et al., 2011). Even if the small sample size of these studies may have precluded the identification of statistically significant differences between groups, negative results may also be attributable to the implication of other biological and psychological factors in methamphetamine and nicotine dependence and craving. In particular, learned contextual associations and context-induced relapse (Crombag et al., 2008) may not be affected by NAC treatment. Indeed, interesting preliminary results in other behavioral disorders including pathological gambling and impulsive-compulsive disorders, which appear alleviated with NAC treatment, may suggest that NAC is not necessarily working to treat these behavioral disorders at the same level of the drug of abuse.

At the neurobiological level this suggests that NAC-induced re-regulation of the homeostatic extrasynaptic glutamate levels in the brain may be affecting the behavioral component of 'seeking' – whether that be drug, a poker game, or the anxiety-alleviation provided by compulsive hair pulling. Preclinical studies using models in rats that specifically address the development of habitual drug seeking behavior, compulsive seeking and taking behavior, or addiction-like behavior (Belin et al., 2011) may help to elucidate the main psychological and associated neural substrate whereby NAC exerts its action and so in the different addictions, as it has been shown, for example, that opiate and stimulants addiction are behaviorally and neurobiologically distinct (for review see Badiani et al., 2011). Studies evaluating the efficacy of NAC on neuropsychological processes that contribute to the development of drug addiction, (e.g., decision-making or impulsivity) may also prove useful. In humans, clinical studies should take interest in assessing efficacy of NAC as a cognitive enhancer (Brady et al., 2011), as it has been shown that improvement of inhibitory control, attentional and decision-making processes may help individuals perform better in face of stressful and complex environmental situations.

6. References

Ahmed SH, Koob GF (1998) Transition from moderate to excessive drug intake: change in hedonic set point. Science 282:298-300.

Amen SL, Piacentine LB, Ahmad ME, Li S-J, Mantsch JR, Risinger RC, Baker DA (2011) Repeated N-acetyl cysteine reduces cocaine seeking in rodents and craving in cocaine-dependent humans. Neuropsychopharmacology 36:871-878.

American Psychiatric Association (2000) Diagnostic and Statistical Manual of Mental Disorders DSM-IV-TR. Washington DC.

Arroyo M, Markou A, Robbins TW, Everitt BJ (1998) Acquisition, maintenance and reinstatement of intravenous cocaine self-administration under a second-order schedule of reinforcement in rats: effects of conditioned cues and continuous access to cocaine. Psychopharmacology 140:331-344.

Badiani A, Belin D, Epstein D, Calu D, Shaham Y (2011) Opiate versus psychostimulant addiction: the differences do matter. Nat Rev Neurosci 12:685-700.

Brady KT, Gray KM, Tolliver BK (2011) Cognitive enhancers in the treatment of substance use disorders: clinical evidence. Pharmacol Biochem Behav 99:285-294.

Baker DA, Xi Z-X, Shen H, Swanson CJ, Kalivas PW (2002) The origin and neuronal function of in vivo nonsynaptic glutamate. J Neurosci 22:9134-9141.

Baker DA, McFarland K, Lake RW, Shen H, Toda S, Kalivas PW (2003a) N-acetyl cystine-induced blockade of cocaine-induced reinstatement. Ann N Y Acad Sci 1003:349-351.

Baker DA, McFarland K, Lake RW, Shen H, Tang X-C, Toda S, Kalivas PW (2003b) Neuroadaptations in cystine-glutamate exchange underlie cocaine relapse. Nat Neuro 6:743-749.

Bannai S (1986) Exchange of cystine and glutamate across plasma membrane of human fibroblasts. J Biol Chem 261:2256-2263.

Belin D, Everitt BJ (2008) Cocaine seeking habits depend upon dopamine-dependent serial connectivity linking the ventral with the dorsal striatum. Neuron 57:432-441.

Belin D, Economidou D, Pelloux Y, Everitt BJ (2011) Habit formation and compulsion. In: Animal Models of drug addiction. Olmstead, MC, ed. pp 337–378. Neuromethods, vol. 53. Springer.

Belin D, Everitt BJ (2010) The Neural and Psychological Basis of a Compulsive Incentive Habit. In: Handbook of basal ganglia structure and function, Steiner, H, tseng, K, eds) Elsvier, ACADEMIC PRESS.

Belin D, Jonkman S, Dickinson A, Robbins TW, Everitt BJ (2009a) Parallel and interactive learning processes within the basal ganglia: Relevance for the understanding of addiction. Behavioural Brain Research, 199(1):89–102.

Belin D, Dalley JW (2012) Animal models in addiction research. In: Drug Abuse & Addiction in Medical Illness: causes, consequences and treatment, Vester, J, ed, Totowa: Humana Press Inc.

Belin D, Besson M, Bari A, Dalley JW (2009b) Multi-disciplinary investigations of impulsivity in animal models of attention-deficit hyperactivity disorder and drug addiction vulnerability. In: Endophenotypes of Psychiatric and Neurodegenerative Disorders in Rodent Models, Granon, S, ed, New York: Oxford University Press.

Berk M, Jeavons S, Dean OM, Dodd S, Moss K, Gama CS, Malhi GS (2009) Nail-biting stuff? The effect of N-acetyl cysteine on nail-biting. CNS Spectr 14:357–360.

Bouton ME (2002) Context, ambiguity, and unlearning: sources of relapse after behavioral extinction. Biol Psychiatry 52:976-986.

Brignori C, Quintavalle C, De Micco F, Condorelli G (2011) Nephrotoxicity of contrast media and protective effects of acetylcysteine. Arch Toxicol 85:165–173.

Chen BT, Bowers MS, Martin M, Hopf FW, Guillory AM, Carelli RM, Chou JK, Bonci A (2008) Cocaine but not natural reward self-administration nor passive cocaine infusion produces persistent LTP in the VTA. Neuron 59:288-297.

Chen BT, Hopf FW, Bonci A (2010) Synaptic plasticity in the mesolimbic system. Ann N Y Acad Sci 1187:129-139.

Crombag HS, Bossert JM, Koya E, Shaham Y (2008) Context-induced relapse to drug seeking: a review. Philos Trans R Soc Lond B Biol Sci 363:3233–3243.

Dauletbaev N, Fischer P, Aulbach B, Gross J, Kusche W, Thyroff-Friesinger U, Wagner TO, Bargon J (2009) A phase II study on safety and efficacy of high-dose N-acetylcysteine in patients with cystic fibrosis. Eur J Med Res 14:352-358.

Dean O, Giorlando F, Berk M (2011) N-Acetylcysteine in psychiatry: current therapeutic evidence and potential mechanisms of action. J Psychiatry Neurosci 36:78-86.

Decramer M, Rutten-van Molken M, Dekhuijzen PN, Troosters T, van Herwaarden C, Pellegrino R, van Schayck CP, Olivieri D, Del Donno M, De Backer W, Lankhorst I, Ardia A (2005) Effects of N-acetylcysteine on outcomes in chronic obstructive pulmonary disease (Bronchitis Randomized on NAC Cost-Utility Study, BRONCUS): a randomised placebo-controlled trial. Lancet 365:1552–1560.

Decramer M, Janssens W (2010) Mucoactive therapy in COPD. Eur Respir Rev 19:134-140.

Dietrich D, Kral T, Clusmann H, Friedl M, Schramm J (2002) Presynaptic group II metabotropic glutamate recepotrs reduce stimulated and spontaneous transmitter release in human dentate gyrus. Neuropharmacology 42:297-305.

de Wit H, Stewart J (1981) Reinstatement of cocaine-reinforced responding in the rat. Psychopharmacology 75:134-143.

Dodd S, Dean O, Copolov DL, Malhi GS, Berk M (2008) N-acetylcysteine for antioxidant therapy: pharmacology and clinical utility. Expert Opin Biol Ther 8:1955–1962.

Dringen R, Hirrlinger J (2003) Glutathione pathways in the brain. Biol Chem 384:505-516.

Economidou D, Dalley JW, Everitt BJ (2011) Selective norepinephrine reuptake inhibition by atomoxetine prevents cue-induced heroin and cocaine seeking. Biol Psychiatry 69:266-274.

EMCDDA (2009) The state of the drugs problem in Europe (annual report 2009).

Everitt BJ, Robbins TW (2000) Second-order schedules of drug reinforcement in rats and monkeys: measurement of reinforcing efficacy and drug-seeking behaviour. Psychopharmacology 153:17-30.

Everitt BJ, Robbins TW (2005) Neural systems of reinforcement for drug addiction: from actions to habits to compulsion. Nat Neurosci, 8:1481–1489.

Goldberg SR (1973) Comparable behavior maintained under fixed-ratio and second-order schedules of food presentation, cocaine injection or D-amphetamine injection in the squirrel monkey. J Pharmacol Exp Ther 186:18-30.

Grant JE, Kim SW, Odlaug BL (2007) N-acetyl cysteine, a glutamate-modulating agent, in the treatment of pathological gambling: a pilot study. Biol Psychiatry 62:652–657.

Grant JE, Odlaug BL, Kim SW (2009) N-acetylcysteine, a glutamate modulator, in the treatment of trichotillomania: a double-blind, placebo-controlled study. Arch Gen Psychiatry 66:756–763.

Grant JE, Odlaug BL, Kim SW (2010) A double-blind, placebo-controlled study of N-acetyl cysteine plus naltrexone for methamphetamine dependence. Eur Neuropsychopharmacol 20:823–828.

Gray KM, Watson NL, Carpenter MJ, Larowe SD (2010) N-acetylcysteine (NAC) in young marijuana users: an open-label pilot study. Am J Addict, 19:187–189.

Hall G (2002) Associative structures in Pavlovian and instrumental conditioning. In Gallistel R & Pashler H (Eds.) Stevens' Handbook of Experimental Psychology 3rd Edition: Learning, Motivation, and Emotion, Volume 3 (pp.1-45) John Wiley & Sons, Inc: New York.

Haugeto O, Ullensvang K, Levy LM, Chaudhry FA, Honoré T, Nielsen M, Lehre KP, Danbolt NC (1996) Brain glutamate transporter proteins form homomultimers. J Biol Chem 271:27715-27722.

Ito R, Dalley JW, Robbins TW, Everitt BJ (2002) Dopamine release in the dorsal striatum during cocaine-seeking behavior under the control of a drug-associated cue. J Neurosci 22:6247-6253.

Janáky R, Ogita K, Pasqualotto BA, Bains JS, Oja SS, Yoneda Y, Shaw CA (1999) Glutathione and signal transduction in the mammalian CNS. J Neurochem 73:889-902.

Kalivas PW (2009) The glutmate homeostasis hypothesis of addiction. Nat Rev Neurosci 10:561-572.

Kampman KM, Volpicelli JR, McGinnis DE, Alterman AI, Weinrieb RM, D'Angelo L, Epperson LE (1998) Reliability and validity of the Cocaine Selective Severity Assessment. Addict Behav 23:449–461.

Kampman KM, Volpicelli JR, Mulvaney F, Rukstalis M, Alterman AI, Pettinati H, Weinrieb RM, O'Brien CP (2002) Cocaine withdrawal severity and urine toxicology results from treatment entry predict outcome in medication trials for cocaine dependence. Addict Behav 27:251–260.

Kau KS, Madayag A, Mantsch JR, Grier MD, Abdulhameed O, Baker DA (2008) Blunted cysteine-glutamate antiporter function in the nucleus accumbens promotes cocaine-induced drug seeking. Neuroscience 155:530-537.

Knackstedt LA, LaRowe S, Mardikian P, Malcolm R, Upadhyaya H, Hedden S, Markou A, Kalivas PW (2009) The role of cystine-glutamate exchange in nicotine dependence in rats and humans. Biol Psychiatry 65:841-845.

Knackstedt LA, Melendez RI, Kalivas PW (2010a) Ceftriaxone restores glutamate homeostasis and prevents relapse to cocaine seeking. Biol Psychiatry 67:81-84.

Knackstedt LA, Moussawi K, LaLumiere R, Schwendt M, Klugmann M, Kalivas PW (2010b) Extinction training after cocaine self-administration induces glutamatergic plasticity to inhibit cocaine seeking. J Neurosci 30:7984-7992.

Koob G, Kreek MJ (2007) Stress, dysregulation of drug reward pathways, and the transition to drug dependence. Am J Psychiatry 164:1149-1159.

Kory RC, Hirsch SR, Giraldo J (1968) Nebulization of N-acetylcysteine combined with a bronchodilator in patients with chronic bronchitis. Dis Chest 54:504-509.

Lafleur DL, Pittenger C, Kelmendi B, Gardner T, Wasylink S, Malison RT, Sanacora G, Krystal JH, Coric V (2006) N-acetylcysteine augmentation in serotonin reuptake inhibitor refractory obsessive-compulsive disorder. Psychopharmacology 184:254–256.

LaRowe SD, Mardikian P, Malcolm R, Myrick H, Kalivas P, McFarland K, Saladin M, McRae A, Brady K (2006) Safety and tolerability of N-acetylcysteine in cocaine-dependent individuals. Am J Addict 15:105–110.

LaRowe SD, Myrick H, Hedden S, Mardikian P, Saladin M, McRae A, Brady K, Kalivas PW, Malcolm R (2007) Is cocaine desire reduced by N-acetylcysteine? Am J Psychiatry 164:1115–1117.

Leshner AI (1997) Addiction is a brain disease, and it matters. Science 278:45-47.

Lüscher C, Malenka RC (2011) Drug-evoked synaptic plasticity in addiction: from molecular changes to circuit remodelling. Neuron 69:650-663.

Madayag A, Lobner D, Kau KS, Mantsch JR, Abdulhameed O, Hearing M, Grier MD, Baker DA (2007) Repeated N-acetylcysteine administration alters plasticity-dependent effects of cocaine. J Neurosci 27:13968-13976.

Manzoni O, Michel J-M, Bockaert J (1997) Metabotropic glutamate recepotrs in the rat nucleus accumbens. Eur J Neurosci 9:1514-1523.

Mardikian PN, LaRowe SD, Hedden S, Kalivas PW, Malcolm RJ (2007) An open-label trial of N-acetylcysteine for the treatment of cocaine dependence: a pilot study. Prog Neuropsychopharmacol Biol Psychiatry 31:389–394.

Martin M, Chen BT, Hopf FW, Bowers MS, Bonci A (2006) Cocaine self-administration selectively abolishes LTD in the core of the nucleus accumbens. Nat Neuro 9:868-869.

McFarland K, Lapish CC, Kalivas PW (2003) Prefrontal glutamate release into the core of the nucleus accumbens mediates cocaine-induced reinstatement of drug-seeking behavior. J Neurosci 23:3531-3537.

Monti PM, MacKillop J (2007) Advances in the treatment of craving for alcohol and tobacco. In, P. M. Miller and D. Kavanagh, Eds. Translation of Addictions Science into Practice, Elsevier Science, New York, pp. 211-237.

Moran MM, McFarland K, Melendez RI, Kalivas PW, Seamans JK (2005) Cystine/glutamate exchange regulates metabotropic glutamate receptor presynaptic inhibition of excitatory transmission and vulnerability to cocaine seeking. J Neurosci 25:6389-6393.

Moussawi K, Pacchioni A, Moran M, Olive MF, Gass JT, Lavin A, Kalivas PW (2009) N-Acetylcysteine reverses cocaine-induced metaplasticity. Nat Neurosci 12:182-189.

Moussawi K, Zhou W, Shen H, Reichel CM, See RE, Carr DB, Kalivas PW (2011) Reversing cocaine-induced synaptic potentiation provides enduring protection from relapse. PNAS 108:385-390.

Murray JE, Belin D, Everitt BJ (in press) Double dissociation of the dorsomedial and dorsolateral striatal control over the acquisition and performance of cocaine seeking. Neuropsychopharmacology.

Murray JE, Everitt BJ, Belin D (2012) N-Acetylcysteine reduces early- and late-stage cocaine seeking without affecting cocaine taking in rats. Addict Biol 17:437-440.

Nguyen-Khac E, Thevenot T, Piquet MA, Benferhat S, Goria O, Chatelain D, Tramier B, Dewaele F, Ghrib S, Rudler M, Carbonell N, Tossou H, Bental A, Bernard-Chabert

B, Dupas JL; AAH-NAC Study Group (2011) Glucocorticoids plus N-acetylcysteine in severe alcoholic hepatitis. N Engl J Med 365:1781-789.

Niaura RS, Rohsenow DJ, Binkoff JA, Monti PM, Pedraza M, Abrams DB (1988) Relevance of cue reactivity to understanding alcohol and smoking relapse. J Abnorm Psychol 97:133-152.

O'Brien CP, Childress AR, Ehrman R, Robbins SJ (1998) Conditioning factors in drug abuse: can they explain compulsion? J Psychopharmacol 12:15-22.

O'Brien CP, Childress AR, McLellan AT, Ehrman R (1992) Classical conditioning in drug-dependent humans. Ann N Y Acad Sci 654:400-415.

O'Connor EC, Chapman K, Butler P, Mead AN (2011) The predictive validity of the rat self-administration model for abuse liability. Neurosci Biobehav Rev 35:912-938.

Olive MF, Cleva RM, Kalivas PW, Malcolm RJ (2012) Glutamatergic medications for the treatment of drug and behavioral addictions. Pharmacol Biochem Behav 100:801-810.

Olmstead MC, Lafond MV, Everitt BJ, Dickinson A (2001) Cocaine seeking by rats is a goal-directed action. Behav Neurosci 115:394-402.

Pallanti S, DeCaria CM, Grant JE, Urpe M, Hollander E (2005) Reliability and validity of the pathological gambling adaptation of the Yale-Brown Obsessive-Compulsive Scale (PG-YBOCS). J Gambl Stud 21:431–443.

Panlilio LV, Goldberg SR (2007) Self-administration of drugs in animals and humans as a model and an investigative tool. Addiction 102:1863-1870.

Panlilio LV, Yasar S, Nemeth-Coslett R, Katz JL, Henningfield JE, Solinas M, Heishman SJ, Schindler CW, Goldberg SR (2005) Human cocaine-seeking behavior and its control by drug-associated stimuli in the laboratory. Neuropsychopharmacology 30:433-443.

Pierce RC, Bell K, Duffy P, Kalivas PW (1996) Repeated cocaine augments excitatory amino acid transmission in the nucleus accumbens only in rats having developed behavioural sensitization. J Neurosci 16:1550-1560.

Pittenger C, Krystal JH, Coric V (2005) Initial evidence of the beneficial effects of glutamate-modulating agents in the treatment of self-injurious behavior associated with borderline personality disorder. J Clin Psychiatry 66:1492–1493.

Prescott LF, Park J, Ballantyne A, Adriaenssens P, Proudfoot AT (1977) Treatment of paracetamol (acetaminophen) poisoning with N-acetylcysteine. Lancet 2:432–434.

Reep GL, Soloway RD (2011) Recent and currently emerging medical treatment options for the treatment of alcoholic hepatitis. World J Hepatol 3:211–214.

Reichel CM, Bevins RA (2009) Forced abstinence model of relapse to study pharmacological treatments of substance use disorder. Curr Drug Abuse Rev 2:184-194.

Reichel CM, Moussawi K, Do PH, Kalivas PW, See RE (2011) Chronic N-Acetylcysteine during abstinence or extinction after cocaine self-administration produces enduring reductions in drug seeking. J Pharmacol Exp Ther 337:487-493.

Rohsenow DJ, Martin RA, Eaton CA, Monti PM (2007) Cocaine craving as a predictor of treatment attrition and outcomes after residential treatment for cocaine dependence. J Stud Alcohol Drugs 68:641–648.

Russo SJ, Dietz DM, Dumitriu D, Morrison JH, Malenka RC, Nestler EJ (2010) The addicted synapse: mechanisms of synaptic and structural plasticity in nucleus accumbens. TINS 33:267-276.

Saal D, Dong Y, Bonci A, Malenka RC (2003) Drugs of abuse and stress trigger a common synaptic adaptation in dopamine neurons. Neuron 37:577-582.

Sandilands EA, Bateman DN (2009) Adverse reactions associated with acetylcysteine. Clin Toxicol (Phila) 47:81–88.

Sansone RA, Sansone LA (2011) Getting a Knack for NAC: N-Acetyl-Cysteine. Innov Clin Neurosci 8:10–14.

Scalley RD, Conner CS (1978) Acetaminophen poisoning: a case report of the use of acetylcysteine. Am J Hosp Pharm 35:964-967.

Schindler CW, Gilman JP, Panlilio LV, McCann DJ, Goldberg SR (2011) Comparison of the effects of methamphetamine, bupropion, and methylphenidate on the self-administration of methamphetamine by rhesus monkeys. Exp Clin Psychopharmacol 19:1-10.

Schindler CW, Panlilio LV, Goldberg SR (2002) Second-order schedules of drug self-administration in animals. Psychopharmacology 163:327-344.

Schmaal L, Berk L, Hulstijn KP, Cousijn J, Wiers RW, van den Brink W (2011) Efficacy of N-acetylcysteine in the treatment of nicotine dependence: a double-blind placebo-controlled pilot study. *Eur Addict Res* 17:211-216.

Schmidt LE, Dalhoff K (2001) Risk factors in the development of adverse reactions to N-acetylcysteine in patients with paracetamol poisoning. Br J Clin Pharmacol 51:87–91.

Seiva FR, Amauchi JF, Rocha KK, Ebaid GX, Souza G, Fernandes AA, Cataneo AC, Novelli EL (2009) Alcoholism and alcohol abstinence: N-acetylcysteine to improve energy expenditure, myocardial oxidative stress, and energy metabolism in alcoholic heart disease. Alcohol 43:649–656.

Shadel WG, Martino SC, Setodji C, Cervone D, Witkiewitz K, Beckjord EB, Scharf D, Shih R (in press) Lapse-induced surges in craving influence relapse in adult smokers: an experimental investigation. Health Psychol. doi: 10.1037/a0023445

Siegel S, Ramos BMC (2002) Applying laboratory research: drug anticipation and the treatment of drug addiction. Exp Clin Psychopharmacol 10:162-183.

Stamm SJ, Docter J (1965) Clinical evaluation of acetylcysteine as a nucolytic agent in cystic fibrosis. Dis Chest 47:414-420.

Steensland P, Simms JA, Holgate J, Richards JK, Bartlett SE (2007) Varenicline, an alpha4beta2 nicotinic acetylcholine receptor partial agonist, selectively decreases ethanol consumption and seeking. Proc Natl Acad Sci U S A 104:12518-12523.

Stuber GD, Hnasko TS, Britt JP, Edwards RH, Bonci A (2010) Dopaminergic terminals in the nucleus accumbens but not the dorsal striatum corelease glutamate. J Neurosci 30:8229-8233.

Substance Abuse and Mental Health Services Administration (2010) Results from the 2009 National Survey on Drug Use and Health: Volume I. Summary of National Findings (Office of Applied Studies, NSDUH Series H-38A, HHS Publication No. SMA 10-4856Findings). Rockville, MD.

Taylor JR, Olausson P, Quinn JJ, Torregrossa MM (2009) Targeting extinction and reconsolidation mechanisms to combat the impact of drug cues on addiction. Neuropharmacology 56:186-195.

Ungless MA, Whistler JL, Malenka RC, Bonci A (2001) Single cocaine exposure in vivo induces long-term potentiation in dopamine neurons. Nature 411:583-587.

Vanderschuren LJ, Di Ciano P, Everitt BJ (2005) Involvement of the dorsal striatum in cue-controlled cocaine seeking. J Neurosci 25:8665-8670.

Weeks, JR (1962) Experimental morphine addiction: method for automatic intravenous injections in unrestrained rats. Science 138:143-144.

Wilson, MC, Hitomi M, Schuster CR (1971) Psychomotor stimulant self administration as a function of dosage per injection in the rhesus monkey. Psychopharmacologia 22:271-281.

Witkiewitz K, Masyn KE (2008) Drinking trajectories following an initial lapse. Psychol Addict Behav 22:157-167.

World Health Organization (2010) *ATLAS on Substance Use – Resources for the Prevention and Treatment of Substance Use Disorders.* WHO Press: Geneva, Switzerland.

Zapata A, Minney VL, Shippenberg TS (2010) Shift from goal-directed to habitual cocaine seeking after prolonged experience in rats. J Neurosci 30:15457-15463.

Zhou W, Kalivas PW (2008) N-Acetylcysteine reduces extinction responding and induces enduring reductions in cue- and heroin-induced drug-seeking. Biol Psychiatry 63:338-340.

Zimmer BA, Dobrin CV, Roberts DCS (2011) Brain-cocaine concentrations determine the dose self-administered by rats on a novel behaviourally dependent dosing schedule. Neuropsychopharmacology 36:2741-2749.

2

Medication Development for the Treatment of Cocaine Addiction – Progress at Preclinical and Clinical Levels

Zheng-Xiong Xi
National Institute on Drug Abuse, Intramural Research Program,
National Institutes of Health, Baltimore, MD
USA

1. Introduction

Cocaine addiction continues to be an important public health problem in the United States and other countries. Acute cocaine produces potent rewarding and psychostimulant effects primarily by blocking dopamine (DA) transporters (DAT) in the brain's reward system – the mesocorticolimbic DA system. However, repeated use of cocaine leads to addiction, persistent craving and a high risk of relapse. To date, there are no proven pharmacotherapies for cocaine addiction. Recent progress in the neurobiology of drug dependence in preclinical animal models has lead to the discovery of various novel compounds that appear to be promising for the treatment of drug addiction. Some have been tested in controlled clinical trials and have produced encouraging results in reducing cocaine use and in increasing abstinence from relapse. In this review article, I will focus on those medication strategies that are well-studied in experimental animals and are currently under clinical trials for the treatment of addiction or for other diseases. These strategies include DAT-based agonist therapy, DA receptor-based antagonist therapy, glutamate-based therapy, GABA-based therapy and endocannabinoid-based therapy. For each treatment, I will first review the rationale and the underlying neurochemical mechanisms of the therapy, and then summarize the major findings of the drugs in each category at both preclinical and clinical levels.

2. Dopamine transporter-based agonist therapies

Rationale: The mesocorticolimbic DA system is thought to be critically involved in drug reward and addiction (Wise, 2005; Sulzer, 2011). This system originates from the DA neurons in the ventral tegmental area (VTA) in the midbrain and projects predominantly to the nucleus accumbens (NAc) and prefrontal cortex (PFC) in the forebrain (Figure 1). Almost all addictive drugs, such as cocaine, heroin, nicotine and alcohol, have been shown to increase extracellular DA in the NAc via different mechanisms (Wise, 2005; Sulzer, 2011). For example, cocaine elevates extracellular DA by blockade of DAT, while heroin increases extracellular DA by inhibition of GABA release in the VTA that disinhibits (activates) DA neurons. Such an increase in NAc DA has been thought to underlie the euphoria associated with drug abuse. Based on this DA hypothesis, much attention in medication development for treatment of addiction has been focused on manipulation of DA transmission in the brain reward circuitry. One strategy is to target DAT (agonist therapy), and another is to target brain DA receptors (antagonist therapy) (Figure 2).

A (Human brain mesocorticolimbic DA system)

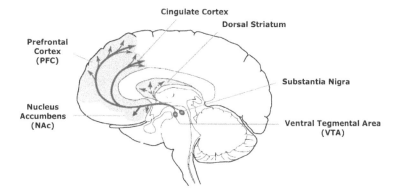

B (Rat brain mesocorticolimbic DA system and modulations)

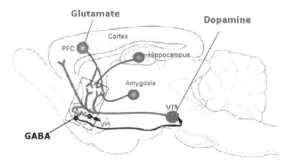

Fig. 1. Schematic diagrams, illustrating the mesocorticolimbic DA reward system in human (A) and rat (B) brains. The mesocorticolimbic DA system originates in the midbrain ventral tegmental area (VTA) and projects predominantly to the nucleus accumbens (NAc) and prefrontal cortex (PFC). Dopaminergic afferents from the VTA and glutamatergic afferents from the PFC, hippocampus and amygdala synapse on NAc medium-spiny (GABAergic) neurons (MSN), which project to the VTA and the ventral pallidum (VP).

Agonist or substitution therapies have been successful in the treatment of opioid (Mattick et al., 2009) and nicotine dependence (Xi et al., 2009; Xi, 2010). As such, drugs that block the DAT, but have lower addictive potential than cocaine, would have potential as 'cocaine-like' agonist therapies for the treatment of cocaine addiction. Indeed, this strategy has been at the forefront of medication development for the treatment of cocaine addiction for more than a decade (Rothman and Baumann, 2006; Howell and Kimmel, 2008). To date, many DAT inhibitors have been developed, and several of them have been tested in human clinical trials (Newman and Kulkarni, 2002; Runyon and Carroll, 2006; Rothman et al., 2006, 2008).

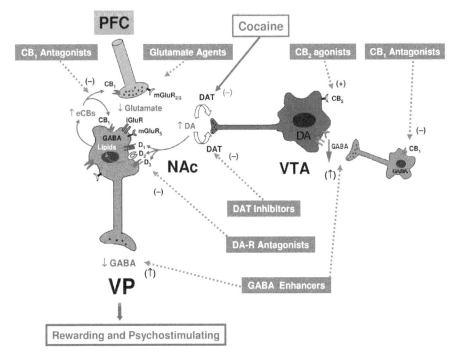

Fig. 2. Schematic diagram of the VTA-NAc-VP reward pathway, illustrating the actions of acute cocaine on extracellular DA, endocannabinoids (eCBs), glutamate and GABA in the NAc and VP, and the sites of action of various mechanism-based pharmacological agents in the brain reward system. Cocaine elevates extracellular DA in the NAc by blocking DAT on presynaptic DA terminals. DA activates postsynaptic DA receptors, in particular D2 and D3 receptors, producing an overall inhibitory effect on NAc medium-spiny (GABAergic) neurons (MSN). In addition, activation of D2 receptors may also increase eCB release from MSNs, which subsequently activates cannabinoid CB1 receptors located on presynaptic glutamatergic terminals and GABAergic MSNs themselves, causing a reduction in glutamate release and in MSN excitability. Thus, increases in NAc DA and eCBs and a reduction in NAc glutamate release lead to a reduction in MSN excitability and GABA release in the VTA (not shown) and VP. Decreased GABA release in the VTA causes an increase in DA neuron activity (via a disinhibition mechanism) and DA release in the NAc. Based upon these neurochemical hypotheses, various pharmacological therapies have been proposed and tested in animal models of drug addiction to interfere with cocaine's action. More details are discussed in the text of this review.

However, none have proven to be successful due to significant abuse liability by those compounds themselves and/or unwanted side-effects. Given the recent finding that rewarding and psychostimulant effects of the drugs are positively correlated with the speed of onset and offset of action on brain DA (Volkow et al., 1995; Kimmel et al., 2007; Xi and Gardner, 2008), it has been proposed that DAT inhibitors (Figure 2), in particular those with a slower-onset longer-acting profile than cocaine, would have lower addictive potential by themselves. In the following sections, we will review several DAT inhibitors with such a slow-onset long-action profile.

2.1 GBR-12909

Preclinical studies: GBR-12909 (Vanoxerine), a phenyl-substituted piperazine derivative, is a relatively slow-onset long-acting DAT inhibitor compared to cocaine (Howell and Wilcox, 2001). To date, it is the most extensively studied DAT inhibitor proposed to be beneficial in the treatment of cocaine addiction (Rothman et al., 2008). GBR-12909 binds at the DAT site with high affinity, and selectively inhibits DA re-uptake. GBR-12909 can also compete with psychostimulants at the DAT site, thus blocking cocaine- or amphetamine-induced increases in extracellular DA. Compared to the same doses of cocaine, GBR-12909-induced increases in striatal DA and locomotion are relatively slow-onset and long-lasting (Baumann et al., 1991, 1994; Kelley and Lang, 1989). Pretreatment with GBR-12909 significantly inhibits cocaine self-administration in rats and nonhuman primates at doses that have little or no effect on food self-administration (Glowa et al., 1995). Repeated treatment with low doses of GBR-12909 sustains the selective suppression of cocaine self-administration *versus* food self-administration (Glowa et al., 1995). Further, a single injection of a slow-release formulation of GBR-12909 produced a prolonged (up to one month) suppression of cocaine self-administration in nonhuman primates (Glowa et al., 1996). These findings support GBR-12909 as a potential candidate for the treatment of cocaine addiction (Rothman et al., 2008).

Clinical trials: GBR-12909 was investigated in clinical trials at NIDA and University of Texas from 2003 to 2008 (Table 1). However, the appearance of cardiovascular side-effects has prevented its further development as an anti-cocaine medicine at NIDA, NIH (Vocci and Elkashef, 2005).

2.2 RTI-336

Preclinical studies: RTI-336 is a novel DAT inhibitor of the 3-phenyltropane class and has a slower-onset (30 min *vs.* < 10 min) longer-acting (4 hrs *vs.* 1-2 hrs) profile than cocaine (Carroll et al., 2006; Kimmel et al., 2007). It has >1000- and >400-fold selectivity for DAT over serotonin transporter (SERT) and norepinepherine transporter (NET), respectively (Carroll et al., 2006). Pretreatment with RTI-336 produced a dose-dependent reduction in cocaine self-administration in both rats and nonhuman primates (Haile et al., 2005; Howell et al., 2007). The ED_{50} dose of RTI-336 for reducing cocaine self-administration resulted in approximately 90% DAT occupancy, suggesting that high levels of DAT occupancy by RTI-336 are required to reduce cocaine self-administration. However, co-administration of the ED_{50} dose of RTI-336 with the SERT inhibitors fluoxetine or citalopram produced more robust reductions in cocaine self-administration in non-human primates than RTI-336 alone (Howell et al., 2007), suggesting that blockade of both DAT and SERT may be more effective in attenuating cocaine's reinforcing effects than selective blockade of DAT alone (Rothman et al., 2007). In addition, at the doses that effectively suppressed cocaine self-administration, RTI-336 also inhibited food-taking behavior (Howell et al., 2007). This differs from GBR-12909, which selectively inhibits cocaine self-administration but not food-taking behavior. RTI-336, like many other DAT inhibitors, reliably maintained self-administration behavior in all non-human primates tested (Howell et al., 2007) and produced locomotor stimulating effects in mice and rats, suggesting abuse potential by itself. However, compared to cocaine, RTI-336 maintained lower rates of responding and lower progressive-ratio (PR) break-points in the self-administration paradigm. It also produced weaker locomotion hyperactivity and drug discriminative stimulus effects, and showed very low sensitization in locomotion (Carroll et al., 2006; Czoty et al., 2010). These data suggest that RTI-336 may have lower abuse potential than cocaine.

Clinical trials: RTI-336 has been investigated in Phase I clinical trials at RTI International (NC, USA) and NIDA (MD, USA) since 2008 (Table 1). It was a double-blind, placebo-controlled Phase I study to evaluate the safety, tolerability, and pharmacokinetics of RTI-336 in healthy, male subjects. The study has been completed, but not yet reported.

Compound	Company	Pharmacology	Indication	Status	Reference
GBR-12909	Antia Lab., China; Others	DAT inhibitor	Safety and PK profiles; Cocaine addiction	Phase I, terminated at NIDA in 2008	http://clinica ltrials.gov
RTI-336	RTI, NC, USA	DAT inhibitor	Safety, tolerability & PK profiles	Phase I,	http://clinica ltrials.gov
Methylpheni date	Shire US, Dublin, Ireland	DAT inhibitor	Substance Abuse (cocaine, methamphetamine)	Phase II	http://clinica ltrials.gov
Modafinil	Cephalon, PA, USA	DAT inhibitor; Glutamate enhancer; GABA inhibitor	Drug Addiction (cocaine, methamphetamine	Phase II	http://clinica ltrials.gov
			Schizophrenia	Phase IV	
Disulfiram	LKT Lab., MN, USA	Aldehyde dehydrogenase inhibitor;	Substance Abuse (cocaine, heroin or methamphetamine)	Phase III	http://clinica ltrials.gov
		Dopamine-β-hydroxylase inhibitor	Others		

Table 1. DAT- or DA-related drug candidates in clinical trials

2.3 CTDP-31,345

Based upon the above finding that a combination of DAT and SERT inhibitors appears to be more potent and effective than DAT inhibitor alone in attenuation of cocaine self-administration (Howell et al., 2007), we studied slow-onset long-acting monamine transporter

(MAT) inhibitors that have higher affinity for both DAT and SERT over to NET. In addition, our interest in non-selective MAT inhibitors as potential anti-cocaine medications originally stems from the fact that cocaine is also a non-selective MAT inhibitor. Thus, it was hypothesized that a 'cocaine-like' MAT inhibitor with slow-onset and long-acting profiles would be able to substitute for cocaine for the treatment of cocaine dependence (Peng et al., 2010c). CTDP-31,345 is such a MAT inhibitor with slow-onset (30-60 min) long-acting (at least 6 hrs) (Peng et al., 2010c) and with higher selectivity for DAT and SERT over NET (K_i = 18, 23 and 81 for DAT, SERT and NET, respectively) (Froimowitz et al., 2000). The "CTDP" terminology derives from the "Cocaine Treatment Discovery Program" of the NIDA Extramural Program. Structurally, it is a *trans*-aminotetralin derivative (Peng et al., 2010c). It is a prodrug, which is metabolized (*N*-demethylated) to CTDP-31,346, a slow-onset long-acting MAT inhibitor. Pretreatment with a single dose of CTDP-31,345 produced a dose-dependent long-term (24-48 h) reduction in cocaine self-administration in rats (Peng et al., 2010c). CTDP-31,345 itself appears to have lower abuse liability than cocaine because it produces weaker brain-stimulation reward and maintains a lower rate of self-administration than cocaine (Peng et al., 2010c). In addition, systemic administration of CTDP-31,345 produces moderate, but long-lasting, increases in NAc DA, which may translate to decreases in drug craving and relapse by restoring reduced synaptic DA in brain reward circuits (Volkow et al., 1999). CTDP-31,345 is not currently in clinical trials.

2.4 Methylphenidate

Preclinical studies: Methylphenidate is a FDA-approved DAT inhibitor for the treatment of attention deficit hyperactivity disorder (ADHD). It binds to presynaptic DAT and NET, but not to SERT, blocking DA and NE re-uptake and increasing synaptic DA and NE (Leonard et al., 2004). Methylphenidate is self-administered in rodents, and pretreatment with methylphenidate significantly shifts the cocaine self-administration dose-response curve to the left (Hiranita et al., 2009, 2011), suggesting that methylphenidate has cocaine-like abuse potential and produces additive effects in combination with cocaine.

Clinical trials: ADHD has high comorbidity with cocaine-dependent patients as much as 30% in some studies (Schubiner et al., 2000). Because of this, its therapeutic effects for the treatment of cocaine addiction in this population have been recently evaluated in clinical trials (Table 1). Placebo-controlled studies produced mixed results with one study reporting no effect (Schubiner et al., 2002) while three studies demonstrating a significant reduction in both cocaine use and the positive subjective effects of cocaine compared to placebo (Winhusen et al., 2006; Collins et al., 2006; Levin et al., 2007). Because the half-life of methylphenidate is short (2-3 hrs in humans), the drug has been made available in sustained-release formulations in addition to the traditional immediate-release formulation. The sustained-release methylphenidate displayed much lower abuse potential than immediate-release, and appears to be more effective than immediate-release in decreasing cocaine use and the positive subjective effects (Arria and Wish, 2006; White et al., 2006).

2.5 CTDP-32,476

Based on the aforementioned findings of sustained-release methylphenidate in clinical trials, we have recently developed a series of methylphenidate analogs with slow-onset long-acting profiles as medication candidates for the treatment of cocaine addiction. CTDP-32,476 is a representative compound in this drug category. Structurally, CTDP-32,476 is a metabolically stable methylphenidate analog, in which the metabolically unstable ester moiety of methylphenidate is removed from methylphenidate's structure (Froimowitz et al. 2007). *In vitro* binding assays suggest that CTDP-32,476 is a selective DAT inhibitor with ~50-fold and ~350-fold selectivity for DAT over NET and SERT (K_i= 16, 5900 and 840 nM for DAT, SERT and NET, respectively) (Froimowitz et al., 2007). Functional reuptake assays reveal that CTDP-32,476 has IC_{50} values of 8.6, 490 and 120 nM for inhibition of DA, 5-HT and NE reuptake, respectively. In addition, it also displays approximately 30-fold higher affinity for the DAT than cocaine (K_i: 16 *vs.* 500 nM; IC_{50}: 8.6 *vs.* 244 nM) (Froimowitz et al., 2007). Systemic administration of CTDP-32,476 produced a slow-onset (20-60 min) long-term (6-12 hrs) increase in locomotion and extracellular DA in the NAc (Xi et al., 2009). Pretreatment with CTDP-32,476 significantly and dose-dependently inhibited intravenous cocaine self-administration under both FR and PR reinforcement, shifted the cocaine dose-response self-administration curves downward and to the right, and attenuated cocaine-induced increases in locomotion and extracellular DA in the NAc (Xi et al., 2011a). These data suggest that pretreatment with CTDP-32,476 produced functional antagonism of cocaine's action, likely by attenuating cocaine's binding to DAT. CTDP-32,476 itself appears to have much lower addictive potential than cocaine. Drug naïve rats selectively self-administer cocaine, but not CTDP-32,476. In rats trained to self-administer cocaine, CTDP-32,476 maintained significantly lower rates of self-administration and lower PR break-points than cocaine. Taken together, these data suggest that CTDP-32,476 appears to be an excellent agonist therapy for cocaine dependence. CTDP-32,476 has not been tested in human clinical trials.

2.6 Modafinil

Preclinical studies: Modafinil is a wake-promoting drug used in the clinic for the treatment of narcolepsy and idiopathic hypersomnia (Wise et al., 2007). However, the neurochemical mechanisms underlying modafinil's action are not fully understood. It is reported that modafinil increases extracellular levels of glutamate in numerous brain regions including striatum, thalamus, hippocampus, and hypothalamus (Ballon and Feifel, 2006; Wise et al., 2007). In addition, it also inhibits brain GABA release (Ballon and Feifel, 2006). Recent studies suggest that modafinil is a DAT inhibitor in humans and primates (Madras et al., 2006; Volkow et al., 2009). This is further supported by the findings that mice lacking DAT or DA (D1 and D2) receptors do not respond to the wake-promoting effects of modafinil (Qu et al., 2008; Wisor et al., 2001). *In vivo* microdialysis studies demonstrated that modafinil increases extracellular DA (Wisor et al., 2001; Ferraro et al., 1997; Murillo-Rodríguez et al., 2007). Neuroimaging studies in both non-human primates and healthy human subjects demonstrated significant occupancy of DAT (and also NET) by intravenously-administered modafinil (Madras et al., 2006; Volkow et al., 2009). Consistent with these findings, modafinil has been shown to have weak cocaine-like discriminative and reinforcing effects in both rodents and non-human primates (Gold and Balster., 1996; Deroche-Gamonet et al., 2002), and weak stimulant-like subjective effects in humans (Kruszewski, 2006; O'Brien et al., 2006). Based on these recent findings, modafinil is categorized as a DAT-based 'agonist therapy' for cocaine dependence.

Clinical studies: Dackis et al (2003) first reported that modafinil's stimulant-like activity may diminish the symptoms of cocaine withdrawal, including hypersomnia, lethargy, dysphoric mood, cognitive impairment, and increased appetite, thereby reducing the desire to use cocaine. The first randomized, double-blind clinical trial involved 62 cocaine-dependent outpatients who received either a single dose of modafinil or placebo daily for 8 weeks (Dackis et al., 2005). Patients treated with modafinil had significantly less cocaine use than patients treated with placebo (Hart et al., 2008). No significant adverse effects were noted. The therapeutic effects of modafinil in cocaine users have been supported by a recently completed multi-site, placebo-controlled clinical trial involving 210 cocaine-dependent outpatients (Anderson et al., 2009). Currently, more than 10 additional clinical trials are under way to further evaluate the efficacy of modafinil treatment for cocaine addiction (Table 1).

2.7 Disulfiram

Preclinical studies: Although disulfiram is not a DAT inhibitor, I list it under this treatment category because it elevates extracellular DA by inhibiting DA metabolism, producing effects similar to DAT inhibitors. In 1937, disulfiram was first reported as a potential treatment for alcoholism by Williams, a plant physician in a chemical company. Unexpectedly, Williams observed that after exposure to disulfram, his laboratory assistants could not drink alcohol in any form because alcohol produced a series of unwanted effects such as flushing, sweating, headaches, nausea, tachycardia, palpitations, arterial hypotension and hyperventilation (Williams, 1937). Since then, disulfiram has been used in the treatment of alcoholism for more than half a century (Suh et al., 2006; Barth and Malcolm, 2010). Disulfiram is an inhibitor of aldehyde dehydrogenase, the enzyme that transforms acetaldehyde into acetate during alcohol metabolism (Weinshenker, 2010). When a person drinks alcohol while taking disulfiram, the resulting acetylaldehyde accumulation causes an aversive reaction as described above, which discourages further drinking. In addition, disulfiram also inhibits dopamine-β-hydroxylase (DBH) (Weinshenker, 2010), the enzyme that transforms DA into norepinephrine. Such DBH inhibition would increase brain DA levels while decreasing brain NE release. This effect could be therapeutic for cocaine dependence since an increase in brain DA may be helpful in attenuating withdrawal syndromes and craving (Volkow et al., 1999), while a decrease in NE may be helpful in attenuating relapse to drug use (Smith and Aston-Jones, 2008; Weinshenker, 2010). In experimental animals, disulfram stimulates DA release and potentiates cocaine-induced increases in extracellular DA in the prefrontal cortex (Devoto et al., 2011). It also facilitates the development and expression of locomotor sensitization to cocaine in rats (Haile et al., 2003). However, in animal models of relapse, pretreatment with disulfram attenuates cocaine-induced reinstatement of drug-seeking behaviour (Schroeder et al., 2010).

Clinical trials: The initial impetus for the use of disulfiram to treat cocaine dependence was the high rate of comorbidity between cocaine abuse and alcohol abuse (Gossop and Carroll, 2006). Thus, it was hypothesized that a reduction in alcohol use would lead to secondary reduction in cocaine use. Additionally, abstinence from alcohol would prevent formation of cocaethylene, a metabolite formed when alcohol and cocaine are present together. Cocaethylene has pharmacological actions similar to cocaine and increases subjective euphoria and heart rate (Hart et al., 2000). Several short-term clinical trials in outpatients using both cocaine and alcohol showed that disulfiram, along with cognitive behavioural therapy (CBT), significantly reduced cocaine and alcohol use (Carroll et al., 1998; Higgins et al., 1993; Grassi et al., 2007). In one study, the reduction in cocaine use was still present one year after treatment (Carroll et al., 2000). An 11-week, double-blind, placebo-controlled trial evaluated the efficacy of disulfiram, naltrexone and their combined treatment in 208 patients with concurrent cocaine and alcohol dependence. Patients taking disulfiram alone or in combination with naltrexone were more likely to achieve combined abstinence from cocaine and alcohol than placebo-treated patients (Pettinati et al., 2008). In several randomized, placebo-controlled trials, disulfiram seemed to directly reduce cocaine use rather than reducing it indirectly by reducing concurrent alcohol use (George et al., 2000; Petrakis et al., 2000; Carroll et al., 2004). In addition, dilsufiram appears to be effective in attenuating cocaine use in comorbid cocaine- and opioid-dependent individuals (Oliveto et al., 2011). As a caveat, disulfiram is reported to inhibit cocaine metabolism, and therefore increases cocaine plasma levels in humans (Baker et al., 2006). Because of this, it should be used cautiously in comorbid cocaine and alcohol patients with severe cardiovascular diseases (Malcolm et al., 2008).

3. Dopamine receptor-based antagonist therapies

Rationale: Cocaine's action is largely mediated by elevation of extracellular DA that activates postsynaptic DA receptors. Thus, blockade of DA receptors is a plausible therapeutic approach for cocaine addiction (Figure 2). There are five DA receptor subtypes identified in the brain that are classified as D1-like (D1, D5) and D2-like (D2, D3, D4) based on their pharmacological profile (Beaulieu and Gainetdinov, 2011). Although both D1 and D2 receptor subtypes have been shown to play predominant roles in mediating actions of DA, clinical trials with selective D1 or D2 receptor antagonists for the treatment of cocaine addiction have failed due to ineffectiveness and/or unwanted side-effects such as sedation and extra pyramidal locomotor syndromes (see review by Platt et al., 2002; Gorelick et al., 2004). In response, efforts have increased to develop relatively low selective D1/2 receptor antagonists or D3 receptor-based antagonist therapies for cocaine dependence.

3.1 *Levo*-tetrahydropalmatine (*l*-THP)

Preclinical studies: Tetrahydropalmatine (THP) is a tetrahydroprotoberberine (THPB) isoquinoline alkaloid and a primary active constituent of the herbal plant species *Stephania rotunda Lour* and *Corydalis ambigua* (Yanhusuo) (Jin et al., 1987). The levo-isomer of THP (*l*-THP) has been shown to contribute to many of the therapeutic effects of these herbs such as sedative, neuroleptic and analgesic effects (Chu et al., 2008; Jin, 1987). Purified or synthetic *l*-THP has been approved in China as a traditional sedative-analgesic agent for the treatment of chronic pain and anxious insomnia for more than 40 years. Pharmacologically, *l*-THP is a non-selective DA receptor antagonist with roughly 3-fold selectivity for D1 *versus* D2 receptor and 10-fold selectivity for D1 *versus* D3 receptor (K_i = 124, 388, or 1420 nM for D1, D2, or D3 receptors, respectively) (Wang and Mantsch, 2012). In addition, it has moderate binding affinity to alpha (α_1, α_{2A}) adrenergic and 5-HT$_{1A}$ (K_i = 340 nM) receptors. Because cocaine is a non-selective MAT inhibitor, which increases brain DA, NE and 5-HT levels, it was hypothesized that blockade of multiple DA, adrenergic and 5-HT$_{1A}$ receptors by *l*-THP would functionally antagonize cocaine's action (Mantsch et al., 2007; Xi et al., 2007). In support of this hypothesis, *l*-THP was found to significantly inhibit intravenous cocaine self-administration under FR and PR reinforcement schedules (Mantsch et al., 2007, 2010; Xi et al., 2007), cocaine-induced conditioned place preference (CPP) (Luo et al., 2003), cocaine-enhanced electrical brain-stimulation reward (Xi et al., 2007), and cocaine-, cue- or stress-induced reinstatement of drug-seeking behaviour in rats (Mantsch et al., 2007, 2010; Figueroa-Guzman et al., 2011). These anti-cocaine effects are unlikely due to *l*-THP-induced sedation or locomotor impairment, since the effective doses that decrease cocaine's effects are much lower (3-10 fold) than those that produce locomotion inhibition (Xi et al., 2007). These data suggest that *l*-THP may have therapeutic potential for treatment of cocaine addiction in humans.

Clinical studies: A pilot study examined the efficacy of *l*-THP in reducing craving and relapse in 120 heroin addicts (Yang et al., 2008). In this randomized, double-blind, placebo-controlled study, patients received 4 weeks of *l*-THP treatment and three months follow-up after *l*-THP treatment. The results showed that *l*-THP significantly lowered opiate withdrawal symptoms and craving and increased abstinence rate. Another study examined the therapeutic effect of *l*-THP combined with methadone for heroin detoxification (Hu et al., 2006), and found that *l*-THP, combined with methadone, significantly elevated detoxification rate, lowered total amount of methadone and decreased time for the detoxification. L-THP is being investigated in human clinical trial for the treatment of cocaine addiction in University of Maryland, Baltimore (Table 2).

Compound	Company	Pharm. Action	Indication	Status	Reference
L-THP	Best & Wide, Nanning, China	D1/D2/D3 Antagonist	Drug abuse (heroin, cocaine)	Phase I, Phase II	Yang et al., 2008; Wang & Mantsch, 2012
BP-897	Bioproject, Paris, France	D3 Partial Agonist	Safety Study	Phase II	Garcia-Ladona & Cox, 2003
Cariprazine	Gideon Richter, Budapest, Hungary	D3-Partial Agonist	Bipolar disorder; Schizophrenia	Phase III	http://clinicaltrials.gov
ABT-925	Abbott, IL, USA	D3 Antagonist	Schizophrenia	Phase II	http://clinicaltrials.gov
ABT-614	Abbott, IL, USA	D3 Antagonist	PK properties D3R binding by PET	Phase I	http://clinicaltrials.gov
GSK598809	GSK, Uxbridge, UK	D3 Antagonist	Substance abuse (nicotine); Food reward	Phase II	http://clinicaltrials.gov
GSK618334	GSK, Uxbridge, UK	D3 Antagonist	Substance abuse (alcoholism)	Phase I	http://clinicaltrials.gov
S33138	Institut de Recherches Servier, Croissy sur Seine, France	D3-Preferring Antagonist	D3R binging by PET; Safety	Phase I	Thomasson-Perret et al., 2008; Millan et al., 2008

Table 2. DA receptor-based drug candidates in clinical trials

3.2 BP-897

Preclinical studies: BP-897 is the first developed D3-selective partial agonist (Pilla et al., 1999) or antagonist (Wicke and Garcia-Ladona, 2001). A series of studies have assessed the efficacy of BP-897 in animal models of drug addiction (see reviews by Garcia-Ladona and Cox, 2003; Le Foll et al., 2005; Heidbreder et al., 2005). BP-897 produces a dose-dependent decrease in cocaine self-administration under second-order reinforcement, cocaine-induced CPP, cocaine's discriminative stimulus properties, and cocaine- or cue-induced reinstatement of cocaine-seeking behaviour. These data support the potential use of BP-897 in the treatment of cocaine addiction, particularly in relapse to drug-seeking behavior.

Clinical trials: BP-897 entered Phase II clinical studies for the treatment of drug addiction in the early 2000s. However, the detailed results about its safety, pharmacokinetics and therapeutic efficacy have not yet been reported.

3.3 Cariprazine

Preclinical studies: Cariprazine (RGH-188) is a novel D3 receptor partial agonist with 10-fold selectivity for D3 over D2 (Gründer, 2010; Kiss et al., 2010). It is also a weak 5-HT$_{1A}$ and 5-HT$_{5C}$ partial agonist. Although limited preclinical data are available, the 'concept-proven' finding with BP-897 suggests that cariprazine might be similarly effective in attenuation of cocaine's actions.

Clinical studies: Cariprazine is currently in Phase III clinical trials for the treatment of schizophrenia and bipolar disorder (Table 2). Data from Phase II trials in patients with schizophrenia and bipolar mania indicate that the drug has antipsychotic and antimanic properties that are superior to placebo. The efficacy of cariprazine for treatment of cocaine addiction has not been evaluated.

3.4 SB-277011A

Preclinical studies: SB-277011A is the most well-characterized D3 receptor antagonist in preclinical animal models of drug addiction to date (Heidebreder et al., 2005; Heidbreder and Newman, 2010). SB-277011A has high affinity for human D3 receptor, and the selectivity for human and rat D3 over D2 receptor is 120 and 80, respectively (Reavill et al., 2000). In experimental animals, SB-277011A significantly and dose-dependently attenuates cocaine-enhanced brain-stimulation reward (Vorel et al., 2002; Spiller et al., 2008), cocaine-induced CPP (Vorel et al., 2002), cocaine self-administration under PR or FR10 (but not FR1 or FR2) reinforcement (Xi et al., 2005), and reinstatement of drug-seeking behavior caused by cocaine priming, cue or footshock stress (Vorel et al., 2002; Xi et al., 2004b; Gilbert et al., 2005). In addition, systemic administration or intracranial microinjections into the NAc or basolateral amygdala significantly and dose-dependently inhibited contextual cue-induced incubation of cocaine craving in rats (Xi et al., 2012). These data suggest that SB-277011A is a promising candidate in medication development for treatment of cocaine addiction.

Clinical trials: Further development of SB-277011A as a medication for treatment of cocaine addiction has been halted by GlaxoSmithKline Pharmaceuticals, due to unexpected poor bioavailability (~2%) and a short half-life (<20 min) in primates (Austin et al., 2001; Remington and Kapue, 2001). Therefore, much effort has been made to develop other D3-

selective antagonists with higher bioavailability and more promising pharmacotherapeutic profiles (Newman et al., 2005).

3.5 GSK598809 and GSK618334

Preclinical studies: Based on the results with SB-277011A, GSK is currently developing other D3 receptor antagonists, such as GSK618334 and GSK598809, for the treatment of substance abuse and addiction. GSK598809 is a novel, potent and selective DA D_3 receptor antagonist (Searle et al., 2010). Functional assays showed that GSK598809 has >100-fold selectivity for D_3 receptors over D_2, histamine H_1, muscarinic M_1, M_2, M_3, M_4, serotonin $5-HT_{1A}$, $5-HT_{1B}$ and $5-HT_{1D}$ receptors (te Beek et al., 2012). CPP experiments in animal models indicated that GSK598809 significantly reduced nicotine- and cocaine-seeking behaviour in a dose-dependent manner (te Beek et al., 2012). In addition, GSK598809 significantly prevented relapse to nicotine-seeking behaviour, although no effect was observed on reducing alcohol consumption in rats.

Clinical studies: GSK618334 is currently under Phase I and Phase II clinical trials (Table 2). A recent PET imaging study suggests that GSK598809 significantly and dose-dependently inhibits [^{11}C]PHNO binding in D3-rich brain regions such as the ventral striatum, globus pallidus and substantia nigra (Searle et al., 2010). In healthy volunteers, single doses of GSK598809 were generally well tolerated. Plasma concentration of GSK598809 increased rapidly after oral administration (T_{max} 2-3 hrs) and subsequently decreased in an apparent bi-exponential manner (terminal half-life of roughly 20 hrs). The CNS effects of GSK598809 alone were limited to elevation of serum prolactin and a small decrease in adaptive tracking performance (te Beek et al., 2012). GSK598809, at a dose (175 mg) that associated >90% D2/3 receptor occupancy, appeared to have no overall effect on attention bias to food-related cues (as measured behaviorally) (Nathan et al., 2011), on subjective hunger or craving ratings and on brain response to food images (as measured by fMRI) in overweight and obese binge eating individuals (Dodds et al., 2012). These findings are consistent with previous findings in experimental animals demonstrating that SB-277011A or NGB-2904 have no significant effects on food-induced CPP and food-taking behavior (Vorel et al., 2002; Ross et al., 2007; Thanos et al., 2008). Contrary to the promising finding in experimental animals, a recent clinical trial with GSK598809 for the treatment of alcoholism demonstrated that it produces an additive, not an expected inhibitory, effect on alcohol intake (te Beek et al., 2012). GSK598809 is currently under Phase II clinic trial for treatment of nicotine dependence (http://clinicaltrials.gov/). The effects of GSK598809 on cocaine dependence have not yet been evaluated.

3.6 ABT-925

ABT-925, also known as A-437203 or BSF-201640, is a selective D3 receptor antagonist developed by Abbott Laboratories. It has an approximately 100-fold selectivity for D3 versus D2 receptors (Geneste et al., 2006). Although the preclinical data for this compound are currently unavailable, proof-of-concept for D3 receptor antagonists in treatment of schizophrenia and drug abuse has been well-established. In Phase I and Phase II clinical trials (Table 2), ABT-925 was safe and generally well tolerated up to the highest dose levels tested (600 mg single dose, 500 mg once daily for 7 days) (Day et al., 2010; Graff-Guerrero et al., 2010; Redden et al., 2011). However, a recent double-blind, placebo-controlled study for the treatment of acute schizophrenia suggest that ABT-925, at 50-150 mg per day, did not produce statistically significant therapeutic effects compared to placebo (Redden et al., 2011).

3.7 NGB-2904

NGB-2904 is another highly selective D3 receptor antagonist with >150-fold or 800-fold selectivity for primate or rat D3 over D2 receptors and 5000-fold selectivity for D3 over D1, D4, and D5 receptors (Yuan et al., 1998). Based upon its high selectivity for DA D3 receptors, we have recently evaluated the pharmacological effects in animal models of drug addiction. We found that systemic administration of NGB-2904 dose-dependently inhibits cocaine self-administration under PR (but not FR2) reinforcement (Xi et al., 2006b), cocaine-enhanced electrical brain reward function (Xi et al., 2006b; Spiller et al., 2008), and cocaine- and cocaine cue-induced reinstatement of cocaine-seeking behavior (Gilbert et al., 2005; Xi et al., 2006b). NGB-2904 alone neither produces dysphorigenic effects in brain-stimulation reward nor substitutes for cocaine in self-administration, suggesting that NGB-2904 itself has no abuse potential (Xi and Gardner, 2007). NGB-2904 is not currently under clinical trials, and detailed data regarding bioavailability and pharmacokinetic properties are presently unavailable.

3.8 YQA-14

YQA-14 is a novel D3 receptor antagonist developed recently (Song et al., 2012). Structurally, YQA-14 is a NGB-2904 analog. *In vivo* pharmacokinetic assays suggest that YQA-14 has improved oral bioavailability (>40%) and a longer half-life (>6 h in humans) compared to SB-277011A (~20 min in primates). In experimental animals, YQA-14 dose-dependently inhibits cocaine self-administration under both FR2 and PR reinforcement schedules, cocaine-induced CPP, cocaine-enhanced brain-stimulation reward, and cocaine- or cue-induced reinstatement of drug-seeking behavior (Song et al., 2012). Strikingly, at the doses that inhibit cocaine's actions, YQA-14 failed to alter oral sucrose self-administration and locomotor activity. YQA-14 is neither self-administered in drug-naïve rats nor substitutes for cocaine in maintenance of self-administration in rats previously trained for cocaine self-administration, suggesting that YQA-14 itself has no abuse liability. Deletion of DA D3 receptors in D3-knockout mice almost completely abolished the inhibitory effect by YQA-14 of cocaine self-administration, suggesting an effect mediated by blocking DA D3 receptors *in vivo* (Song et al., 2012). YQA-14 is currently not under clinical trials.

3.9 S33138

Preclinical studies: S33138 is a preferential D3 *versus* D2 receptor (~25-fold selectivity) antagonist (Millan et al., 2008). It was hypothesized that blockade of D3 plus partial blockade of D2 receptors may produce additive anti-cocaine therapeutic effects, but have fewer unwanted side-effects such as sedation and extrapyramidal locomotor impairment due to partial blockade of D2 receptors (Peng et al., 2009). In experimental animals, we found that S33138 produced biphasic effects – low doses increase, while high doses inhibit, cocaine self-administration under FR2 reinforcement. We interpret this increase in cocaine self-administration as a compensatory response to a reduction in cocaine's rewarding efficacy at low doses. In addition, S33138 also dose-dependently inhibits cocaine-enhanced brain-stimulation reward and cocaine-induced reinstatement of drug-seeking behavior (Peng et al., 2009). S33138, at low-to-moderate doses, has no effect on brain reward function by itself, while at high doses, produces an aversive-like effect as assessed by electrical brain-stimulation reward experiments, suggesting a D2 receptor-mediated effect at high doses. Further high doses of S33138 also inhibit oral sucrose self-administration, suggesting possible unwanted effects on nature reward at high doses.

Clinical trials: S33138 is currently under clinical trials as an anti-psychotic agent for the treatment of schizophrenia and other psychiatric diseases (Millan and Brocco, 2008; Thomasson-Perret et al., 2008). The efficacy of S33138 for treatment of cocaine addiction has not been evaluated in human clinical trials.

4. Glutamate-based medication strategies

Rationale: L-glutamate is the major excitatory neurotransmitter in the brain and acts through two heterogeneous families of glutamate receptors: ionotropic (iGluR) and metabotropic (mGluR) glutamate receptors. While iGluRs (i.e. NMDA, AMPA and kainite) are ligand-gated ion channels and responsible for fast excitatory neurotransmission, mGluRs (mGluR$_{1-8}$) are G-protein-coupled receptors linked to intracellular second messenger pathways. The eight subtypes of mGluRs have been classified into three groups on the basis of sequence similarities and pharmacological properties. Group I (mGluR$_{1,5}$) receptors activate phospholipase C via G$_q$ proteins, whereas group II (mGluR$_{2,3}$) and group III (mGluR$_{4,6,7,8}$) receptors inhibit adenylate cyclase via G$_{\alpha i/o}$ proteins (see review by Cartmell and Schoepp, 2000).

Although the role of glutamate in mediating cocaine's rewarding effects remains unclear (see review by Xi and Gardner, 2008), growing evidence suggests that glutamate is critically involved in relapse to drug-seeking behavior (Figure 3) (Kalivas, 2009; Bowers et al., 2010). In brief, chronic cocaine produces a reduction in basal levels of extracellular glutamate or glutamate transmission in the NAc during cocaine withdrawal, while cocaine priming or re-exposure to cocaine-associated cues stimulate glutamate release in both the VTA and NAc. These findings suggest that both a reduction in basal glutamate transmission and enhanced glutamate responding to cocaine or cocaine-associated cues may constitute a neurobiological substrate of relapse to drug-seeking behavior (Kalivas, 2009). Based on this hypothesis, a number of pharmacotherapeutic strategies have been proposed. These include, first, normalization (increase) of reduced basal glutamate neurotransmission during abstinence, and second, antagonism of enhanced glutamate responses to cocaine or cocaine-associated cues (Figure 3).

4.1 *N*-acetylcysteine

Preclinical studies: N-acetylcysteine (NAC) is a cystine prodrug. It is approved for the treatment of pulmonary complications of cystic fibrosis and paracetamol (acetaminophen) overdose. By providing a source of extracellular cysteine, which is converted to cystine, NAC can exchange extracellular cystine for intracellular glutamate. This restores (renormalizes) decreased basal levels of extracellular glutamate (Baker et al., 2003). The increased extracellular glutamate may subsequently attenuate cocaine-induced increases in glutamate release by activation of presynaptic mGluR2/3 receptors, and therefore inhibits cocaine- or cocaine cue-induced reinstatement of drug-seeking behaviour (Figure 3). NAC did not decrease cocaine self-administration or acute cocaine-induced hyperactivity, while it decreased repeated cocaine-induced escalation of drug intake and behavioural sensitization (Madayag et al., 2007). In addition, repeated NAC treatments also attenuated cocaine-induced increases in drug seeking in rats (Baker et al., 2003; Amen et al., 2010). Interestingly, NAC is also a prodrug for the synthesis of the endogenous antioxidant glutathione, and that NAC pretreatment protects animals from high dose methamphetamine or amphetamine induced DA neurotoxicity and behavioural changes by lowering oxidative stress levels (Fukami et al., 2004; Achat-Mendes et al., 2007).

Clinical trials: NAC is currently under clinical trials (Table 3). In double-blind, placebo-controlled clinic trials, NAC was well tolerated and produced a significant reduction in cocaine-related withdrawal symptoms and/or cravings triggered by exposure to cocaine-related cues or by an experimenter-delivered intravenous injection of cocaine (LaRowe et al., 2006, 2007; Amen et al., 2010). A 4-week open-label clinical trial demonstrated that NAC significantly reduced cocaine use in 16 of 23 human cocaine-dependent subjects (Mardikian et al., 2007). More clinical trials are currently underway (http://clinicaltrials.gov/).

Compound	Company	Pharm. Action	Indication	Status	Reference
N-acetylcysteine (NAC)	TwinLab, NY, USA; Others	Cystine prodrug	Substance abuse (cocaine, nicotine, methamphetamine)	Phase II	http://clinicaltrials.gov
AZD8529	AntraZeneca, London, UK	mGluR2/3 PAM	Schizophrenia	Phase II	http://clinicaltrials.gov
ADX71149	Janssen, USA	mGluR2 PAM	Schizophrenia; Anxiety	Phase II	http://www.addexpharma.com/pipline/
LY214023	Eli Lilly, USA	mGluR2/3 PAM	PK study	Phase I	http://clinicaltrials.gov
LY404039	Eli Lilly, USA	mGluR2/3 PAM	Schizophrenia	Phase II	Patil et al., 2007
LY354740	Eli Lilly, USA	mGluR2 PAM	Schizophrenia; Anxiety	Phase II	Dunayevich et al., 2008
JNJ-40411813	Johnson & Johnson, USA	mGluR2 PAM	Schizophrenia	Phase II	http://clinicaltrials.gov
GPI-5633	Guiford, USA	mGluR3 PAM	Safety & PK profile	Phase I	Van der Post et al., 2005
Fenobam	Enzo Life Sci. USA; Others	mGluR5 NAM	Anxiety; Fragile X syndrome	Phase II	http://clinicaltrials.gov
ADX10059	Addex Switzerland	mGluR5 NAM	Gastro-oesophageal reflux	Phase II	http://clinicaltrials.gov
STX107	Seaside, USA	mGluR5 NAM	Fragile X Syndrome	Phase II	http://clinicaltrials.gov

Table 3. Glutamate-based drug candidates in clinical trials

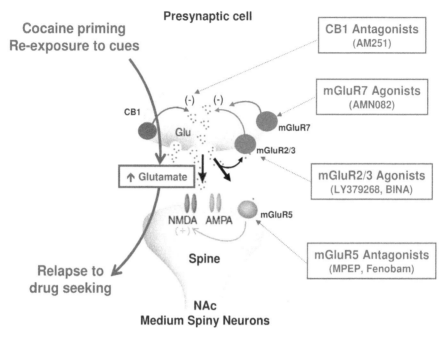

Fig. 3. Schematic diagram of glutamatergic synaptic transmission in the NAc, illustrating that cocaine priming or re-exposuse to cocaine-associated cues evokes an increase in glutamate release and relapse to drug-seeking behaviour in rats. Various compounds that target CB1 and mGluRs may attenuate cocaine- or cue-induced increase in glutamate release or in postsynaptic glutamate receptor signalling, and therefore, inhibit relapse to drug-seeking behaviour.

4.2 MPEP

Preclinical studies: MPEP is a selective mGluR5 negative allosteric modulator (NAM) or antagonist (Gasparini et al., 1999). The first study to examine the role of mGluR5 in drug addiction reported that deletion of mGluR5 subtype abolishes cocaine self-administration in mice, while systemic administration of MPEP significantly inhibited cocaine self-administration in mice (Chiamulera et al., 2001). Since then, a large number of studies suggest that systemic administration of MPEP or its analog MTEP (a more selective mGluR5 NAM) (Lea and Faden, 2006) significantly and dose-dependently inhibits cocaine self-administration in rats (Xi et al., 2004a, 2004c; Tessari et al., 2004; Paterson and Markou, 2005; Kenny et al., 2005; Lee et al., 2005), cocaine-induced CPP (McGeehan and Olive, 2003; Herzig and Schmidt, 2004), cocaine-induced hyperactivity (McGeehan et al., 2004), and cocaine-, cue- or stress-induced reinstatement of cocaine-seeking behaviour (Xi et al., 2004a, 2004c; Lee et al., 2005; Backstrom and Hyytia, 2006; Kumaresan et al., 2009; Martin-Fardon and Weiss, 2011; Wang et al., 2012). These data strongly suggest that mGluR5 antagonists may be promising in the treatment of cocaine addiction.

Clinical trials: MPEP and MTEP have not been tested in clinical trials. Relatively poor selectivity of MPEP for mGluR5 over other targets (NET, NR2B-containing NMDA receptor, monoamine oxidase A and mGluR4) may have prevented its use in human clinical trials.

4.3 Fenobam

Preclinical studies: Fenobam (McN-3377) was originally developed as a nonbenzodiazepine anxiolytic in the 1980s with an unknown molecular target until 2005 when it was reported that fenobam is a selective mGluR5 NAM or antagonist (Porter et al., 2005). Fenobam was reported to have improved mGluR5 selectivity compared to MPEP, as assessed by the use of mGluR5-KO mice, and rapidly penetrate brain-blood barrier to concentrate in the brain (Montana et al., 2009). Systemic administration of fenobam dose-dependently elevates stimulation threshold for brain-stimulation reward in rats, suggesting a reduction in brain reward function (Cleva et al., 2012). In addition, our pilot experimental data also suggest that oral administration of fenobam significantly inhibits cocaine self-administration and cocaine- or cue-, induced cocaine-seeking behaviour.

Clinical trials: Fenobam was investigated in Phase II clinical trials in the 1980s for the treatment of anxiety and depression (Table 3). Earlier single- or double-blind, placebo-controlled clinical trials demonstrated that fenobam was effective in attenuating severe anxiety with good safety profiles (Pecknold et al., 1982; Pecknold et al., 1980; Lapierre and Oyewumi, 1982). However, in another report, it was reported to be inactive and have psychostimulant effects by itself (Friedmann et al., 1980). At the time, fenobam was discontinued from further development as an anxiolytic. In 2006, it was granted orphan drug designation by the FDA for clinical trials in the treatment of Fragile X syndrome, an inherited mental retardation disorder. The efficacy of fenobam in the treatment of cocaine addiction has not yet been evaluated.

4.4 ADX10059

ADX10059 is another novel mGluR5-selective NAM or antagonist with an IC_{50} of 17.1 nM at human mGluR5, showing good selectivity for mGluR5 over > 65 other receptors, transporters, ion channels and enzymes (Marin and Goadsby, 2010). Although limited preclinical data are available, it has been under Phase I and Phase II clinical trials for the treatment of gastro-oesophageal reflux disease (Zerbib et al., 2010, 2011) and migraine (Marin and Goadsby, 2010) (Table 3). To date, ADX10059 has been studied in at least 10 clinical trials. However, Addex Pharmaceuticals announced the discontinuation of development of ADX10059 in December 2009 due to liver enzyme changes. The efficacy of ADX10059 in the treatment of cocaine addiction has not been evaluated.

4.5 LY379268

Preclinical studies: LY379268 is a systemically effective $mGluR_{2/3}$ orthosteric (competitive) agonist (Marek, 2004). The $mGluR_{2/3}$ receptors have become attractive targets in medication development for the treatment of drug addiction because $mGluR_{2/3}$ receptors function as glutamate autoreceptors, modulating presynaptic glutamate release (Xi et al., 2002a) (Figure 3). In addition, $mGluR_{2/3}$ modulates DA and other neurotransmitter release in the NAc. Since cocaine-induced increases in NAc DA and glutamate are critically involved in drug reward and relapse, it was proposed that $mGluR_{2/3}$ agonists might be useful for the treatment of cocaine addiction (Xi et al., 2002a). Systemic administration of LY379268 inhibits cocaine self-administration and cocaine cue-induced reinstatement of drug-seeking behaviour (Baptista et al., 2004; Peters and Kalivas, 2006). Microinjections of LY369268 into the NAc or central amygdala also inhibit cocaine- or food-triggered reinstatement of reward-seeking behaviour (Peters and Kalivas, 2006) or incubation of cocaine craving in rats (Lu et al., 2007). These data suggest that LY369268 may be useful for the treatment of cocaine addiction.

Clinical studies: LY379268 is not currently under clinical trials. This may be related to its intrinsic competitive agonist properties that may produce unwanted side-effects by itself and/or reduce efficacy due to competitive binding inhibition by excessive glutamate release under pathological conditions. In contrast to LY379268, several other mGluR2/3 positive allosteric modulators (PAMs) are being investigated in Phase I and Phase II clinical trials for the treatment of schizophreria and anxiety (Mezler et al., 2010; Patil., et al., 2007). These compounds include AZD8529, LY404039, LY354740, and LY2140023 (Table 3). The potential effects of these mGluR2/3 agonists in treatment of cocaine addiction have not been evaluated.

4.6 BINA

Preclinical studies: Biphenylindanone A (BINA) is a selective mGluR2 PAM or agonist (Johnson et al., 2003; Galici et al., 2006). Recent studies suggest that the pharmacological effects of LY379268 (a competitive mGluR2/3 orthosteric agonist) in animal models relevant to neuropsychiatric diseases could be mediated predominantly by activation of mGluR2, not mGluR3 receptor (Woolley et al., 2008), suggesting that mGluR2-selective agonists may produce similar therapeutic effects but have fewer unwanted effects than LY379268. Recently, Markou and her colleagues have compared the pharmacotherapeutic effects of BINA and LY379268 in animal models of drug addiction. They found that BINA selectively inhibits cocaine self-administration and cue-induced reinstatement of cocaine-seeking behaviour without affecting behaviours motivated by food reinforcement, while LY379268 nonselectively inhibits both cocaine- and food-taking and –seeking behaviour (Jin et al., 2010). These data suggest that selective mGluR2 PAMs (BINA) might have better therapeutic potential than dual mGluR2/3 agonists (LY379268) for the treatment of cocaine addiction.

Clinical trials: BINA is currently not under clinical trials. However, other mGluR2 PAMs such as AZD71149, LY354740 and JNJ-40411813 are currently under clinical trials for safety and *in vivo* binding property in healthy volunteers (Table 3).

4.7 2-PMPA and GPI-5693

Preclinical studies: 2-PMPA and GPI-5693 (also called 2-MPPA) are inhibitors of NAALADase (N-acetylated-α-linked acidic dipeptidase, also called glutamate carboxypeptidase II, GCPII), an enzyme that hydrolyzes N-acetylaspartate-glutamate (NAAG) to N-acetylaspartate (NAA) and glutamate (Neal et al., 2000, 2011). NAAG is an endogenous mGluR3 agonist, which negatively modulates the release of glutamate and other neurotransmitters (Neale et al., 2000, 2011). Given the important role of NAc glutamate in relapse to drug seeking as stated above, it was hypothesized that inhibition of NAALADase by 2-PMPA and GPI-5693 would increase extracellular NAAG and decrease extracellular glutamate levels (due to decreased glutamate release from NAAG degradation), while the increase in NAAG would further inhibit glutamate release from neuronal terminals and/or glial cells by activating mGluR3 receptors (Xi et al., 2002a, 2010b). In addition, NAAG also inhibits DA release by activating mGluR3 receptors located on DA terminals in the NAc (Xi et al., 2010b). Thus, the endogenous NAALADase-NAAG-mGluR3 signal system may constitute a novel important target in medication development for the treatment of cocaine addiction. Earlier studies have shown that systemic administration of 2-PMPA inhibits cocaine-induced CPP (Slusher et al., 2001) and cocaine-induced behavioural sensitization (Shippenberg et al., 2000). Recently, we reported that systemic administration of 2-PMPA or GPI-5693 inhibited cocaine self-administration, cocaine-enhanced brain-stimulation reward, and cocaine-triggered reinstatement of drug-seeking behaviour (Xi et al., 2010a, 2010b; Peng et al., 2010b). This action was blocked by pretreatment with LY341495, a selective mGluR2/3 antagonist. In addition, 2-PMPA dose-dependently attenuated cocaine-induced increases in extracellular DA and glutamate in the NAc (Xi et al., 2010a; 2010b). Taken together, these data suggest that inhibition of NAALADase by 2-PMPA or GPI-5693 produces an inhibitory effect on cocaine-taking and cocaine-seeking behaviour

Clinical trials: GPI-5693 was investigated in a Phase I clinical trial for its safety, pharmacokinetics and efficacy for treatment of neuropathic pain (Table 3) (van der Post et al., 2005). It was reported to be safe and tolerable in healthy subjects.

4.8 AMN082

AMN082 is a novel systemically active mGluR7 PAM or agonist (Mitsukawa et al., 2005). The mGluR7 receptor subtype has attracted much attention in medication development for treatment of addiction for several reasons (Li et al., 2012). First, mGluR7 is the most abundant subtype of the group III mGluR subtypes in reward-related brain regions such as striatum, hippocampus and olfactory tubercles (Ferraguti and Shigemoto, 2006). Second, activation of group III mGluRs (including mGluR7) by L-AP4 inhibits DA and glutamate release in the NAc (Hu et al., 1999; Xi et al., 2003b). Third, it is the most conserved mGluR subtype across different mammalian species (Makoff et al., 1996), suggesting that selective mGluR7 ligands that are effective in experimental animals are more likely to be effective in humans. And fourth, the development of AMN082 has allowed us to explore the role of mGluR7 in drug reward and addiction.

Based on the above, we and others have recently reported that systemic administration of AMN082 inhibits cocaine self-administration behaviour under both FR2 and PR reinforcement, cocaine-enhanced brain reward function, and cocaine-induced reinstatement of drug-seeking behaviour. In addition, AMN082 also decreases, while the selective mGluR7 antagonist MMPIP increases, alcohol intake and preference (Salling et al., 2008; Bahi et al., 2011). Importantly, the same doses of AMN082 neither alters locomotion or sucrose self-administration (Li et al., 2010; Bahi et al., 2011; but see Salling et al., 2008) nor alters brain reward function (Li et al., 2008), suggesting that AMN082 produces therapeutic anti-cocaine effects without significant unwanted effects such as sedation, dysphoria or natural reward depression. Further mechanistic studies suggest that a NAc-VP GABAergic mechanism underlies its antagonism of cocaine reward (Li et al., 2008, 2009), while a glutamate-mGluR2/3 mechanism underlies its antagonism of relapse to drug-seeking behaviour (Li et al., 2008, 2010, 2012). Together, these preclinical data suggest a potential utility of AMN082 in the treatment of cocaine addiction. AMN082 has not yet been tested in clinical trials.

5. GABA-based medication strategies

Rationale: It is well known that the mesolimbic DA system is critically involved in drug reward and addiction. However, it remains unclear how increased NAc DA underlies these actions. Anatomically, the majority of neurons in the striatum are medium-spiny GABAergic output neurons, which receive DA projections from the VTA and glutamatergic projections predominantly from the prefrontal cortex, and project to the dorsal globus pallidus (from the dorsal striatum) and the ventral pallidum (VP) and VTA (from the ventral striatum, i.e. the NAc) (Bennett and Bolam, 1994; Groenewegen et al., 1996). Overall, DA produces a net inhibitory effect on striatal medium-spiny GABAergic neurons (Nicola and Malenka, 1997; Umemiya and Raymond, 1997), predominantly by activation of D2-like DA receptors (Centonze et al., 2002). Similarly, cocaine also produces an overall inhibitory effect on VTA GABAergic neurons (Cameron and Williams, 1994), striatal GABAergic neurons (Uchimura and North, 1990; White et al., 1993; Centonze et al., 2002; Schramm-Sapyta et al., 2006), and GABA release in the VP (Tang et al., 2005; Li et al., 2010). Based on this, the NAc-VP/VTA GABAergic projection constitutes common final pathway underlying drug reward and addiction (Figure 2). Thus, it has been hypothesized that a pharmacological strategy that enhances GABAergic transmission in the VTA and/or the VP would produce an inhibitory effect on cocaine- or DA-induced reductions in GABA release, therefore antagonizing cocaine's rewarding effects. Based on this, several GABAergic compounds have been studied extensively in experimental animals.

5.1 Gamma-vinyl GABA

Preclinical studies: Gamma-vinyl GABA (GVG) (also called vigabatrin) is an irreversible GABA transaminase inhibitor. GABA transaminase is an enzyme that breaks down GABA, causing an increase in brain GABA after GVG administration (Peng et al., 2010a). In the 1990s, Dewey and colleagues first proposed that GVG might be useful for the treatment of drug addiction (Dewey et al., 1998). Since then, many preclinical studies appear to support this hypothesis (Xi and Gardner, 2008). Systemic administration of GVG inhibits cocaine self-administration, cocaine-enhanced brain-stimulation reward, cocaine-induced CPP and behavioural sensitization (see review by Xi and Gardner, 2008). Similarly, it also dose-dependently inhibits cocaine-induced reinstatement of drug-seeking behaviour (Peng et al., 2008). All these data support the use of GVG in the treatment of cocaine addiction.

Clinical trials: GVG is currently under clinical trials for treatment of cocaine addiction (Table 4). In three open-labeled studies, GVG was well-tolerated and produced a significant increase in cocaine abstinence rate (Brodie et al., 2003, 2005; Fechtner et al., 2006). In a more recent randomized, double-blind, placeto-controled trial, short-term GVG treatment significantly increased abstinence rate compared to placebo (Brodie et al., 2009). However, in another clinical trial for the treatment of methamphetamine dependence, GVG was not effective (De La Garza et al., 2009). GVG is not marketed in the USA because of concerns over ophthalmological side-effects, but none were observed during these short-term studies (Fechtner et al., 2006). More studies are underway to confirm its efficacy for cocaine dependence (http://clinicaltrials.gov).

Compound	Company	Pharm. Action	Indication	Status	Reference
GVG	Aventis, Quebec, Canada	GABA transaminase inhibitor	Substance abuse (cocaine, methamphetamine)	Phase II	http://clinicaltrials.gov
Topiramate	Meliapharm, Montreal, Canada	GABA$_A$ PAM	Substance abuse (cocaine)	Phase II	http://clinicaltrials.gov
	VIVUS, CA, USA				
Tiagabine	Cephalon, PA, USA	GABA transporter inhibitor	Substance abuse (cocaine);	Phase II	http://clinicaltrials.gov
			Anxiety Schizophrenia	Phase III	
Baclofen	Remedy Repack, PA, USA	GABA$_B$ receptor agonist	Substance abuse (cocaine, nicotine, alcohol)	Phase II	http://clinicaltrials.gov
Gabapentin	Meliapharm, Montreal, Canada	GABA enhancer, Alpha2delta-Ca^{++} channel blocker	Substance abuse (cocaine, nicotine, alcohol)	Phase II	http://clinicaltrials.gov

Table 4. GABA receptor-based drug candidates in clinical trials

5.2 Tiagabine

Preclinical studies: Tiagabine is a selective type 1 GABA transporter (GAT1) inhibitor, which increases extracellular GABA levels (Eriksson et al., 1999). It has been approved as an antiepileptic medication (Schousboe et al., 2011). Preclinical studies suggest that tiagabine inhibited intravenous cocaine self-administration in rats (Filip et al., 2007) or baboons (Weerts et al., 2005), but had no significant effect on cocaine-induced reinstatement of drug-seeking behaviour (Filip et al., 2007; Weerts et al., 2007). Our experimental data suggest that tiagabine, at much higher doses (10-20 mg/kg) than those used in the above-cited studies, selectively inhibited cocaine self-administration, but had no effect on cocaine-induced reinstatement of drug-seeking behaviour in rats (Yang et al., 2012).

Clinical trials: The results of clinical trials with tiagabine are mixed. Two small-scale (45 and 76 subjects, respectively) placebo-controlled clinical trials indicated that tiagabine produced a moderate reduction (~30%) in cocaine use in methadone-treated cocaine addicts (González et al., 2003, 2007), while other studies demonstrated that the same doses of tiagabine neither altered the acute effects of cocaine (Lile et al., 2004), nor lowered cocaine use in cocaine addicts (Winhusen et al., 2005; 2007).

5.3 Topiramate

Preclinical studies: Topiramate is a positive modulator of GABA$_A$ receptors (acting at non-benzodiazepine sites) and a licensed antiepileptic drug (Czuczwar and Patsalos, 2001). In addition, topiramate has other pharmacological actions, including antagonism of AMPA/kainate glutamate receptors, inhibition of voltage-gated sodium and calcium channels and inhibition of carbonic anhydrase (Johnson, 2005). In animal studies, topiramate was reported to inhibit cocaine self-administration and attenuate NAc DA response to cocaine or cocaine-associated cues (Johnson, 2005).

Clinical studies: In a double-blind, placebo-controlled clinical trial (40 subjects), topiramate significantly increased abstinence rates compared to placebo (Kampman et al., 2004). A recent 12-week, open-label pilot study showed a significant reduction in craving intensity and duration in 25% of the sample group (Reis et al., 2008). Evidence for a beneficial role of topiramate in the treatment of cocaine dependence is promising but is limited by small sample sizes (Cubells, 2006; Minozzi et al., 2008). More studies are currently underway (Table 4).

5.4 Baclofen

Preclinical studies: Baclofen is a selective GABA$_B$ receptor agonist, licensed as an antispasmodic for patients with spinal cord injuries or multiple sclerosis. In rodents, pretreatment with baclofen dose-dependently attenuates cocaine self-administration under FR and PR reinforcement (Roberts et al., 1996; Brebner et al., 2000), cocaine-enhanced brain-stimulation reward (Slattery et al., 2005), and cocaine-induced increases in NAc DA (Fadda et al., 2003). It also inhibited cocaine- or cue-induced cocaine-taking and cocaine-seeking behaviour (Di Ciano and Everitt, 2003; Campbell et al., 1999; Weerts et al., 2007).

Clinical trials: In an initial open-label clinical trial, baclofen reduced self-reports of craving and cocaine use in 10 cocaine abusers (Ling et al., 1998). In a subsequent 16-week double-blind study in 35 cocaine-dependent subjects, baclofen reduced cocaine use and increased the number of cocaine-free urines (Shoptaw et al., 2003), but did not alter cocaine craving. In a recent placebo-controlled, double-blind study, baclofen lowered cocaine intake, decreased cocaine craving, and attenuated cocaine's cardiovascular effects in both cocaine- and opioid-dependent subjects (Haney et al., 2006). However, a more recent large scale (160 cocaine addicts), double-blind, placebo-controlled clinical trial demonstrated that baclofen was not effective in attenuating cocaine use (Kahn et al., 2009). Thus, more studies are required to determine its efficacy in relapse prevention.

5.5 Gabapentin

Preclinical studies: Gabapentin is structurally analogous to GABA but, unlike the latter, it crosses the blood–brain barrier and can be administered systemically. Pharmacologically, gabapentin is a GABAmimetic drug that increases extracellular GABA levels, possibly by increasing the synthesis and nonvesicular release of GABA as well as by preventing GABA catabolism (Taylor et al., 1998). In addition, gabapentin also inhibits alpha2delta subunit-composed voltage-dependent Ca^{++} channels (Gee et al., 1996). Early studies suggest that gabapentin (1-30 mg/kg, i.p.) significantly inhibited cocaine-induced hyperactivity and locomotor sensitization (Filip et al., 2006; but see Itzhak and Martin, 2000). However, other studies demonstrate that gabapentin, at a broad dose range (10-200 mg/kg i.p.), neither inhibited cocaine self-administration nor altered cocaine-induced reinstatement of drug-seeking behaviour in rats (Filip et al., 2007; Peng et al., 2008b). *In vivo* microdialysis studies demonstrate that gabapentin, at 100-200 mg/kg, produced a significant increase (~50 %) in extracellular GABA in the NAc, but failed to alter either basal or cocaine-enhanced NAc DA (Peng et al., 2008b). These data suggest that gabapentin is a weak GABA enhancer and may have limited potential in the treatment of cocaine addiction.

Clinical trials: Early clinical studies and small-scale, open-label outpatient trials demonstrated that gabapentin reduced cocaine craving and use (Raby and Coomaraswamy, 2004; Myrick et al., 2001; Hart et al., 2004, 2005). However, this finding was not repeated by larger-scale, double-blind, placebo-controlled clinical trials demonstrating that gabapentin, at doses up to 2400-3200 mg/day for 6-12 weeks, had no effect on abstinence rate, craving or subjective effects of cocaine (Bisaga et al., 2006; Berger et al., 2005; González et al., 2007; Hart et al., 2007). More clinical trials are currently under way to evaluate the effects of gabapentin or gabapentin combined with the antidepressant sertraline on cocaine or other addictive drug dependence (Table 4).

6. Cannabinoid-based medication strategies

Rationale: Marijuana is the most widely used illicit drug in the United States. Δ^9-tetrahydrocannabinol (Δ^9-THC) is the major psychoactive ingredient in marijuana. Two major types of cannabinoid receptors, CB_1 and CB_2, have been cloned. Since CB_1 receptors are found in both brain and peripheral tissues, whereas CB_2 receptors are found predominantly in peripheral immune system, it is generally belived that the psychoactive effects of Δ^9-THC or marijuana are mediated by activation of brain CB1, not CB2, receptors (Tanda and Goldberg, 2003). However, growing evidence suggests that functional CB_2 receptors are also found in the brain (Van Sickle et al., 2005; Gong et al., 2006; Xi et al., 2011), suggesting that brain CB_2 receptors may be also involved in marijuana's actions.

As stated above, the mesolimbic DA and the downstream NAc-VP GABAergic transmission have been thought to underlie cocaine reward and addiction. Growing evidence suggests that similar mechanisms may also underlie the action produced by Δ^9-THC or marijuana. It was reported that Δ^9-THC elevates extracellular DA in the NAc (Chen et al., 1990; Tanda et al., 1997). This action could be mediated by a GABAergic mechanism, i.e., Δ^9-THC may initially activate CB1 receptors located on VTA GABAergic interneurons and produce a decrease in GABA release, which subsequently disinhibits (or activates) VTA DA neurons (Figure 2) (Fernandez-Ruiz et al., 2010). In addition, CB_1 receptors are also highly expressed on presynaptic glutamatergic terminals in the NAc (Lupica et al., 2004). Thus, activation of CB1 receptors located on glutamatergic terminals decreases glutamate inputs onto medium-spiny GABAergic neurons in the NAc and decrease GABA release in their projection areas – the VP and VTA. Further, CB1 receptors are also expressed on striatal GABAergic neurons, and activation of the CB1 receptors produces a direct inhibitory effect on medium-spiny GABAergic neurons and decreases GABA release in the VP and the VTA (Maldonado et al., 2011). Lastly, cocaine or DA has been shown to increase endocannabinoid release in the striatum (Giuffrida et al., 1999; Centonze et al., 2004; Caille et al., 2007), which subsequently increases endocannabinoid binding to CB1 receptors located on presynaptic glutamatergic terminals and postsynaptic GABAergic neurons (Figure 2). Taken together, activation of

CB1 receptors located on both GABAergic and glutamatergic neurons causes an increase in NAc DA and a decrease in GABA release in both the VTA and VP. This decrease in NAc-VP GABAergic transmission constitutes a final common pathway underlying drug reward and addiction. Accordingly, blockade of CB_1 receptors in both the VTA and NAc would attenuate the actions of cocaine on NAc DA and VP GABA release, and therefore attenuate cocaine reward and addiction.

6.1 SR141716A

Preclinical studies: SR141716A (also called rimonabant) is the first developed CB_1 receptor antagonist (also an inverse agonist) (Rinaldi-Carmona et al., 1994). SR141716A was reported to inhibit cocaine self-administration under PR reinforcement (Soria et al., 2005; Xi et al., 2008), decrease cocaine-enhanced NAc DA (Cheer et al., 2007; Soria et al., 2005), and inhibit cocaine- and cue-induced reinstatement of drug-seeking behaviour (De Vries et al., 2001), while other studies suggest that it has no effect on cocaine self-administration under low FR reinforcement, cocaine-induced CPP, or cocaine-induced behavioural sensitization (Arnold, 2005). These data suggest that SR141716A may have therapeutic effects in attenuating relapse to drug-seeking behaviour, but is limited in terms of attenuating cocaine's acute rewarding effects (Beardsley and Thomas, 2005; Xi and Gardner, 2008).

Clinical trials: SR141716A was the first CB1 receptor antagonist to be approved for clinical trials for the treatment of obesity and cigarette smoking. However, there are some safety concerns with rimonabant – increased risk of anxiety, depression, and suicide tendency, which had led it to being withdrawn from the market in Europe and North America in 2008. Since then, many pharmaceutical companies (Sanofi-Aventis, Merck, Pfizer, Solvay) have announced that they will stop further clinical research on this class of drug.

6.2 AM251

Preclinical studies: AM251 is a more potent and selective CB_1 receptor antagonist than SR141716A (Krishnamurthy et al., 2004). In animal models of drug addiction, AM251 appears to be more potent and effective than SR141716A in attenuating cocaine's action (Xi et al., 2006, 2008). For example, AM251 significantly and dose-dependently inhibited cocaine self-administration (under PR, but not FR reinforcement) (Xi et al., 2008), cocaine-enhanced brain-stimulation reward (Xi et al., 2008), and cocaine-induced behavioural sensitization (Corbille et al., 2007), as well as cocaine-triggered reinstatement of drug-seeking behaviour (Xi et al., 2006). Further, a glutamate-mGluR2/3 mechanism has been shown to underlie the antagonism of reinstatement of drug seeking (Xi et al., 2006). That is, blockade of CB1 receptors by AM251 elevates extracellular glutamate in the NAc, which subsequently increased glutamate binding to presynaptic mGluR2/3 receptors, inhibiting cocaine-induced increases in glutamate release and relapse to drug-seeking behaviour (Xi et al., 2006) (Figure 3). These findings suggest that AM251 may be more potent and effective than SR141716A for treatment of cocaine addiction.

Clinical trials: Since the above mentioned side-effects of SR141716A have been linked to its inverse agonist property, it is generally believed that AM251, a CB1 receptor antagonist with similar inverse agonist property might have the same unwanted side-effects. It is not under clinical trials.

6.3 JWH133

Preclinical studies: In addition to CB1 receptors, recent breakthrough findings suggest that brain CB_2 receptors are also involved in drug reward and addiction (Onaivi et al., 2008; Xi et al., 2011; Aracil-Fernández, et al., 2012). JWH133 and GW405833 are highly selective CB2 receptor agonists. We have recently reported that systemic, intranasal or intra-NAc administration of JWH133 or GW405833 significantly and dose-dependently inhibits cocaine self-administration, cocaine-induced increases in locomotion and extracellular DA in wild-type and CB1-KO mice, but not in CB2-KO mice. Similarly, overexpression of CB2 receptors in mouse brain decreases intravenous cocaine self-administration and cocaine-induced locomotor sensitization (Aracil-Fernández, et al., 2012). These data suggest that CB2 receptor agonists may have therapeutic potential for the treatment of cocaine addiction (Figure 2) (Xi et al., 2011).

Clinical trials: JWH133 and GW405833 are currently not under clinical trials. However, many other selective CB2 receptor agonists, such as cannabinor, GW842166, GRC-10693, LY-2828360, ABT-521, and KHK-6188, are currently under Phase I and Phase II clinical trials for the treatment of pain or other diseases (Table 5). In addition, several dual CB1/CB2

Compound	Company	Pharm. Action	Indication	Status	Reference
Cannabinor	Pharmos, NJ, USA	CB2 agonist	Pain	Phase II	http://www.pharmoscorp.com/development/cannabinor.html
GW842166	GSK, London, UK	CB2 agonist	Pain	Phase II	http://clinicaltrials.gov
GRC 10693	Glenmark, Munbai, India	CB2 agonist	Pain	Phase I	http://www.evaluatepharma.com/Universal/View.aspx?type=Story&id=183092
LY-2828360	Eli Lilly, USA	CB2 agonist	Pain	Phase II	http://clinicaltrials.gov
ABT-521	Abbott, USA	CB2 agonist	Pain	Phase I	http://www.pharmalive.com/special_reports/sample.cfm?reportID=283
KHK-6188	Kyowa Hakka Kirin, Japan	CB2 agonist	Pain	Phase I	http://clinicaltrials.gov
Nabilone (Cesamet): Δ^9-THC analog	NEMA Research, USA	CB1/CB2 agonist	Cannabis addiction; Pain	Phase III Phase IV	http://clinicaltrials.gov
Marinol (Dronabinol): Δ^9-THC	UNIMED, USA	CB1/CB2 agonist	Substance abuse (opioid, marijuana, alcohol), PTSD	Phase II Phase IV	http://clinicaltrials.gov
Sativex: Δ^9-THC + Cannabidiol	GW, London, UK	CB1/CB2 agonist	Cannabis abuse, Pain	Phase II	http://clinicaltrials.gov

Table 5. Cannabinoid-based drug candidates in clinical trials

receptor agonists such as Nabilone (a Δ^9-THC analog), Marinol (Δ^9-THC), Sativex (a mixture of THC and cannabidiol) have been approved for the treatment of pain and chemotherapy-induced nausea and vomiting (Table 5). Based upon the recent findings that activation of CB2 receptors in primary afferents and spinal cord produces analgesic effects (Anand et al., 2009; Beltramo, 2009), and that activation of CB2 receptors in the brainstem inhibits morphine-6-glucuronide–induced emesis (vomiting) (Van Sickle et al., 2005), it is likely that the therapeutic effects of these dual CB1/CB2 receptor agonists may at least in part be mediated by activation of brain CB2 receptors.

7. Conclusion

In this review article, I first briefly reviewed the neurochemical mechanisms underlying cocaine reward and addiction, and then provided the rationale for development of various pharmacological therapies for the treatment of cocaine addiction. Lastly, I summarized the major findings of multiple pharmacological agents in each drug catagory in animal models of drug addiction and the current status in clinical trials for the treatment of drug addiction and/or other neuropsychiatric diseases. In summary, the VTA-NAc-VP pathway, including the mesolimbic DA and the NAc-VP GABAergic transimission, appears to play a critical role in mediating cocaine's rewarding effects (Figure 2), while a NAc glutamate-mGluR2/3 mechanism plays an important role in controlling relapse to drug-seeking behaviour (Figure 3). Accordingly, various pharmacological agents have been proposed and tested in animal models of drug addiction to interfere with the pharmacological actions produced by cocaine. Among those compounds discussed above, the DAT inhibitors (modafinil, RTI-335, CTDP31,345, CTDP-32,476), the DA receptor antagonists (*l*-THP, S33138, GSK598809, YQA-14) and the glutamatergic ligands (NAC, MPEP, LY369268, 2-PMPA) appear to be promising in preclinical animal models of drug addiction. In addition, several compounds (such as modafinil, disulfram, topiramate) were initially found to be effective in humans with unknown mechanisms, while subsequent preclinical studies helped to uncover the mechanisms of the actions. Although many compounds are currently or at some point were, under clinical trials, most of them have been used to evaluate their safety and efficacy for other neuropsychiatric diseases such schizophrenia, anxiety, obesity or smoking, rather than for cocaine addiction. Clearly, more translational studies from preclinical research to human clinical trials are required to promote the medication discovery for the treatment of cocaine dependence.

8. Acknowledgements

This research was supported by the NIDA/IRP, National Institutes of Health. I thank Jennifer Bossert and Tomas Keck of the NIDA/IRP for their proof-reading of on this manuscript.

9. References

Achat-Mendes C, Anderson KL, Itzhak Y. Impairment in consolidation of learned place preference following dopaminergic neurotoxicity in mice is ameliorated by N-acetylcysteine but not D1 and D2 dopamine receptor agonists. Neuropsychopharmacology 2007; 32: 531-41.

Amen SL, Piacentine LB, Ahmad ME, et al., Repeated N-acetyl cysteine reduces cocaine seeking in rodents and craving in cocaine-dependent humans. Neuropsychopharmacology 2010; 36:871-8.

Anand P, Whiteside G, Fowler CJ, Hohmann AG. Targeting CB2 receptors and the endocannabinoid system for the treatment of pain. Brain Res Rev. 2009; 60:255-66.

Anderson AL, Reid MS, Li SH, et al. Modafinil for the treatment of cocaine dependence. Drug Alcohol Depend. 2009; 104:133-9.

Aracil-Fernández A, Trigo JM, García-Gutiérrez MS, et al.,. Decreased cocaine motor sensitization and self-administration in mice overexpressing cannabinoid CB(2) receptors. Neuropsychopharmacology. 2012 37:1749-63.

Arnold JC. The role of endocannabinoid transmission in cocaine addiction. Pharmacol Biochem Behav 2005; 81: 396-406.

Arria, AM, Wish, ED. Nonmedical use of prescription stimulants among students. Pediatric Annals 2006; 35: 565–571.

Austin NE, Baldwin SJ, Cutler L, et al. Pharmacokinetics of the novel, high-affinity and selective dopamine D3 receptor antagonist SB-277011 in rat, dog and monkey: in vitro/in vivo correlation and the role of aldehyde oxidase. Xenobiotica 2001; 31: 677-86.

Backstrom P, Hyytia P. Ionotropic and metabotropic glutamate receptor antagonism attenuates cue-induced cocaine seeking. Neuropsychopharmacology 2006; 31: 778-86.

Bahi A, Fizia K, Dietz M, Gasparini F, Flor PJ. Pharmacological modulation of mGluR7 with AMN082 and MMPIP exerts specific influences on alcohol consumption and preference in rats. Addict Biol. 2012; 17:235-47.

Baker DA, McFarland K, Lake RW, Shen H, Tang XC, Toda S, Kalivas PW. Neuroadaptations in cystine-glutamate exchange underlie cocaine relapse. Nat Neurosci 2003; 6: 743-49.

Baker, JR, Jatlow, P, McCance-Katz, EF. Disulfiram effects on responses to intravenous cocaine administration. Drug and Alcohol Dependence 2006; 87: 202–209

Ballon JS, Feifel D. A systematic review of modafinil: Potential clinical uses and mechanisms of action. J Clin Psychiatry 2006; 67:554-566.

Baptista MA, Martin-Fardon R, Weiss F. Preferential effects of the metabotropic glutamate 2/3 receptor agonist LY379268 on conditioned reinstatement versus primary reinforcement: comparison between cocaine and a potent conventional reinforcer. J Neurosci 2004; 24: 4723-7.

Barth KS, Malcolm RJ. Disulfiram: an old therapeutic with new applications. CNS Neurol Disord Drug Targets 2010; 9:5-12

Baumann MH, Char GU, de Costa BR, Rice KC, Rothman RB. GBR 12909 attenuates cocaine-induced activation of mesolimbic dopamine neurons in the rat. J Pharmacol Exp Ther 1994; 271: 1216-22.

Beardsley PM, Thomas BF. Current evidence supporting a role of cannabinoid CB1 receptor (CB1R) antagonists as potential pharmacotherapies for drug abuse disorders. Behav Pharmacol 2005, 16. 275-96.

Beaulieu JM, Gainetdinov RR. The physiology, signaling, and pharmacology of dopamine receptors. Pharmacol Rev. 2011; 63:182-217.

Beltramo M. Cannabinoid type 2 receptor as a target for chronic - pain. Mini Rev Med Chem. 2009; 9:11-25.

Bennett BD, Bolam JP. Synaptic input and output of parvalbumin-immunoreactive neurons in the neostriatum of the rat. Neuroscience 1994; 62:707-19.

Berger SP, Winhusen TM, Somoza EC, et al. A medication screening trial evaluation of reserpine, gabapentin and lamotrigine pharmacotherapy of cocaine dependence. Addiction 2005; 100 (Suppl 1): 58-67.

Berger UV, Luthi-Carter R, Passani LA, Elkabes S, Black I, Konradi C, Coyle JT. Glutamate carboxypeptidase II is expressed by astrocytes in the adult rat nervous system. J Comp Neurol 1999; 415: 52-64.

Bisaga A, Aharonovich E, Garawi F, Levin FR, Rubin E, Raby WN, Nunes EV. A randomized placebo-controlled trial of gabapentin for cocaine dependence. Drug Alcohol Depend 2006; 81: 267-74.

Bowers MS, Chen BT, Bonci A. AMPA receptor synaptic plasticity induced by psychostimulants: the past, present, and therapeutic future. Neuron. 2010;67:11-24.

Brebner K, Phelan R, Roberts DC. Effect of baclofen on cocaine self-administration in rats reinforced under fixed-ratio 1 and progressive-ratio schedules. Psychopharmacology 2000; 148: 314-21.

Brodie JD, Case BG, Figueroa E, et al., Randomized, double-blind, placebo-controlled trial of vigabatrin for the treatment of cocaine dependence in Mexican parolees. Am J Psychiatry 2009; 166:1269-77.

Brodie JD, Figueroa E, Dewey SL. Treating cocaine addiction: from preclinical to clinical trial experience with γ-vinyl GABA. Synapse 2003; 50: 261-5.

Brodie JD, Figueroa E, Laska EM, Dewey SL. Safety and efficacy of γ-vinyl GABA (GVG) for the treatment of methamphetamine and/or cocaine addiction. Synapse 2005; 55: 122-5.

Caille S, Alvarez-Jaimes L, et al. Specific alterations of extracellular endocannabinoid levels in the nucleus accumbens by ethanol, heroin, and cocaine self-administration. J Neurosci 2007; 27: 3695-702.

Cameron DL, Williams JT. Cocaine inhibits GABA release in the VTA through endogenous 5-HT. J Neurosci 1994; 14: 6763-7.

Campbell UC, Lac ST, Carroll ME. Effects of baclofen on maintenance and reinstatement of intravenous cocaine self-administration in rats. Psychopharmacology 1999; 143: 209-14.

Carroll FI, Howard JL, Howell LL, Fox BS, Kuhar MJ. Development of the dopamine transporter selective RTI-336 as a pharmacotherapy for cocaine abuse. AAPS J 2006; 8:E196-203.

Carroll, KM, Fenton, LR, Ball, SA, et al. Efficacy of disulfiram and cognitive behavior therapy in cocaine-dependent outpatients: a randomized placebo-controlled trial. Arch Gen Psychiatry 2004; 61: 264–272.

Carroll, KM, Nich, C, Ball, SA, et al. One-year follow-up of disulfiram and psychotherapy for cocaine-alcohol users: sustained effects of treatment. Addiction 2000; 95: 1335–1349.

Carroll, KM, Nich, C, Ball, SA, McCance, E, Rounsavile, BJ. Treatment of cocaine and alcohol dependence with psychotherapy and disulfiram. Addiction 1998; 93: 713–727.

Cartmell J, Schoepp DD. Regulation of neurotransmitter release by metabotropic glutamate receptors. J Neurochem 2000; 75: 889-907.

Centonze D, Battista N, Rossi S, et al. A critical interaction between dopamine D2 receptors and endocannabinoids mediates the effects of cocaine on striatal GABAergic transmission. Neuropsychopharmacology 2004; 29: 1488-97.

Centonze D, Picconi B, Baunez C. Cocaine and amphetamine depress striatal GABAergic synaptic transmission through D2 dopamine receptors. Neuropsychopharmacology 2002; 26: 164-75.

Cheer JF, Wassum KM, Sombers LA, et al. Phasic dopamine release evoked by abused substances requires cannabinoid receptor activation. J Neurosci 2007; 27: 791-5.

Chen J, Paredes W, Li J, Smith D, Lowinson J, Gardner EL. Δ9-Tetrahydrocannabinol produces naloxone-blockable enhancement of presynaptic basal dopamine efflux in nucleus accumbens of conscious, freely-moving rats as measured by intracerebral microdialysis. Psychopharmacology 1990; 102: 156-62.

Chiamulera C, Epping-Jordan MP, Zocchi A, et al. Reinforcing and locomotor stimulant effects of cocaine are absent in mGluR5 null mutant mice. Nat Neurosci 2001; 4: 873-4.

Chu H, Jin G, Friedman E, Zhen X. Recent development in studies of tetrahydroprotoberberines: mechanism in antinociception and drug addiction. Cell Mol Neurobiol. 2008; 28:491-9.

Cleva RM, Watterson LR, Johnson MA, Olive MF. Differential Modulation of Thresholds for Intracranial Self-Stimulation by mGlu5 Positive and Negative Allosteric Modulators: Implications for Effects on Drug Self-Administration. Front Pharmacol. 2012; 2:93.

Collins, SL, Levin, FR, Foltin, RW, et al. Response to cocaine, alone and in combination with methylphenidate, in cocaine abusers with ADHD. Drug and Alcohol Dependence 2006; 82: 158-167.

Corbille AG, Valjent E, Marsicano G, et al. Role of cannabinoid type 1 receptors in locomotor activity and striatal signaling in response to psychostimulants. J Neurosci 2007; 27: 6937-47.

Cubells JF. Topiramate for cocaine dependence. Curr Psychiatry Rep 2006; 8: 130-1.

Czoty PW, Martelle JL, Carroll FI, Nader MA. Lower reinforcing strength of the phenyltropane cocaine analogs RTI-336 and RTI-177 compared to cocaine in nonhuman primates. Pharmacol Biochem Behav. 2010; 96:274-8.

Czuczwar SJ, Patsalos PN. The new generation of GABA enhancers. Potential in the treatment of epilepsy. CNS Drugs. 2001; 15:339-50.

Dackis CA, Kampman KM, Lynch KG, Pettinati HM, O'Brien CP. A double-blind, placebo-controlled trial of modafinil for cocaine dependence. Neuropsychopharmacology 2005; 30:205-211.

Dackis CA, Lynch KG, Yu E, et al. Modafinil and cocaine: a double-blind, placebo-controlled drug interaction study. Drug Alcohol Depend 2003; 70:29-37.

Day M, Bain E, Marek G, Saltarelli M, Fox GB. D3 receptor target engagement in humans with ABT-925 using [11C](+)-PHNO PET. Int J Neuropsychopharmacol. 2010, 13:291-2.

De La Garza R 2nd, Zorick T, Heinzerling KG, et al. The cardiovascular and subjective effects of methamphetamine combined with gamma-vinyl-gamma-aminobutyric acid (GVG) in non-treatment seeking methamphetamine-dependent volunteers. Pharmacol Biochem Behav. 2009; 94:186-93.

De Vries TJ, Shaham Y, Homberg JR, et al. A cannabinoid mechanism in relapse to cocaine seeking. Nat Med 2001; 7: 1151-4.

Deroche-Gamonet V, Darnaudéry M, Bruins-Slot L, et al. Study of the addictive potential of modafinil in naive and cocaine-experienced rats. Psychopharmacology 2002; 161:387-395.

Devoto P, Flore G, Saba P, Cadeddu R, Gessa GL. Disulfiram stimulates dopamine release from noradrenergic terminals and potentiates cocaine-induced dopamine release in the prefrontal cortex. Psychopharmacology 2012; 219(4):1153-64.

Dewey SL, Morgan AE, Ashby CR Jr, et al. Brodie JD. A novel strategy for the treatment of cocaine addiction. Synapse 1998; 30: 119-29.

Di Ciano P, Everitt BJ. The GABA(B) receptor agonist baclofen attenuates cocaine- and heroin-seeking behavior by rats. Neuropsychopharmacology 2003a; 28: 510-8.

Dodds CM, O'Neill B, Beaver J, et al. Effect of the dopamine D(3) receptor antagonist GSK598809 on brain responses to rewarding food images in overweight and obese binge eaters. Appetite. 2012 Mar 21. [Epub ahead of print]

Eriksson IS, Allard P, Marcusson J. [3H]tiagabine binding to GABA uptake sites in human brain. Brain Res 1999; 851:183-8.

Fadda P, Scherma M, Fresu A, Collu M, Fratta W. Baclofen antagonizes nicotine-, cocaine-, and morphine-induced dopamine release in the nucleus accumbens of rat. Synapse 2003; 50:1-6.

Fechtner RD, Khouri AS, Figueroa E, et al. Short-term treatment of cocaine and/or methamphetamine abuse with vigabatrin: ocular safety pilot results. Arch Ophthalmol. 2006; 124:1257-62.

Fernández-Ruiz J, Hernández M, Ramos JA. Cannabinoid-dopamine interaction in the pathophysiology and treatment of CNS disorders. CNS Neurosci Ther. 2010; 16:e72-91.

Ferraro L, Antonelli T, O'Connor WT, et al. Modafinil: an antinarcoleptic drug with a different neurochemical profile to d-amphetamine and dopamine uptake blockers. Biol Psychiatry 1997; 42:1181–1183.

Figueroa-Guzman Y, Mueller C, Vranjkovic O, et al. Oral administration of levo-tetrahydropalmatine attenuates reinstatement of extinguished cocaine seeking by cocaine, stress or drug-associated cues in rats. Drug Alcohol Depend 2011; 116:72-9.

Filip M, Frankowska M, Golda A, et al. Various GABA-mimetic drugs differently affect cocaine-evoked hyperlocomotion and sensitization. Eur J Pharmacol 2006; 541: 163-70.

Filip M, Frankowska M, Zaniewska M, et al. Diverse effects of GABA-mimetic drugs on cocaine-evoked self-administration and discriminative stimulus effects in rats. Psychopharmacology 2007; 192: 17-26.

Friedmann CTH, Davis LJ, Ciccone PE, and Rubin RT. Phase II double blind controlled study of a new anxiolytic, fenobam (McN-3377) vs placebo. Curr Ther Res 1980; 27: 144-151.

Froimowitz M, Gu Y, Dakin LA, et al. Slow-onset, long-duration, alkyl analogues of methylphenidate with enhanced selectivity for the dopamine transporter. J Med Chem. 2007; 50:219-32.

Froimowitz M, Wu KM, Moussa A, et al. Slow-onset, long-duration 3-(3',4'-dichlorophenyl)-1-indanamine monoamine reuptake blockers as potential medications to treat cocaine abuse. J Med Chem 2000; 43: 4981-92.

Fukami G, Hashimoto K, Koike K, et al. Effect of antioxidant N-acetyl-L-cysteine on behavioral changes and neurotoxicity in rats after administration of methamphetamine. Brain Res 2004; 1016: 90-5.

Galici R, Jones CK, Hemstapat K, et al. Biphenyl-indanone A, a positive allosteric modulator of the metabotropic glutamate receptor subtype 2, has antipsychotic- and anxiolytic-like effects in mice. J Pharmacol Exp Ther 2006; 318:173-85.

Garcia-Ladona FJ, Cox BF. BP 897, a selective dopamine D3 receptor ligand with therapeutic potential for the treatment of cocaine-addiction. CNS Drug Rev 2003; 9: 141-58.

Gasparini F, Lingenhöhl K, Stoehr N, , et al. 2-Methyl-6-(phenylethynyl)-pyridine (MPEP), a potent, selective and systemically active mGlu5 receptor antagonist. Neuropharmacology 1999; 38:1493-503.

Gee NS, Brown JP, Dissanayake VU, et al. The novel anticonvulsant drug, gabapentin (Neurontin), binds to the alpha2delta subunit of a calcium channel. J Biol Chem 1996; 271: 5768-76.

Geneste H, Amberg W, Backfisch G, et al. (2006). Synthesis and SAR of highly potent and selective dopamine D3-receptor antagonists : variations on the 1H-pyrimidin-2-one theme. Bioorganic & Medicinal Chemistry Letters 2006; 16: 1934–1937.

George, TP, Chawarski, MC, Pakes, J, et al. Disulfiram versus placebo for cocaine dependence in buprenorphine-maintained subjects: a preliminary trial. Biological Psychiatry 2000; 47: 1080–1086.

Gilbert JG, Newman AH, Gardner EL, Ashby CR Jr, Heidbreder CA, Pak AC, Peng XQ, Xi ZX. Acute administration of SB-277011A, NGB 2904, or BP 897 inhibits cocaine cue-induced reinstatement of drug-seeking behavior in rats: role of dopamine D3 receptors. Synapse 2005; 57: 17-28.

Giuffrida A, Parsons LH, Kerr TM, et al. Dopamine activation of endogenous cannabinoid signaling in dorsal striatum. Nat Neurosci 1999; 2: 358-363.

Glowa JR, Fantegrossi WF, Lewis DB, et al. Sustained decrease in cocaine-maintained responding in rhesus monkeys with 1-[2-[bis(4-fluorophenyl)methyoxy]ethyl]-4-(3-hydroxy-3-phenylpropyl)piperazinyl decanoate, a long-acting ester derivative of GBR 12909. J Med Chem 1996; 39: 4689-91.

Glowa JR, Wojnicki FHE, Matecka D, et al. Effects of dopamine reuptake inhibitors on food- and cocaine-maintained responding: I. Dependence on unit dose of cocaine. Exp Clin Psychopharmacol 1995; 3: 219-31.

Gold LH, Balster RL. Evaluation of the cocaine-like discriminative stimulus effects and reinforcing effects of modafinil. Psychopharmacology 1996; 126:286-292.

Gong JP, Onaivi ES, Ishiguro H, Liu QR, Tagliaferro PA, Brusco A, Uhl GR. Cannabinoid CD2 receptors. immunohistochemical localization in rat brain. Brain Res. 2006;1071:10-23.

González G, Desai R, Sofuoglu M, et al. Clinical efficacy of gabapentin versus tiagabine for reducing cocaine use among cocaine dependent methadone-treated patients. Drug Alcohol Depend 2007; 87: 1-9.

González G, Sevarino K, Sofuoglu M, et al. Tiagabine increases cocaine-free urines in cocaine-dependent methadone-treated patients: results of a randomized pilot study. Addiction 2003; 98: 1625-32.

Gorelick DA, Gardner EL, Xi ZX. Agents in development for the management of cocaine abuse. Drugs 2004, 64:1547-73.

Gossop M, Carroll KM. Disulfiram, cocaine, and alcohol: two outcomes for the price of one? Alcohol Alcohol 2006; 41: 119-20.

Graff-Guerrero A, Redden L, Abi-Saab W, et al. Blockade of [11C](+)-PHNO binding in human subjects by the dopamine D3 receptor antagonist ABT-925. Int J Neuropsychopharmacol. 2010; 13:273-87.

Grassi, MC, Cioce, AM, Giudici, FD, Antonilli, L, Nencini, P. Short-term efficacy of Disulfiram or Naltrexone in reducing positive urinalysis for both cocaine and cocaethylene in cocaine abusers: a pilot study. Pharmacology Research 2007; 55: 117–121.

Groenewegen HJ, Wright CI, Beijer AV. The nucleus accumbens: gateway for limbic structures to reach the motor system? Prog Brain Res 1996; 107: 485-511.

Gründer G. Cariprazine, an orally active D2/D3 receptor antagonist, for the potential treatment of schizophrenia, bipolar mania and depression. Curr Opin Investig Drugs. 2010; 11:823-32.

Haile CN, During MJ, Jatlow PI, Kosten TR, Kosten TA. Disulfiram facilitates the development and expression of locomotor sensitization to cocaine in rats. Biol Psychiatry. 2003; 54:915-21.

Haile CN, Zhang XY, Carroll FI, Kosten TA. Cocaine self-administration and locomotor activity are altered in Lewis and F344 inbred rats by RTI 336, a 3-phenyltropane analog that binds to the dopamine transporter. Brain Res 2005; 1055:186-195.

Haney M, Hart C, Collins ED, Foltin RW. Smoked cocaine discrimination in humans: effects of gabapentin. Drug Alcohol Depend 2005; 80: 53-61.

Haney M, Hart CL, Foltin RW. Effects of baclofen on cocaine self-administration: opioid- and nonopioid-dependent volunteers. Neuropsychopharmacology 2006; 31: 1814-21.

Hart C, Jatlow P, Sevarino K, Cance-Katz E. Comparison of intravenous cocaethylene and cocaine in humans. . Psychopharmacology 2000; 149: 153-62.

Hart CL, Haney M, Collins ED, Rubin E, Foltin RW. Smoked cocaine self-administration by humans is not reduced by large gabapentin maintenance doses. Drug Alcohol Depend 2007; 86: 274-7.

Hart CL, Haney M, Vosburg SK, Rubin E, Foltin RW. Smoked cocaine self-administration is decreased by modafinil. Neuropsychopharmacology 2008; 33:761-768.

Hart CL, Ward AS, Collins ED, Haney M, Foltin RW. Gabapentin maintenance decreases smoked cocaine-related subjective effects, but not self-administration by humans. Drug Alcohol Depend 2004; 73: 279-87.

Heidbreder CA, Gardner EL, Xi ZX, et al. The role of central dopamine D3 receptors in drug addiction: a review of pharmacological evidence. Brain Res Rev 2005; 49: 77-105.

Heidbreder CA, Newman AH. Current perspectives on selective dopamine D(3) receptor antagonists as pharmacotherapeutics for addictions and related disorders. Ann N Y Acad Sci. 2010; 1187:4-34.

Herzig V, Schmidt WJ. Effects of MPEP on locomotion, sensitization and conditioned reward induced by cocaine or morphine. Neuropharmacology 2004; 47: 973-84.

Higgins, ST, Budney, AJ, Bickel, WK, Hughes, JR, Foerg, F. Disulfiram therapy in patients abusing cocaine and alcohol. American Journal of Psychiatry 1993; 150: 675–676.

Hiranita T, Soto PL, Kohut SJ, et al. Decreases in Cocaine Self Administration with Dual Inhibition of Dopamine Transporter and {sigma} Receptors. J Pharmacol Exp Ther 2011; 339:662-77.

Hiranita T, Soto PL, Newman AH, Katz JL. Assessment of reinforcing effects of benztropine analogs and their effects on cocaine self-administration in rats: comparisons with monoamine uptake inhibitors. J Pharmacol Exp Ther 2009; 329:677-86.

Howell LL, Carroll FI, Votaw JR, Goodman MM, Kimmel HL. Effects of combined dopamine and serotonin transporter inhibitors on cocaine self-administration in rhesus monkeys. J Pharmacol Exp Ther 2007; 320:757-765.

Howell LL, Kimmel HL. Monoamine transporters and psychostimulant addiction. Biochem Pharmacol 2008; 75: 196-217.

Howell LL, Wilcox KM. The dopamine transporter and cocaine medication development: drug self-administration in nonhuman primates. J Pharmacol Exp Ther 2001; 298: 1-6.

Hu G, Duffy P, Swanson C, Ghasemzadeh MB, Kalivas PW. The regulation of dopamine transmission by metabotropic glutamate receptors. J Pharmacol Exp Ther 1999; 289: 412-6.

Hu Y, Qiu Y, Zhong Y, He H. Therapeutic effects of rotundine combined with methadone in treatment of heroin dependence. Chinese Journal of Drug Abuse Prevention and Treatment. 2006; 12:270-271.

Itzhak Y, Martin JL. Effect of riluzole and gabapentin on cocaine- and methamphetamine-induced behavioral sensitization in mice. Psychopharmacology 2000; 151: 226-233.

Jin G-Z. (-)-Tetrahydropalmatine and its analogues as new dopamine receptor antagonists. Trends Pharmacol Sci 1987; 8: 81–82.

Jin X, Semenova S, Yang L, Ardecky R, et al. The mGluR2 positive allosteric modulator BINA decreases cocaine self-administration and cue-induced cocaine-seeking and counteracts cocaine-induced enhancement of brain reward function in rats. Neuropsychopharmacology 2010; 35:2021-36.

Johnson BA. Recent advances in the development of treatments for alcohol and cocaine dependence: focus on topiramate and other modulators of GABA or glutamate function. CNS Drugs 2005; 19: 873-96.

Johnson MP, Baez M, Jagdmann Jr GE, et al. Discovery of allosteric potentiators for the metabotropic glutamate 2 receptor: synthesis and subtype selectivity of N-(4-(2-methoxyphenoxy)phenyl)-N-(2,2,2-trifluoroethylsulfonyl)pyrid-3-ylmethylamine. J Med Chem 2003; 46: 3189–3192.

Kahn R, Biswas K, Childress AR, Shoptaw S, Fudala PJ, Gorgon L, et al. Multi-center trial of baclofen for abstinence initiation in severe cocaine-dependent individuals. Drug Alcohol Depend 2009; 103:59-64.

Kalivas PW. The glutamate homeostasis hypothesis of addiction. Nat Rev Neurosci. 2009; 10:561-72.

Kampman KM, Pettinati H, Lynch KG, et al. A pilot trial of topiramate for the treatment of cocaine dependence. Drug Alcohol Depend 2004; 75: 233-240.

Kelley AE, Lang CG. Effects of GBR 12909, a selective dopamine uptake inhibitor, on motor activity and operant behavior in the rat. Eur J Pharmacol 1989; 167: 385-95.

Kenny PJ, Boutrel B, Gasparini F, Koob GF, Markou A. Metabotropic glutamate 5 receptor blockade may attenuate cocaine self-administration by decreasing brain reward function in rats. Psychopharmacology 2005; 179: 247-54.

Kimmel HL, O'Connor JA, Carroll FI, Howell LL Faster onset and dopamine transporter selectivity predict stimulant and reinforcing effects of cocaine analogs in squirrel monkeys. Pharmacol Biochem Behav 2007; 86:45-54.

Kiss B, Horváth A, Némethy Z, Schmidt E, Laszlovszky I, et al. Cariprazine (RGH-188), a dopamine D(3) receptor-preferring, D(3)/D(2) dopamine receptor antagonist-partial agonist antipsychotic candidate: in vitro and neurochemical profile. J Pharmacol Exp Ther. 2010; 333:328-40.

Krishnamurthy M, Li W, Moore BM 2nd. Synthesis, biological evaluation, and structural studies on N1 and C5 substituted cycloalkyl analogues of the pyrazole class of CB1 and CB2 ligands. Bioorg Med Chem 2004; 12: 393-404.

Kruszewski SP. Euphorigenic and abusive properties of modafinil. Am J Psychiatry. 2006; 163:549.

Kumaresan V, Yuan M, Yee J, Famous KR, et al. Metabotropic glutamate receptor 5 (mGluR5) antagonists attenuate cocaine priming- and cue-induced reinstatement of cocaine seeking. Behav Brain Res. 2009; 202:238-44.

Lapierre YD and Oyewumi LK. Fenobam: another anxiolytic? Curr Ther Res 1982; 31: 95-101.

LaRowe SD, Mardikian P, Malcolm R, et al. Safety and tolerability of N-acetylcysteine in cocaine-dependent individuals. Am J Addict 2006; 15: 105-10.

LaRowe SD, Myrick H, Hedden S, et al. Is cocaine desire reduced by N-acetylcysteine? Am J Psychiatry 2007; 164: 1115-7.

Le Foll B, Goldberg SR, Sokoloff P. The dopamine D3 receptor and drug dependence: effects on reward or beyond? Neuropharmacology 2005; 49: 525-41.

Lea PM 4th, Faden AI. Metabotropic glutamate receptor subtype 5 antagonists MPEP and MTEP. CNS Drug Rev 2006; 12: 149-66.

Lee B, Platt DM, Rowlett JK, Adewale AS, Spealman RD. Attenuation of behavioral effects of cocaine by the Metabotropic Glutamate Receptor 5 Antagonist 2-Methyl-6-(phenylethynyl)-pyridine in squirrel monkeys: comparison with dizocilpine. J Pharmacol Exp Ther 2005; 312: 1232-40.

Leonard BE, McCartan D, White J, King DJ. Methylphenidate: a review of its neuropharmacological, neuropsychological and adverse clinical effects. Hum Psychopharmacol. 2004; 19:151-80.

Levin, FR, Evans, SM, Brooks, DJ, Garawi, F. Treatment of cocaine dependent treatment seekers with adult ADHD: double-blind comparison of methylphenidate and placebo. Drug and Alcohol Dependence 2007; 87: 20–29.

Li X, Gardner EL, Xi ZX. The metabotropic glutamate receptor 7 (mGluR7) allosteric agonist AMN082 modulates nucleus accumbens GABA and glutamate, but not dopamine, in rats. Neuropharmacology 2008; 54: 542-551.

Li X, Li J, Gardner EL, Xi ZX. Activation of mGluR7s inhibits cocaine-induced reinstatement of drug-seeking behavior by a nucleus accumbens glutamate-mGluR2/3 mechanism in rats. J Neurochem 2010; 114:1368-1380.

Li X, Li J, Peng XQ, Spiller K, Gardner EL, Xi ZX. Metabotropic glutamate receptor 7 modulates the rewarding effects of cocaine in rats: involvement of a ventral pallidal GABAergic mechanism. Neuropsychopharmacology 2009; 34:1783-1796.

Li X, Xi ZX, Markou A. Metabotropic glutamate receptor 7 (mGluR7): A new target in medication development for treatment of cocaine addiction. Neuropharmacology, 2012, Apr 21. [Epub ahead of print].

Lile JA, Stoops WW, Glaser PE, Hays LR, Rush CR. Acute administration of the GABA reuptake inhibitor tiagabine does not alter the effects of oral cocaine in humans. Drug Alcohol Depend 2004; 76: 81-91.

Ling W, Shoptaw S, Majewska D. Baclofen as a cocaine anti-craving medication: a preliminary clinical study. Neuropsychopharmacology 1998; 18: 403-4.

Lu L, Uejima JL, Gray SM, Bossert JM, Shaham Y. Systemic and central amygdala injections of the mGluR(2/3) agonist LY379268 attenuate the expression of incubation of cocaine craving. Biol Psychiatry 2007; 61: 591-8.

Luo J-Y, Ren Y-H, Zhu R, Lin D-Q, Zheng J-W. The effect of l-tetrahydropalmatine on cocaine induced conditioned place preference, Chin J Drug Depend 2003; 12: 177-9.

Lupica CR, Riegel AC, Hoffman AF. Marijuana and cannabinoid regulation of brain reward circuits. Br J Pharmacol 2004; 143:227-34.

Madayag A, Lobner D, Kau KS, Mantsch JR, et al. Repeated N-acetylcysteine administration alters plasticity-dependent effects of cocaine. J Neurosci. 2007; 27:13968-76.

Madras BK, Xie Z, Lin Z, Jassen A, Panas H, et al. Modafinil occupies dopamine and norepinephrine transporters in vivo and modulates the transporters and trace amine activity in vitro. J Pharmacol Exp Ther 2006; 319:561-569.

Makoff A, Pilling C, Harrington K, Emson P. Human metabotropic glutamate receptor type 7: molecular cloning and mRNA distribution in the CNS. Mol Brain Re. 1996; 40: 165-70.

Malcolm R, Olive MF, Lechner W. The safety of disulfiram for the treatment of alcohol and cocaine dependence in randomized clinical trials: guidance for clinical practice. Expert Opin Drug Saf 2008; 7: 459-72.

Maldonado R, Berrendero F, Ozaita A, Robledo P. Neurochemical basis of cannabis addiction. Neuroscience. 2011; 181:1-17.

Mantsch JR, Li SJ, Risinger R, et al. Levo-tetrahydropalmatine attenuates cocaine self-administration and cocaine-induced reinstatement in rats. Psychopharmacology 2007; 192: 581-91.

Mantsch JR, Wisniewski S, Vranjkovic O, et al. Levo-tetrahydropalmatine attenuates cocaine self-administration under a progressive-ratio schedule and cocaine discrimination in rats. Pharmacol Biochem Behav. 2010, 97.310-6.

Mardikian PN, LaRowe SD, Hedden S, et al. An open-label trial of N-acetylcysteine for the treatment of cocaine dependence: a pilot study. Prog Neuropsychopharmacol Biol Psychiatry 2007; 31: 389-94.

Marek GJ. Metabotropic glutamate 2/3 receptors as drug targets. Curr Opin Pharmacol 2004; 4: 18-22.

Marin JC, Goadsby PJ. Glutamatergic fine tuning with ADX-10059: a novel therapeutic approach for migraine? Expert Opin Investig Drugs. 2010; 19:555-61.

Martin-Fardon R, Weiss F. (-)-2-oxa-4-aminobicylco[3.1.0]hexane-4,6-dicarboxylic acid (LY379268) and 3-[(2-methyl-1,3-thiazol-4-yl)ethynyl]piperidine (MTEP) similarly attenuate stress-induced reinstatement of cocaine seeking. Addict Biol. 2012; 17:557-64.

Mattick RP, Breen C, Kimber J, Davoli M. Methadone maintenance therapy versus no opioid replacement therapy for opioid dependence. Cochrane Database Syst Rev 2009:CD002209.

McGeehan AJ, Janak PH, Olive MF. Effect of the mGluR5 antagonist 6-methyl-2-(phenylethynyl)pyridine (MPEP) on the acute locomotor stimulant properties of cocaine, D-amphetamine, and the dopamine reuptake inhibitor GBR12909 in mice. Psychopharmacology 2004; 174: 266-73.

McGeehan AJ, Olive MF. The mGluR5 antagonist MPEP reduces the conditioned rewarding effects of cocaine but not other drugs of abuse. Synapse 2003; 47: 240-2.

Mezler M, Geneste H, Gault L, Marek GJ. LY-2140023, a prodrug of the group II metabotropic glutamate receptor agonist LY-404039 for the potential treatment of schizophrenia. Curr Opin Investig Drugs 2010; 11:833-45.

Millan MJ, Brocco M. Cognitive impairment in schizophrenia: a review of developmental and genetic models, and pro-cognitive profile of the optimised D(3) > D(2) antagonist, S33138. Therapie. 2008; 63:187-229.

Millan MJ, Mannoury la Cour C, et al. S33138 [N-[4-[2-[(3aS,9bR)-8-cyano-1,3a,4,9b-tetrahydro[1]-benzopyrano[3,4-c]pyrrol-2(3H)-yl)-ethyl]phenylacetamide], a preferential dopamine D3 versus D2 receptor antagonist and potential antipsychotic agent: I. Receptor-binding profile and functional actions at G-protein-coupled receptors. J Pharmacol Exp Ther 2008; 324:587-99.

Minozzi S, Amato L, Davoli M, et al. Anticonvulsants for cocaine dependence. Cochrane Database Syst Rev. 2008; (2):CD006754.

Mitsukawa K, Yamamoto R, Ofner S, et al. A selective metabotropic glutamate receptor 7 agonist: activation of receptor signaling via an allosteric site modulates stress parameters in vivo. Proc Natl Acad Sci USA 2005; 102: 18712-7.

Montana MC, Cavallone LF, Stubbert KK, et al. The metabotropic glutamate receptor subtype 5 antagonist fenobam is analgesic and has improved in vivo selectivity compared with the prototypical antagonist 2-methyl-6-(phenylethynyl)-pyridine. J Pharmacol Exp Ther. 2009; 330:834-43.

Murillo-Rodríguez E, Haro R, Palomero-Rivero M, et al. Modafinil enhances extracellular levels of dopamine in the nucleus accumbens and increases wakefulness in rats. Behav Brain Res. 2007; 176:353–357.

Myrick H, Henderson S, Brady KT, Malcolm R. Gabapentin in the treatment of cocaine dependence: a case series. J Clin Psychiatry 2001; 62: 19-23.

Nathan PJ, O'Neill BV, Mogg K, et al. The effects of the dopamine D3 receptor antagonist GSK598809 on attentional bias to palatable food cues in overweight and obese subjects. Int J Neuropsychopharmacol. 2011; 12:1-13.

Neale JH, Bzdega T, Wroblewska B. N-Acetylaspartylglutamate: the most abundant peptide neurotransmitter in the mammalian central nervous system. J Neurochem 2000; 75: 443-52.

Neale JH, Olszewski RT, Zuo D, et al. Advances in understanding the peptide neurotransmitter NAAG and appearance of a new member of the NAAG neuropeptide family. J Neurochem. 2011; 118:490-8.

Newman AH, Grundt P, Nader MA. Dopamine D3 receptor partial agonists and antagonists as potential drug abuse therapeutic agents. J Med Chem 2005; 48: 3663-79.

Newman AH, Kulkarni S. Probes for the dopamine transporter: new leads toward a cocaine-abuse therapeutic--A focus on analogues of benztropine and rimcazole. Med Res Rev 2002; 22:429-464.

Nicola SM, Malenka RC. Dopamine depresses excitatory and inhibitory synaptic transmission by distinct mechanisms in the nucleus accumbens. J Neurosci 1997; 17: 5697-710.

O'Brien CP, Dackis CA, Kampman K. Does modafinil produce euphoria? Am J Psychiatry 2006; 163:1109.

Oliveto A, Poling J, Mancino MJ, et al. Randomized, double blind, placebo-controlled trial of disulfiram for the treatment of cocaine dependence in methadone-stabilized patients. Drug Alcohol Depend. 2011; 113:184-91.

Onaivi ES, Ishiguro H, Gong JP, et al. Functional expression of brain neuronal CB2 cannabinoid receptors are involved in the effects of drugs of abuse and in depression. Ann N Y Acad Sci. 2008; 1139:434-49.

Paterson NE, Markou A. The metabotropic glutamate receptor 5 antagonist MPEP decreased break points for nicotine, cocaine and food in rats. Psychopharmacology 2005; 179: 255-61.

Patil ST, Zhang L, Martenyi F, et al. Activation of mGlu2/3 receptors as a new approach to treat schizophrenia: a randomized Phase 2 clinical trial. Nat Med. 2007; 13:1102-7.

Pecknold JC, McClure DJ, and Appeltauer L. Fenobam in anxious outpatients. Curr Ther Res 1980; 27:119-123.

Pecknold JC, McClure DJ, Appeltauer L, Wrzesinski L, Allan T. Treatment of anxiety using fenobam (a nonbenzodiazepine) in a double-blind standard (diazepam) placebo-controlled study. J Clin Psychopharmacol. 1982; 2:129-33.

Peng XQ, Ashby CR, Jr., Spiller K, Li X, Li J, Thomasson N, Millan MJ, Mocaer E, Munoz C, Gardner EL, Xi ZX. The preferential dopamine D3 receptor antagonist S33138 inhibits cocaine reward and cocaine-triggered relapse to drug-seeking behavior in rats. Neuropharmacology 2009; 56:752-760.

Peng XQ, Gardner EL, Xi ZX. Gamma-vinyl GABA increases nonvesicular release of GABA and glutamate in the nucleus accumbens in rats via action on anion channels and GABA transporters. Psychopharmacology 2010a; 208:511-519.

Peng XQ, Li J, Gardner EL, Ashby CR, Jr., Thomas A, Wozniak K, Slusher BS, Xi ZX. Oral administration of the NAALADase inhibitor GPI-5693 attenuates cocaine-induced reinstatement of drug-seeking behavior in rats. Eur J Pharmacol 2010b; 627:156-161.

Peng XQ, Li X, Gilbert JG, Pak AC, Ashby CR, Jr., Brodie JD, Dewey SL, Gardner EL, Xi ZX. Gamma-vinyl GABA inhibits cocaine-triggered reinstatement of drug-seeking behavior in rats by a non-dopaminergic mechanism. Drug Alcohol Depend 2008a; 97:216-225.

Peng XQ, Li X, Li J, Ramachandran PV, Gagare PD, Pratihar D, Ashby CR, Jr., Gardner EL, Xi ZX (2008b) Effects of gabapentin on cocaine self-administration, cocaine-triggered relapse and cocaine-enhanced nucleus accumbens dopamine in rats. Drug Alcohol Depend 2008b; 97:207-215.

Peng XQ, Xi ZX, Li X, Spiller K, Li J, Chun L, Wu KM, Froimowitz M, Gardner EL. Is slow-onset long-acting monoamine transport blockade to cocaine as methadone is to heroin? Implication for anti-addiction medications. Neuropsychopharmacology 2010c; 35:2564-2578.

Peters J, Kalivas PW. The group II metabotropic glutamate receptor agonist, LY379268, inhibits both cocaine- and food-seeking behavior in rats. Psychopharmacology 2006; 186: 143-9.

Petrakis, IL, Carroll, KM, Nich, C, et al. Disulfiram treatment for cocaine dependence in methadone-maintained opioid addicts. Addiction 2000; 95: 219–228.

Pettinati HM, Kampman KM, Lynch KG, et al. A double blind, placebo-controlled trial that combines disulfiram and naltrexone for treating co-occurring cocaine and alcohol dependence. Addict Behav. 2008; 33:651-67.

Pilla M, Perachon S, Sautel F, et al. Selective inhibition of cocaine-seeking behaviour by a partial dopamine D3 receptor agonist. Nature 1999; 400:371-5.

Platt DM, Rowlett JK, Spealman RD. Behavioral effects of cocaine and dopaminergic strategies for preclinical medication development. Psychopharmacology 2002; 163: 265-82.

Porter RH, Jaeschke G, Spooren W, et al. Fenobam: a clinically validated nonbenzodiazepine anxiolytic is a potent, selective, and noncompetitive mGlu5 receptor antagonist with inverse agonist activity. J Pharmacol Exp Ther. 2005; 315:711-21.

Qu WM, Huang ZL, Xu XH, Matsumoto N, Urade Y. Dopaminergic D1 and D2 receptors are essential for the arousal effect of modafinil. J Neurosci. 2008; 28:8462–8469.

Raby WN, Coomaraswamy S. Gabapentin reduces cocaine use among addicts from a community clinic sample. J Clin Psychiatry 2004; 65: 84-86.

Reavill C, Taylor SG, Wood MD, et al. Pharmacological actions of a novel, high-affinity, and selective human dopamine D3 receptor antagonist, SB-277011-A. J Pharmacol Exp Ther 2000; 294: 1154-65.

Redden L, Rendenbach-Mueller B, Abi-Saab WM, et al. A double-blind, randomized, placebo-controlled study of the dopamine D3 receptor antagonist ABT-925 in patients with acute schizophrenia. J Clin Psychopharmacol. 2011; 31:221-5.

Reis AD, Castro LA, Faria R, Laranjeira R. Craving decrease with topiramate in outpatient treatment for cocaine dependence: an open label trial. Rev Bras Psiquiatr 2008; 30: 132-5.

Remington G, Kapur S. SB-277011 GlaxoSmithKline. Curr Opin Investig Drugs 2001; 2:946-9.

Rinaldi-Carmona M, Barth F, Heaulme M, et al. SR141716A, a potent and selective antagonist of the brain cannabinoid receptor. FEBS Lett 1994; 350: 240-4.

Roberts DC, Andrews MM, Vickers GJ. Baclofen attenuates the reinforcing effects of cocaine in rats. Neuropsychopharmacology 1996; 15: 417-23.

Ross JT, Corrigall WA, Heidbreder CA, LeSage MG. Effects of the selective dopamine D3 receptor antagonist SB-277011A on the reinforcing effects of nicotine as measured by a progressive-ratio schedule in rats. Eur J Pharmacol. 2007; 559:173-9.

Rothman RB, Baumann MH, Prisinzano TE, Newman AH. Dopamine transport inhibitors based on GBR12909 and benztropine as potential medications to treat cocaine addiction. Biochem Pharmacol 2008; 75: 2-16.

Rothman RB, Baumann MH. Therapeutic potential of monoamine transporter substrates. Curr Top Med Chem 2006; 6:1845-1859.

Rothman RB, Blough BE, Baumann MH. Dual dopamine/serotonin releasers as potential medications for stimulant and alcohol addictions. AAPS J 2007; 9:E1-10.

Rothman RB, Mele A, Reid AA, et al. GBR 12909 antagonizes the ability of cocaine to elevate extracellular levels of dopamine. Pharmacol Biochem Behav 1991; 40: 387-97.

Runyon SP, Carroll FI. Dopamine transporter ligands: recent developments and therapeutic potential. Curr Top Med Chem 2006; 6:1825-1843.

Salling MC, Faccidomo S, Hodge CW. Nonselective suppression of operant ethanol and sucrose self-administration by the mGluR7 positive allosteric modulator AMN082. Pharmacol Biochem Behav 2008; 91(1):14-20.

Schousboe A, Madsen KK, White HS. GABA transport inhibitors and seizure protection: the past and future. Future Med Chem. 2011; 3:183-7.

Schramm-Sapyta NL, Olsen CM, Winder DG. Cocaine self-administration reduces excitatory responses in the mouse nucleus accumbens shell. Neuropsychopharmacology 2006; 31: 1444-51.

Schroeder JP, Cooper DA, Schank JR, et al. Disulfiram attenuates drug-primed reinstatement of cocaine seeking via inhibition of dopamine β-hydroxylase. Neuropsychopharmacology. 2010; 35:2440-9.

Schubiner H, Saules KK, Arfken CL, et al. Double-blind placebo-controlled trial of methylphenidate in the treatment of adult ADHD patients with comorbid cocaine dependence. Exp Clin Psychopharmacol. 2002; 10:286-94.

Schubiner H, Tzelepis A, Milberger S, Lockhart N, Kruger M, Kelley BJ, Schoener EP. Prevalence of attention-deficit/hyperactivity disorder and conduct disorder among substance abusers. J Clin Psychiatry 2000; 61:244-51.

Searle G, Beaver JD, Comley RA, et al. Imaging dopamine D3 receptors in the human brain with positron emission tomography, [11C]PHNO, and a selective D3 receptor antagonist. Biol Psychiatry 2010; 68:392-9.

Shippenberg TS, Rea W, Slusher BS. Modulation of behavioral sensitization to cocaine by NAALADase inhibition. Synapse 2000; 38: 161-6.

Shoptaw S, Yang X, Rotheram-Fuller EJ, et al. Randomized placebo-controlled trial of baclofen for cocaine dependence: preliminary effects for individuals with chronic patterns of cocaine use. J Clin Psychiatry 2003; 64: 1440-8.

Slattery DA, Markou A, Froestl W, Cryan JF. The GABAB receptor-positive modulator GS39783 and the GABAB receptor agonist baclofen attenuate the reward-facilitating effects of cocaine: intracranial self-stimulation studies in the rat. Neuropsychopharmacology 2005; 30: 2065-72.

Slusher BS, Thomas A, Paul M, Schad CA, Ashby CR Jr. Expression and acquisition of the conditioned place preference response to cocaine in rats is blocked by selective inhibitors of the enzyme N-acetylated-alpha-linked-acidic dipeptidase (NAALADASE). Synapse 2001; 41: 22-8.

Smith RJ, Aston-Jones G. Noradrenergic transmission in the extended amygdala: role in increased drug-seeking and relapse during protracted drug abstinence. Brain Struct Funct. 2008; 213:43-61.

Song R, Yang RF, Wu N, Su RB, Li J, Peng XQ, Li X, Gaál J, Xi ZX, Gardner EL. YQA14: a novel dopamine D(3) receptor antagonist that inhibits cocaine self-administration in rats and mice, but not in D(3) receptor-knockout mice. Addict Biol. 2012; 17:259-73.

Soria G, Mendizabal V, Tourino C, et al. Lack of CB1 cannabinoid receptor impairs cocaine self-administration. Neuropsychopharmacology 2005; 30: 1670-80.

Spiller K, Xi ZX, Peng XQ, et al. The putative dopamine D3 receptor antagonists SB-277011A, NGB 2904 or BP 897 inhibit methamphetamine-enhanced brain stimulation reward in rats. Psychopharmacology 2008; 196:533-542.

Suh JJ, Pettinati HM, Kampman KM, O'Brien CP. The status of disulfiram: a half of a century later. J Clin Psychopharmacol 2006; 26: 290-302.

Sulzer D (2011) How addictive drugs disrupt presynaptic dopamine neurotransmission. Neuron 69:628-649.

Tanda G and Goldberg SR. Cannabinoids: reward, dependence, and underlying neurochemical mechanisms - a review of recent preclinical data. Psychopharmacology 2003; 169: 115-134.

Tanda G, Pontieri FE, Di Chiara G. Cannabinoid and heroin activation of mesolimbic dopamine transmission by a common μ1 opioid receptor mechanism. Science 1997; 276: 2048-50.

Tang X-C, McFarland K, Cagle S, Kalivas PW. Cocaine-induced reinstatement requires endogenous stimulation of μ-opioid receptors in the ventral pallidum. J Neurosci 2005; 25: 4512-20.

Taylor CP, Gee NS, Su T-Z, et al. Summary of mechanistic hypotheses of gabapentin pharmacology. Epilepsy Res 1998; 29: 233-49.

te Beek ET, Zoethout RW, Bani MS, et al. Pharmacokinetics and central nervous system effects of the novel dopamine D3 receptor antagonist GSK598809 and intravenous alcohol infusion at pseudo-steady state. J Psychopharmacol. 2012 26:303-14.

Tella SR. Effects of monoamine reuptake inhibitors on cocaine self-administration in rats. Pharmacol Biochem Behav 1995; 51: 687-92.

Tessari M, Pilla M, Andreoli M, Hutcheson DM, Heidbreder CA. Antagonism at metabotropic glutamate 5 receptors inhibits nicotine- and cocaine-taking behaviours and prevents nicotine-triggered relapse to nicotine-seeking. Eur J Pharmacol. 2004; 499: 121-33.

Thanos PK, Michaelides M, Ho CW, et al. The effects of two highly selective dopamine D3 receptor antagonists (SB-277011A and NGB-2904) on food self-administration in a rodent model of obesity. Pharmacol Biochem Behav 2008; 89:499-507.

Thomasson-Perret N, Pénélaud PF, Théron D, Gouttefangeas S, Mocaër E. Markers of D(2) and D(3) receptor activity in vivo: PET scan and prolactin. Therapie 2008; 63:237-42

Uchimura N, North RA. Actions of cocaine on rat nucleus accumbens neurones in vitro. Br J Pharmacol 1990; 99: 736-40.

Umemiya M, Raymond LA. Dopaminergic modulation of excitatory postsynaptic currents in rat neostriatal neurons. J Neurophysiol 1997; 78: 1248-55.

van der Post JP, de Visser SJ, de Kam ML, et al. The central nervous system effects, pharmacokinetics and safety of the NAALADase-inhibitor GPI 5693. Br J Clin Pharmacol 2005; 60:128-36

Van Sickle MD, Duncan M, Kingsley PJ et al. Identification and functional characterization of brainstem cannabinoid CB2 receptors. Science 2005; 310:329-32.

Vocci FJ, Elkashef A. Pharmacotherapy and other treatments for cocaine abuse and dependence. Curr Opin Psychiatry 2005; 18: 265-70.

Volkow ND, Ding Y-S, Fowler JS, et al. Is methylphenidate like cocaine? Studies on their pharmacokinetics and distribution in the human brain. Arch Gen Psychiatry 1995; 52: 456-63

Volkow ND, Fowler JS, Logan J, et al. Effects of modafinil on dopamine and dopamine transporters in the male human brain: clinical implications. JAMA. 2009; 301:1148-54.

Volkow ND, Fowler JS, Wang G-J. Imaging studies on the role of dopamine in cocaine reinforcement and addiction in humans. J Psychopharmacol 1999; 13: 337-45.

Vorel SR, Ashby CR Jr, Paul M, et al. Dopamine D3 receptor antagonism inhibits cocaine-seeking and cocaine-enhanced brain reward in rats. J Neurosci 2002; 22: 9595-603.

Wang JB, Mantsch JR. L-tetrahydropalamatine: a potential new medication for the treatment of cocaine addiction. Future Med Chem. 2012; 4:177-86.

Wang X, Moussawi K, Knackstedt L, Shen H, Kalivas PW. Role of mGluR5 neurotransmission in reinstated cocaine-seeking. Addict Biol. 2012 Feb 17. [Epub ahead of print].

Weerts EM, Froestl W, Griffiths RR. Effects of GABAergic modulators on food and cocaine self-administration in baboons. Drug Alcohol Depend 2005; 80: 369-76.

Weerts EM, Froestl W, Kaminski BJ, Griffiths RR. Attenuation of cocaine-seeking by GABAB receptor agonists baclofen and CGP44532 but not the GABA reuptake inhibitor tiagabine in baboons. Drug Alcohol Depend 2007; 89: 206-13.

Weinshenker D. Cocaine sobers up. Nat Med. 2010; 16:969-70.

White FJ, Hu X-T, Henry DJ. Electrophysiological effects of cocaine in the rat nucleus accumbens: microiontophoretic studies. J Pharmacol Exp Ther 1993; 266: 1075-84.

White, BP, Becker-Blease, KA, Grace-Bishop, K. Stimulant medication use, misuse, and abuse in an undergraduate and graduate student sample. Journal of American College Health 2006; 54, 261–268.

Wicke K, Garcia-Ladona J. The dopamine D3 receptor partial agonist, BP-897, is an antagonist at human dopamine D3 receptors and at rat somatodendritic dopamine D3 receptors. Eur J Pharmacol 2001; 424: 85-90.

Williams E. Effects of alcohol on workers with carbon disulfide JAMA 1937; 109: 1472-3.

Winhusen T, Somoza E, Ciraulo DA, et al. A double-blind, placebo-controlled trial of tiagabine for the treatment of cocaine dependence. Drug Alcohol Depend 2007; 91:141-148.

Winhusen TM, Somoza EC, Harrer JM, et al. A placebo-controlled screening trial of tiagabine, sertraline and donepezil as cocaine dependence treatments. Addiction 2005; 100: 68-77.

Winhusen, T, Somoza, E, Singal, BM, Harrer, J, Apparaju, S, Mezinskis, J, Desai, P, Elkashef, A, Chiang, CN, Horn, P. Methylphenidate and cocaine: a placebo-controlled drug interaction study. Pharmacology, Biochemistry and Behavior 2006; 85: 29–38.

Wise MS, Arand DL, Auger RR, Brooks SN, Watson NF; American Academy of Sleep Medicine. Treatment of narcolepsy and other hypersomnias of central origin. Sleep 2007; 30:1712-1727.

Wise RA. Forebrain substrates of reward and motivation. J Comp Neurol 2005; 493: 115-21.

Wisor JP, Nishino S, Sora I, et al. Dopaminergic role in stimulant-induced wakefulness. J Neurosci. 2001; 21:1787-94.

Woolley ML, Pemberton DJ, Bate S, Corti C, Jones DN. The mGlu2 but not the mGlu3 receptor mediates the actions of the mGluR2/3 agonist, LY379268, in mouse models predictive of antipsychotic activity. Psychopharmacology 2008; 196: 431–440.

Xi Z-X, Baker DA, Shen H, Kalivas PW. Group II metabotropic glutamate receptors modulate glutamate release in the nucleus accumbens. J Pharmacol Exp Ther 2002a; 300: 162-72.

Xi ZX, Gardner EL. Hypothesis-driven medication discovery for the treatment of psychostimulant addiction. Curr Drug Abuse Rev 2008; 1:303-327.

Xi ZX, Gardner EL. Pharmacological actions of NGB 2904, a selective dopamine D3 receptor antagonist, in animal models of drug addiction. CNS Drug Reviews 2007; 13:240-259.

Xi Z-X, Gilbert J, Campos A, Ashby CR Jr, Gardner EL. The metabotropic glutamate receptor 5 antagonist MPEP blocks reinstatement of drug-seeking triggered by cocaine, but not by stress or cues. Abstract at the 66th Annual Meetings of the College on Problems of Drug Dependence, San Juan, Puerto Rico, June 2004a.

Xi Z-X, Gilbert J, Campos AC, Kline N, et al. Blockade of mesolimbic dopamine D3 receptors inhibits stress-induced reinstatement of cocaine-seeking in rats. Psychopharmacology 2004b; 176: 57-65.

Xi Z-X, Gilbert J, Campos AC, Peng X-Q, Ashby CR Jr, Gardner EL. The mGluR5 antagonist MPEP lowers the progressive-ratio break-point for cocaine self-administration, and inhibits reinstatement of drug-seeking triggered by cocaine but not by stress or cues. Abstract at the 34th Annual Meeting of the Society for Neuroscience, San Diego, CA, Oct 23-27, 2004c, Abstract# 691.9.

Xi Z-X, Gilbert JG, Pak AC, Ashby CR Jr, Heidbreder CA, Gardner EL. Selective dopamine D3 receptor antagonism by SB-277011A attenuates cocaine reinforcement as assessed by progressive-ratio and variable-cost--variable-payoff fixed-ratio cocaine self-administration in rats. Eur J Neurosci 2005; 21: 3427-38.

Xi Z-X, Gilbert JG, Peng XQ, Pak AC, Li X, Gardner EL. Cannabinoid CB1 receptor antagonist AM251 inhibits cocaine-primed relapse in rats: role of glutamate in the nucleus accumbens. J Neurosci 2006a; 26: 8531-6.

Xi ZX, Kiyatkin M, Li X, Peng XQ, Wiggins A, Spiller K, Li J, Gardner EL. N-acetylaspartylglutamate (NAAG) inhibits intravenous cocaine self-administration and cocaine-enhanced brain-stimulation reward in rats. Neuropharmacology 2010a; 58:304-313.

Xi ZX, Li X, Li J, Peng XQ, Froimowitz M, Gardner EL. CTDP 32,476: a low addictive slow-onset long-acting dopamine transporter inhibitor that may act as a methadone-like agonist therapy for cocaine addiction. Abstract, 41st Annual Meeting of the Society for Neuroscience, Washington D.C., Nov. 11-16, 2011a;

Xi ZX, Li Y, Li J, Peng XQ, Song R, Gardner EL. Dopamine D3 receptors in the nucleus accumbens and central amygdala underlie incubation of cocaine craving in rats. Addiction Biology. 2012; in press.

Xi ZX, Li X, Peng XQ, Gardner EL. Potential use of slow-onset long-acting dopamine transporter inhibitors in the treatment of cocaine addiction. Chinese Journal Drug Depend 2009; 18:268-270.

Xi ZX, Li X, Peng XQ, Li J, Chun L, Gardner EL, Thomas AG, Slusher BS, Ashby CR, Jr. Inhibition of NAALADase by 2-PMPA attenuates cocaine-induced relapse in rats: a NAAG-mGluR2/3-mediated mechanism. J Neurochem 2010b; 112:564-576.

Xi Z-X, Newman AH, Gilbert JG, Pak AC, Peng X-Q, Ashby CR Jr, Gitajn L, Gardner EL. The novel dopamine D3 receptor antagonist NGB 2904 inhibits cocaine's rewarding effects and cocaine-induced reinstatement of drug-seeking behavior in rats. Neuropsychopharmacology 2006b; 31: 1393-405.

Xi ZX, Peng XQ, Li X, Song R, Zhang HY, Liu QR, Yang HJ, Bi GH, Li J, Gardner EL. Brain cannabinoid CB2 receptors modulate cocaine's actions in mice. Nat Neurosci 2011; 14:1160-1166.

Xi ZX, Shen H, Baker DA, Kalivas PW. Inhibition of non-vesicular glutamate release by group III metabotropic glutamate receptors in the nucleus accumbens. J Neurochem 2003b; 87:1204-12.

Xi ZX, Spiller K, Gardner EL. Mechanism-based medication development for the treatment of nicotine dependence. Acta Pharmacol Sin. 2009; 30:723-39.

Xi ZX, Spiller K, Pak AC, Gilbert J, Dillon C, Li X, Peng XQ, Gardner EL. Cannabinoid CB1 receptor antagonists attenuate cocaine's rewarding effects: Experiments with self-administration and brain-stimulation reward in rats. Neuropsychopharmacology 2008; 33:1735-45.

Xi ZX, Yang Z, Li SJ, Li X, Dillon C, Peng XQ, Spiller K, Gardner EL. Levo-tetrahydropalmatine inhibits cocaine's rewarding effects: experiments with self-administration and brain-stimulation reward in rats. Neuropharmacology 2007; 53:771-782.

Xi ZX. Preclinical Pharmacology, Efficacy and Safety of Varenicline in Smoking Cessation and Clinical Utility in High Risk Patients. Drug Health Patient Saf 2010: 39-48.

Yang Z, Shao YC, Li SJ, Qi JL, Zhang MJ, Hao W, Jin GZ. Medication of l-tetrahydropalmatine significantly ameliorates opiate craving and increases the abstinence rate in heroin users: a pilot study. Acta Pharmacol Sin. 2008; 29:781-8.

Yang HJ, Gardner EL, Xi ZX. Tiagabine inhibits cocaine taking, but not cocaine-seeking in rats. Neurosci Lett 2012, in press.

Yuan J, Chen X, Brodbeck R, et al. Highly selective dopamine D3 receptor antagonists. Bioorg Med Chem Lett 1998; 8: 2715-8.

Zerbib F, Bruley des Varannes S, et al. Randomised clinical trial: effects of monotherapy with ADX10059, a mGluR5 inhibitor, on symptoms and reflux events in patients with gastro-oesophageal reflux disease. Aliment Pharmacol Ther 2011; 33:911-21.

Zerbib F, Keywood C, Strabach G. Efficacy, tolerability and pharmacokinetics of a modified release formulation of ADX10059, a negative allosteric modulator of metabotropic glutamate receptor 5: an esophageal pH-impedance study in healthy subjects. Neurogastroenterol Motil 2010; 22: 859-6.

3

Polydrug Use in Adolescence

Marta Rodríguez-Arias and María Asunción Aguilar
University of Valencia
Spain

1. Introduction

1.1 Drug and polydrug use among adolescents

The 2010 Monitoring the Future survey conducted by the US government raises concerns about an increase in drug use among teenagers, particularly those of a younger age. A similar trend has been reflected by European surveys, such as the 2010 Annual report on the state of the drugs problem in Europe, EMCDDA. According to this study, commissioned by the European Council, the use of multiple substances — polydrug use — is widespread and represents a major challenge. A recent survey by the Spanish government (EDADES 2009/2010) revealed that approximately 50% of drug users consumed two or more substances simultaneously. The objective of users is to increase or reverse the effects of the different drugs taken, but greater health risks and problems and a poor treatment response are also inherent in polydrug consumption. Almost all patterns of polydrug use include alcohol, and the use of amphetamines or ecstasy among frequent or heavy alcohol consumers is much higher than the average. A study by the Spanish government (Encuesta Estatal sobre uso de drogas en estudiantes de enseñanzas secundarias, ESTUDES, 2008) revealed that Spanish students between 14-18 years old who used drugs generally consumed more than one drug at the same time. 96.2% of students who had taken ecstasy in the previous year had simultaneously consumed alcohol and 86.1% had simultaneously consumed cannabis. An association between consumption of stimulants and hallucinogen drugs was also reported. For example, among students who had used ecstasy in the previous year, 71.4% had also consumed cocaine, while 38.5% of those who had used cocaine in the same period had also consumed ecstasy.

2. The adolescent brain

Adolescence is the period of gradual physiological, cognitive, behavioural and psychosocial transition from childhood to adulthood (Pickles et al., 1998) during which individuals experience physical changes, new interests, greater independence and heightened responsibility. Since adolescence is a process, it is difficult to characterize its ontogenetic time course, and no single event signals its onset or termination. In humans, adolescence is often considered to begin with the onset of the biological changes associated with puberty (the period during which an individual becomes sexually mature), although the timing of puberty within the adolescent period varies notably among humans. Adolescence ends when the individual assumes adult social roles, with a change in the sleep pattern having been proposed as a physiological marker of its termination (Abbott, 2005). The adolescent age span in humans is commonly considered to be from 12 to 18 years, although the entire second decade is sometimes considered adolescence, with up to 25 years being considered late adolescence (Baumrind, 1987).

Adolescent subjects exhibit certain characteristic behaviours (some of which are common among adolescents across species), including hyperphagia, shorter periods of sleep, increases in peer-directed social interactions and affiliation with peers, an increase in the number of conflicts with parents, egocentrism, a lack of 'common sense' in decision-making, rigidity in reasoning, impulsivity, including a preference for actions that offer immediate rewards (cognitive impulsivity), reduced self-control, enhanced novelty-seeking and risk-taking behaviours (Spear, 2011a; Sturman & Moghaddam, 2011). All of these behaviours can lead to a higher incidence of risky behaviours such as misconduct at school, drink driving, unsafe sex, use of illegal drugs, and antisocial behaviours (Doremus-Fitzwater et al., 2010; Eaton et al., 2010; Spear, 2011b). Although cognitive control improves throughout adolescence (Luna et al., 2010), youths show differences in cognitive strategies in relation to adults. According to the "fuzzy trace theory" adolescents process the risk and benefits of choices more explicitly than adults, which, paradoxically, leads to greater risk-taking (Rivers et al., 2008). The characteristic irresponsibility of adolescents may be due to differences in the way in which they experience risk and reward, especially under conditions of heightened emotional arousal (Sturman & Moghaddam, 2011). Thus, the risk-taking behaviour of adolescents is probably related to the fact that their decision-making capacity is more vulnerable to disruption by stress. Adolescence is generally considered to be a stressful stage of life, and individuals are more likely to perceive events as stressful at this age, with adolescents exhibiting higher rates of depressed mood, sleep problems, emotional instability, anxiety and self-consciousness (Buchanan et al., 1992). Moreover, some aspects of neurobehavioural and hormonal responses to stressors also vary when adolescents are compared to younger or older individuals (Allen & Matthews, 1997). Similarly, behavioural experiments in laboratory animals have revealed that adolescents are more disrupted by stressors than younger or older counterparts and that they differ behaviourally and physiologically in their response to stressors when compared to animals of other ages (Buwalda et al., 2011; Stone & Quartermain, 1998; Vázquez, 1998). For example, the rise in plasma corticosterone levels induced by restraint stress is prolonged in adolescent rats in comparison with adult animals. Moreover, while adult male rats, which are repeatedly exposed to daily restraint stress, show a clear habituation in their neuroendocrine response, adolescent male rats actually exhibit a facilitation of this response (Romeo, 2010).

The characteristic behaviour of adolescence can be explained in neurobiological terms (Brenhouse & Andersen, 2011; Casey et al., 2011; Sturman & Moghaddam, 2011). Indeed, the features of an adolescent brain predispose individuals to behaving in the way referred to above. Maturational alterations of the brain contribute to these age-specific behavioural characteristics, including the increase in risk-taking and propensity to use drugs of abuse (Doremus-Fitzwater et al., 2010). Recent research has demonstrated the importance of gonadal hormones for neurobehavioural maturation during adolescence in laboratory animals and an association between gonadal hormones and adolescent behaviour/mood in humans (see Vigil et al., 2011, for review). Adolescence represents a stage of development of the nervous system (as does embryonic development) in which steroid hormones trigger various organizational phenomena related to structural brain circuit remodelling:

myelination, apoptosis, neural pruning, and dendritic spine remodelling, thus determining the adult behavioural response to steroids or sensory stimuli (Vigil et al., 2011).

The adolescent brain undergoes dramatic changes in gross morphology. During this phase there is a massive loss of gray matter and synapses in neocortical brain regions (Gogtay et al., 2004), and the most characteristic ontogenetic change, which occurs across a variety of species, is an alteration of the prefrontal cortex. Throughout human adolescence there is a marked increase in hemispheric asymmetry and in the degree to which the two cerebral hemispheres can process information independently (Merola & Liederman, 1985). In the primate cortex, the density of receptors of different neurotransmitter systems (dopamine, serotonine, acetylcholine, and GABA) decreases as adolescence progresses (Lidow et al., 1991; Brenhouse & Andersen, 2011). Most of the synapses that undergo pruning during adolescence are excitatory, which results in a decline in N-methyl-D-aspartate (NMDA) receptors and the extension of glutaminergic excitatory stimulation to the cortex (Insel et al., 1990). There is a body of evidence to show that the balance of excitatory and inhibitory neurotransmission varies between adolescents and adults, suggesting that the increased inhibition associated with development of the prefrontal cortex promotes greater neural coordination (Sturman & Moghaddam, 2011).

Maturational changes are also evident during adolescence in limbic regions such as the hippocampus (Insel et al., 1990; Wolfer and Lipp, 1995), and gray matter reductions also take place in the striatum and other subcortical structures (Sowell et al., 2002). Conversely, white matter increases in cortical and subcortical fiber tracts (Paus et al., 2001) and in circuits connecting the amygdala and striatum with the prefrontal cortex (Asato et al 2010). A decrease is observed in glutamate receptors in the hippocampus (Insel et al., 1990) and DA receptors in the striatum (Seeman et al., 1987; Teicher et al, 1995). Cannabinoid binding peaks in the limbic forebrain of rats during adolescence before declining to adult levels (Rodriguez de Fonseca et al., 1993). Experimental evidence supports a shift during adolescence from a relative balance between subcortical and cortical DA systems toward a greater predominance of cortical DA. In contrast to this enhanced DA tone in the prefrontal cortex during adolescence, DA activity in the accumbens and other subcortical DA terminal regions seems to be less noticeable in adolescents than in adults (Andersen & Gazzara, 1993). Basal levels of synaptic DA are lower during this phase of development, although adolescents show a greater and faster increase in drug-induced DA release (Badanich et al. 2006; Laviola et al. 2001). Consistent with this, adolescents are generally subject to a less positive impact from stimuli with moderate to low incentive value, and thus seek additional appetitive reinforcers (Spear, 2000).

Neuroimaging studies have shown variations in human adolescent functional activity in different forebrain regions, including the amygdala, orbitofrontal cortex and striatum (Bjork et al., 2010). For example, the amygdala and accumbens of adolescents exhibit more activity than those of adults (Ernst et al., 2002). Similarly, in comparison to adults, adolescents show a lower response to reward in the lateral orbitofrontal cortex and a higher activity in the nucleus accumbens (Galvan et al., 2006). Neural coordination within and between brain regions as well as processing efficiency are reduced in adolescents due to a less-effective information transfer between regions, incomplete myelination, and imbalances in neuronal inhibition/excitation within critical brain regions (Sturman & Moghaddan, 2011). Human and animal studies have revealed a differential development of subcortical limbic systems related to top-down control systems during adolescent brain development, with subcortical limbic systems developing earlier than control systems. It has been proposed that the mechanisms underlying adolescent changes in behaviour (impulsiveness, risky choices, drug taking, etc.) could underlie an imbalance between an increased sensitivity to motivational cues and immature cognitive control (Casey et al., 2011). In summary, immature neuronal processing in the prefrontal cortex and other cortical and subcortical regions, and their interaction, lead to a behaviour that is biased toward risk and emotional reactivity during the adolescent period (Sturman & Moghaddan, 2011).

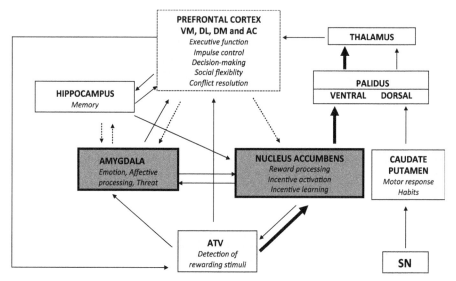

Fig. 1. Neural circuit involved in motivated behaviour. Thick lines represent hyperactive brain areas or connections and faint and dashed lines represent brain areas that are more hypoactive in adolescent subjects than in adults.

The adolescent brain operates in a promotivational state due to the combination of three factors:

a. limited inhibitory capacity and poor regulatory control (due to the lack of cortical maturation)
b. DA hyperactivity in the nucleus accumbens when processing appetitive stimuli
c. Amygdala hyperactivity, which explains affective intensity and liability, and a weaker harm-avoidance system (Ernst et al., 2009).

The relatively early development of bottom-up limbic regions (nucleus accumbens and amygdala), along with an immaturity of top-down regulatory systems (PFC), biases behavior toward risk-taking, risk-seeking, impulsive choice, sensation-seeking and novelty preference.

3. Effects of drugs on adolescents

In addition to increases in sensation- and novelty-seeking, drug use is more common during adolescence (2010 Annual report on the state of the drugs problem in Europe, EMCDDA;

Doremus-Fitzwater et al., 2010; Spear, 2011b). Youngsters differ from adults in their response to a variety of drugs (Schramm-Sapyta et al., 2009). These ontogenetic variations in drug responsiveness may be related with age differences in pharmacokinetics, particularly with respect to the functioning of the neural substrates upon which these drugs act, and also with social enhancement. As discussed previously, the neural systems involved in the effects exerted by drugs (mesolimbic DA system) differ considerably between adolescents and adults. These ontogenetic differences in drug responsiveness may have significant consequences for adolescents, who exhibit a reduced sensitivity to various drugs of abuse. This insensitivity can promote greater use per occasion in relation to more mature individuals (Schramm-Sapyta et al., 2009). After peer substance use, the next most powerful predictor of adolescent alcohol and drug use is perceived stress (Wagner et al., 1999). In animal models, stress has been shown to increase the rewarding effects of drugs of abuse (Piazza & LeMoal, 1998; Ribeiro Do Couto et al., 2006). On the other hand, experimental data suggest that drugs of abuse induce stronger effects in adolescents than in adults, although the literature is not conclusive regarding these differences (for review see Schramm-Sapyta et al., 2009). The developmental stage of adolescence can promote early experimentation with drugs, as addictive substances are generally more rewarding and less aversive (Schramm-Sapyta et al., 2009).

Moreover, adolescent substance use disrupts the normal development of an adolescent brain. Exposure to drugs of abuse can induce neurobehavioural, neurochemical and neuroendocrinal effects in the adolescent rat brain, thereby affecting the growth process and systems involved in plasticity and cognition (Jain & Balhara, 2010). Since adolescents undergo structural and functional dynamic changes in brain areas implicated in the reinforcing properties of drugs of abuse (prefrontal cortex and ventral striatum) and habit formation (dorsal striatum), drug-taking during this period could increase susceptibility to drug dependence, although there is a lack of studies that demonstrate causality.

4. Animal models of drug addiction

The use of animal models to study drug addiction has the advantage of experimental control of variables (age of initial exposure, drug, dose, duration, timing of exposure, etc.) and has provided much valuable information. The main drawback to animal studies is that no model completely reproduces all the stages in the development of drug addiction. Results obtained with multiple behavioural and neurobiological models are necessary to achieve a deeper understanding of this disorder (Ahmed, 2010; Belin et al. 2010; Sanchis-Segura & Spanagel, 2006; Schramm-Sapyta et al., 2009; Shippenberg & Koob, 2002; Weiss, 2010).

There are several animal models with a high predictive value, though most studies are performed with one of two paradigms: self-administration or conditioned place preference (CPP) (Aguilar et al., 2009). The most direct procedure for evaluating the reinforcing properties of a substance is self-administration (the animal works to obtain the substance: for example by pressing a lever), which assesses the intrinsic rewarding properties of a substance; and both oral and intravenous routes have been used to assess the relevance of age in voluntary intake. Animals that acquire drug-taking behaviour more quickly or indulge in it more frequently can be considered to resemble human drug addicts. However, drug taking, even when acquired quickly, is not equivalent to drug dependence (Ahmed, 2010). Another shortcoming of the self-administration paradigm is the complexity of the technique and the lack of a standardized procedure for evaluating substances with different potencies, reinforcement properties and pharmacokinetics. The choice of training substance, species and procedural parameters can radically affect the results obtained (Moser et al., 2011). Variations of the self-administration model have been developed to study the main features of addiction. For example, the progressive ratio method designed by Hodos (1961), in which the sweetness and volume of a milk is varied in order to measure reward strength, has been used to assess motivation to seek a drug (Depoortere et al., 1993). On the other hand, extinction and reinstatement paradigms are employed to model relapse. Following acquisition of self-administration, animals undergo a process by which the response is extinguished and reinstatement is induced by drug priming, stress or drug-associated cues (Shaham et al., 2003; Epstein et al., 2006). Time-out and punished responding model compulsive use (Deroche-Gamonet et al., 2004; Vanderschuren and Everitt, 2004) and long-access training schedules model high-level use (Knackstedt & Kalivas, 2007). Additionally, models of habitual drug-seeking have also been developed (Everitt et al., 2008).

The CPP paradigm (in which rodents repeatedly exposed to a distinct environment in the presence of a positively reinforcing substance show preference for that environment) evaluates the conditioned rewarding properties of a substance, and is also frequently used due to its procedural simplicity and rapidity. This model is dose-sensitive, and drugs of abuse are typically rewarding at low to moderate doses and aversive at high doses. CPP is sensitive to a wide range of substances. In general, CPP is useful for measuring the level and persistence of drug-induced reward (Tzschentke, 1998), but not for modelling pathological drug-seeking or taking. For this reason, variations of this procedure (adding an extinction and reinstatement of the extinguished conditioned preference) have been developed to model addiction-like behaviours (Aguilar et al., 2009).

Other animal models are employed to study motor behaviour, conditioned aversion, withdrawal, sensitization and compulsive drug-seeking (Belin et al., 2009; Schramm-Sapyta et al., 2009; Weiss, 2010). Most drugs of abuse stimulate locomotor behaviour through activation of the dopaminergic circuits that contribute to their reinforcing effects. At lower doses locomotor activity is generally increased, whereas at higher doses, locomotion falls and stereotypical behaviour can emerge. Conditioned place and taste aversion are designed to assess the aversive effects of drugs of abuse (which are assumed to discourage intake). Animals are trained to associate a place or a palatable flavour with the aversive sensations induced by a drug injected by the experimenter (generally lithium), which causes the place or flavour to be subsequently avoided. These tests measure the use-limiting effects of drugs of abuse but do not model pathological drug-seeking or taking (Schramm-Sapyta et al., 2009), since experimenter-delivered injections greatly differ from volitional intake even for the aversive effects of the drug (Galici et al., 2000).

Withdrawal is a constellation of affective and physiological changes that occurs after cessation of intake of some drugs of abuse and is used to evaluate dependence. Symptoms generally reflect the reversal of initial drug effects, although they vary with the drug, duration and extent of exposure. This, together with the kind of observations made and the choice of end points, can obstruct the interpretation of withdrawal effects (Moser et al., 2011). In the case of ethanol or opioids, withdrawal effects (including autonomic and behavioural activation) can be easily quantified in animal models. Withdrawal from psychostimulants and most other drugs of abuse results in a generalized "negative motivational state" which can be assessed using an intracranial self-stimulation procedure (Bauzo & Bruijnzeel, 2012) or an anxiety-like state which can be assessed using many models, including the social interaction test and elevated plus maze (Hall et al. 2010). Repeated exposure to any of the aforementioned drugs can lead to a phenomenon called sensitization, in which the ambulatory, stereotypic or rewarding effect of a repeated low dose is augmented. Sensitization reflects lasting neuroplastic changes in response to repeated exposure, and is hypothesized to be a behavioural correlate of increased drug craving and development of dependence (Robinson and Berridge, 2008), though its relevance to drug dependence is debatable. However, since data from sensitization studies have led to the development of pharmacotherapies that have been tested in animal models of relapse and in human addicts, some authors support sensitisation as a useful model for determining the neural basis of addiction (Steketee & Kalivas, 2011). Compulsive drug-seeking is analysed by the more complex methods of self-administration (progressive ratio, extinction, reinstatement, punishment, long-access, etc.), which tend to be more informative regarding vulnerability to addiction. However, it is difficult to employ these new techniques in developmental studies that aim to examine the behaviour of adolescent vs adult rodents, partly due to the prolonged duration of the experimental procedures.

5. Animal models of adolescent polydrug consumption

Recent advances in imaging have made it easier to study the human brain, but many questions about the effect of drugs in the adolescent brain require experimental manipulation in experimental animals in order to be answered. Given the across-species similarities in neurobehavioural features of adolescence, non-human animals undergoing this developmental transition can be used as models of human adolescence (Spear, 2000). There is growing evidence that adolescent humans and rodents experience many similar structural and functional changes in the brain as they progress towards adulthood. Behavioural changes characteristics of adolescence (increased social behaviour, novelty- and sensation-seeking, risk-taking, emotional instability and impulsivity) are also observed in rodents (Jain & Balhara, 2010). However, the use of adolescent rodent models does have some limitations. There are numerous areas of adolescent functioning in humans that cannot be addressed using animal models (peer pressure and self esteem, impact of parenting styles, obsession about weight, etc.). Moreover, the increases in adrenal hormones/neuroactive steroids during adrenarche in humans are generally not evident in other mammalian species. Furthermore, forebrain systems of rodents are less prominent than in humans, their social organization is simpler, and the time course of adolescence is briefer. The time frame of adolescence in non-human animals such as the rat is even more difficult to characterize than in humans. Among researchers who study adolescence in rats, opinions differ somewhat (Spear, 2000). The problem is further magnified by the limited amount of research to have focused on adolescence in laboratory animals. Animals of both genders exhibit neurobehavioural characteristics typical of adolescence during the period between postnatal days 28 and 42. According to hormonal, physical and social criteria, this development phase corresponds with age 12-18 in humans (Spear 2000). Moreover, different physiological changes (growth spurt, loss of excitatory input to prefrontal cortex, vaginal opening in females and increases in maturing spermatids in males) occur during this period. Indeed, some ontogenetic changes that signal the early onset of adolescence in female rats can emerge as early as 20 days of age, with later development taking place up until 55-60 days of age in males. Taking into account the abovementioned limitations, adolescent rodent models can be considered to possess good face and construct validity, since there are strong similarities between human adolescents and various animal models of adolescence in terms of developmental history, behavioural traits and neural and hormonal characteristics (Spear, 2011a). As more information is generated, stronger evidence of these forms of validity, and of predictive validity, will no doubt be obtained.

Moreover, there are several methodological difficulties that are encountered when using experimental animals to model the complex pattern of drug abuse observed in humans. A polydrug animal model of drug abuse allows a situation that is closer to reality than the simple effect produced by one drug. However, a number of variables need to be taken into account when using such a model. Comparison of the studies published in the literature is difficult, since practically each one of them represents a different model of polydrug administration. This is to be expected given the high number of variables involved in this kind of study (Schensul et al., 2005). The first variable to bear in mind is the combination of drugs employed. In most studies only two drugs are employed; in many cases cocaine or alcohol. Another important aspect is the temporal pattern of drug administration employed. Until now, most studies have focused on acute administration (Braida & Sala, 2002; Daza-Losada et al., 2009a; Diller et al., 2007; Manzanedo et al., 2010; Robledo et al., 2007), though there is a growing number of studies employing repeated administration and studying long-term effects (Achat-Mendes et al., 2003; Daza-Losada et al., 2008a, 2008b, 2009; Estelles et al., 2006; Jones et al., 2010; Ribeiro Do Couto et al., 2011a, 2011b; Rodriguez-Arias et al., 2011). This is another point of discrepancy; some studies have measured effects after very short periods post-administration (only 2 or 3 days), while others have assessed effects weeks or even months after the last administration. Finally, the effect under evaluation can vary considerably between purely physiological studies and those focusing exclusively on behavioural changes. All these discrepancies point to the fact that polydrug models simplify the complex reality of human consumption, in which each the pattern of drug use of each individual is unique.

Most of the studies that have assessed polydrug use have employed adult animals and acute administration. Thus, it is necessary to design models of adolescent polydrug consumption that reflect the human reality, despite the intrinsic difficulties they may pose. Our research group has been working for several years in this field during which we have studied different drug combinations and different patterns of drug administration.

The aim of the present chapter is to offer a detailed review of the experiments performed in this area. With this purpose in mind we will discuss not only the key results obtained in our experiments but also those of other studies of adolescent polydrug use. In an attempt to provide a clear overview of the evidence obtained to date, studies have been classified according to the pattern of drug administration employed. In this way, studies employing acute administration of drugs and studying immediate effects have been grouped together. Studies evaluating the binge pattern of drug administration, commonly employed by users of psychostimulants, constitute a second group. This section also represents a recently employed model developed with the aim of replicating the binge drinking that is so common among adolescents and young people of many cultures. Finally, we will discuss several studies in which a specific drug has triggered the reinstatement of drug-seeking behaviour of a different pharmacological kind of drug, known as the cross-reinstatement phenomenon and also the phenomenon of sensitization.

6. Principal results

6.1 Acute polydrug studies

6.1.1 MDMA plus cocaine

Preclinical studies have until now focused mainly on the long-term consequences of drug pre-treatment in terms of subsequent changes in spontaneous behaviour or in the response to other drugs of abuse. For instance, a substantial number of studies have focused on the long-term consequences of MDMA pre-treatment on subsequent cocaine administration (Achat-Mendes et al., 2003; Åberg et al., 2007; Daza-Losada et al., 2008, 2009b). However, hardly any have examined the interactive profile of concomitant exposure to MDMA and cocaine. Diller and coworkers (2007) studied the effects of concurrent administration of MDMA and cocaine on CPP in adult rats, finding that both drugs induced CPP when administered alone. Co-administration, on the other hand, produced an antagonism, except when higher doses were employed. These results highlight how the neurochemical and behavioural effects of MDMA and cocaine consumed separately are dramatically altered when taken together. Based on the inverse relation between serotonin and DA activity (in general, decreases in serotonin neurotransmission produce an increase of DA function) (Di Giovanni et al., 2010), these authors speculated that cocaine had undermined MDMA-mediated serotonin release more than MDMA-mediated DA release, thereby increasing the overall reward.

In a more recent study, we focused on the interaction of acute MDMA and cocaine administration in adolescent mice (Daza-Losada et al., 2009a), studying the acute interaction of both drugs on motor activity, anxiety, memory and brain monoamines. One of the most important results of this study was that acutely administered cocaine plus MDMA induced an anxiolytic response in the elevated plus maze that was not present when the drugs were administered separately. Mice treated with cocaine and MDMA spent significantly more time in the open arms of the plus maze than controls or animals treated with just one of the drugs. This result was not due to an unspecific increase of motor activity, as no increase in the number of total or closed entries was observed in animals treated with both drugs. Although numerous studies have indicated that MDMA causes anxiety problems in drug users (for review see Baylen et al., 2006), our results revealed that MDMA alone does not exert a strong effect on levels of anxiety in adolescent mice. The few studies performed in the plus maze with mice have shown that acute MDMA administration induces anxiogenic or anxiolytic effects that vary depending on the dose employed (Navarro et al. 2002). Although all the available evidence supports an anxiogenic effect of acute cocaine administration in adult mice (Erhardt et al., 2006), cocaine did not affect the behaviours studied in the plus maze in our study. One possible explanation could be the different experimental conditions of the studies compared or a different dose-response curve to cocaine in adolescent versus adult mice. These results endorse the hypothesis that adolescent animals are more "protected" from adverse psychostimulant-related properties than older subjects (Laviola et al., 1999), and highlight the importance of employing adolescent animals in studies.

Another important observation of our study was that an increase in DA turnover in the striatum was observed only when both drugs were administered together, due to a substantial increase in DOPAC concentration that was not accompanied by alterations of

DA levels. Neither serotonin nor its metabolites were altered in the striatum, but there was an increase in the concentration of serotonin in the cortex (total cortex, including the frontal cortex), which led to a decrease in its turnover. Although MDMA and cocaine act on the same neurotransmitter systems, the mechanisms involved differ, as do the effects produced. MDMA provokes an acute release of both serotonin and dopamine from nerve terminals (review in Colado et al., 2004) and is more potent in inhibiting serotonin and norepinephrine than dopamine transporters, while cocaine blocks these three monoamine transporters at similar concentrations (Han et al., 2006). One report suggested that serotonin plays a more prominent role in the psychotropic effects of MDMA than in those of cocaine (Itzhak et al., 2006). As in our study, both drugs were administered together, cocaine appeared to block MDMA entry into the nerve terminals, thereby inhibiting MDMA-mediated monoamine release, which mainly affects serotonin. On the other hand, the reuptake-blocking effects of these compounds may have been an added factor that made DA more available to the synapse, which could have been responsible for the increase in dopaminergic turnover observed. This DA/serotoninergic balance, which occurred only in the groups treated with both drugs, could be, in part, responsible for the anxiolytic effect observed when cocaine and MDMA were administered together. Our results endorse the hypothesis of Diller and coworkers (2007), since we have observed an increase in DA turnover and lower levels of serotonin turnover in the striatum and cortex. These findings point to an increase in DA availability in conjunction with the release of serotonin in small amounts or at a slow rate, leading to a decrease in its turnover. These studies demonstrate that the combined use of MDMA and cocaine produces a specific neurochemical and behavioural profile different to that observed when each drug is administered alone.

6.1.2 MDMA plus cannabinoids

Several studies have highlighted that the prolonged combined use of MDMA and cannabis is associated with a variety of psychological problems, including elevated impulsiveness, anxiety and psychotic behaviour (Daumann et al., 2004). The cannabinoid system interacts with a variety of neurotransmitters, including DA and serotonin (Nakazi et al., 2000), and represents a common neurobiological substrate for the addictive properties of different drugs of abuse (Maldonado et al., 2006). In line with this, many of the physiological responses provoked by MDMA are modulated by the endocannabinoid system (Piomelli et al., 2005).

Few studies have clarified the effects of exposure to cannabinoids on liability to MDMA abuse, and most of them suggest that cannabinoid agonists potentiate the rewarding effects of MDMA (Braida & Sala, 2002). However, studies performed recently have demonstrated that cannabinoid agonists modify sensitivity to the behavioural effects of MDMA in different ways (increase/decrease) depending on the dose employed. We have observed that a low dose of the specific CB1 agonist WIN 55212-2 increases the rewarding effects of an ineffective dose of MDMA administered during acquisition of the CPP. However, higher doses of the cannabinoid agonist weaken the preference induced by effective doses of MDMA (Manzanedo et al., 2010). Our results are in accordance with those of Robledo and co-workers (2007), who reported that a sub-threshold dose of THC produced CPP in mice when combined with a non-rewarding dose of MDMA but decreased the CPP induced by an effective dose of MDMA.

Cannabinoids participate in the regulation of DA synthesis, release and turnover (Gardner et al., 1998). The overlapping expression of cannabinoid and dopamine receptors in some brain areas such as the nucleus accumbens (Hermann et al., 2002) may represent a neuroanatomical substrate for such an interaction. At doses that neither WIN 55212-2 nor MDMA alter brain monamines, animals treated with both drugs exhibited decreases of striatal DA and serotonin in the cortex (Manzanedo et al., 2010). Despite the anti-inflammatory and anti oxidative properties of cannabinoids (Pazos et al., 2008; Aggarwal et al., 2009), animal studies have revealed that chronic administration of THC causes hippocampal damage (Fisk et al., 2006) and that exposure to low concentrations of cannabinoids over a prolonged period is likely to have a neurotoxic effect (Rubovitch et al., 2002; Sarne & Keren, 2004). This evidence points to the capacity of cannabinoids to increase the neurotoxic potential of MDMA. We must keep in mind that, due to the crucial role that the DA system plays in the reinforcing effects of drugs of abuse, the neurotoxic effect of MDMA on mice could modulate the response of lesioned brains to these drugs. For instance, mice pre-exposed to neurotoxic doses of MDMA exhibit a higher consumption of, and a preference for, EtOH than saline-treated animals (Izco et al. 2007).

6.2 Binge pattern

6.2.1 MDMA plus cocaine

Epidemiological data reveal that the majority of MDMA users cease taking the drug spontaneously in their twenties (von Sydow et al., 2002), which highlights the relevance of using adolescent subjects in animal models. In addition to presenting a distinctive behavioural profile (Spear, 2000; Adriani & Laviola, 2003), young rats and mice are highly sensitive to the administration of psychostimulant agents (Laviola et al., 1999; Spear, 2000).

Both MDMA and cocaine have been proved to induce long-term response after their consumption. MDMA users present weeks after discontinuation of intake, a reduced hormonal response to drug challenge and a combination of depressive pattern, dysphoria, high levels of aggressiveness and elevated scores of novelty-seeking behaviour (Gerra et al., 1998). These long-term effects have also been described in mice and rats exposed to MDMA during adolescence, among which changes in social behaviour (Morley-Fletcher et al., 2002), motor activity (Balogh et al., 2004) and anxiety levels (Faria et al., 2006; Clemens et al., 2007) have been detected. On the other hand, cocaine administration also induces long-term effects in adolescent mice, which are expressed through increased flee and avoidance behaviour and fewer social contacts (Estelles et al., 2006). However, the long-lasting effect of the combination of two drugs taken during adolescence has received little attention. Furthermore, it should be taken into consideration that human MDMA and cocaine consumers commonly adhere to a binge pattern, which has been associated with a higher occurrence of stimulant-induced psychosis and addiction (Gawin, 1991; Segal & Kuczenski, 1997; Belin et al., 2011). To explore these effects, we performed a series of studies using a model that mimics a binge pattern of MDMA and cocaine consumption. This model consists of two daily injections (at 8 am and 8 pm) of an identical dose of MDMA alone or plus cocaine, for 3 days (6 administrations), between postnatal day 28 and 30. Mice were evaluated three weeks after the last treatment, on postnatal day 51. MDMA administration decreased the concentration of striatal DA when administered at high doses (20 mg/kg) in agreement with previous reports (for review see Colado et al., 2004), but cocaine inhibited this decrease in DA concentration three weeks later (Daza-Losada et al., 2008a). In accordance with these results, pretreatment with the dopamine uptake inhibitor GBR 12909 prevented long-term loss in the striatal concentration of DA (O'Shea et al., 2001). This lack of neurotoxicity could have been due to the effect exerted on body temperature by the two drugs together, as cocaine is known to counteract the increase produced by neurotoxic doses of MDMA. Most evidence suggests that merely preventing MDMA-induced hyperthermia is enough to produce significant neuroprotection (Colado et al., 2001). Although a rise in temperature is an important element in MDMA-induced neurotoxicity, this phenomenon appears to involve more than MDMA metabolites, including dopamine deamination and/or autooxidation (Sprague & Nichols, 2005). As we administered both drugs together, it is also feasible that cocaine interfered with the dopamine uptake system by inhibiting the entry of MDMA into the nerve terminal. By affecting one or several of these processes, cocaine is capable of blocking dopamine neurodegeneration in the mouse brain.

Since many MDMA users employ opiates in order to relieve the psychostimulant effects of ecstasy, it is of relevance to evaluate whether such individuals are subject to an increase in the well-known rewarding properties of morphine. We have observed that, following MDMA binges during adolescence, sensitivity to reinstatement of an extinguished preference is increased, as a morphine-induced preference was reinstated with lower priming doses in MDMA–treated mice than in non-treated animals (Daza-Losada et al., 2008b). In the literature regarding learning, reinstatement refers to the recovery of a learned response when a subject is non-contingently exposed to either a conditioned or an unconditioned stimulus after extinction. This recovery of a learned response, which represents a return to drug seeking, occurs when rats or mice are exposed to drugs, drug cues or stressors following extinction. In the CPP version of the reinstatement model, an extinguished CPP is robustly reinstated by non-contingent administration of a priming dose of the drug (Aguilar et al., 2009). Contrasting results were obtained when adolescent mice were treated with cocaine alone or plus MDMA. These animals need higher priming doses of morphine than non-treated mice in order to reinstate the preference. The ability of repeated treatment with psychomotor stimulants to enhance the response to subsequent challenge by an opiate seems to be affected by the route and timing of administration of each drug. Prenatal treatment with cocaine decreases the rewarding actions of morphine in adult offspring (Estelles et al., 2006), while, in adult rats, doses of morphine that fail to produce CPP have been shown to induce a marked preference in those which have previously received cocaine (Shippenberg et al., 1998). However, when acute challenge with heroin takes place 3 weeks after daily systemic injections of cocaine, locomotor cross-sensitization does not occur (DeVries et al., 1998). When cocaine is administered during gestational development, the development of brain reward systems can be altered, resulting in a long-term attenuation of the rewarding properties of morphine. Nevertheless, the possibility that such animals are unable to form the necessary association between a particular environment and morphine cannot be ruled out (Heyser et al., 1990; Inman-Wood et al., 2000). Additionally, prenatal exposure to cocaine can reduce the duration of pregnancy, gestational weight gain and food intake in the dams, factors that can contribute to an abnormal response to morphine. Finally, an association between prenatal cocaine exposure and the effect of altered maternal behaviour on later cognitive functions cannot be ruled out.

Thus, MDMA-treated mice are more vulnerable to relapse after receiving a priming administration of morphine, but this tendency is completely blocked in animals exposed to cocaine, in which an opposite effect is exhibited. Cocaine induces modifications in DA receptor function and transduction events mainly in the mesocorticolimbic dopamine pathway, where it induces an up-regulation of the cAMP-signalling pathway (Nestler, 2004) and augments the activity of the transcription factor cAMP response element-binding protein (CREB) (Walters et al., 2003). Increased CREB expression in the nucleus accumbens undermines the rewarding effects of both cocaine (Carlezon et al., 1998) and morphine (Barrot et al., 2002). In addition, repeated exposure to cocaine upregulates DYN/KOPr systems (Shippenberg et al., 2007).. This increase may initially serve as a homeostatic response that opposes the alteration in neurotransmission that occurs after exposure to this drug use. However, following the discontinuation of drug use, the unopposed actions of this system are likely to result in dysregulation of basal DA and glutamate transmission, thereby contributing to aberrant activity within the prefrontal-cortico-striatal loop (Shippenberg et al., 2007). These could represent some of the mechanisms responsible for the way in which cocaine affects the response of the dopaminergic system by altering the intensity of the response to priming.

MDMA and cocaine are often first consumed at an early age, and the response to MDMA of users in their twenties can be affected by previous exposure to these or other drugs. Similarly to the observations reported with morphine, Achat-Mendes and co-workers (2003) found that a priming injection of cocaine after extinction reinstated a significantly higher CPP in mice previously exposed during adolescence to a comparable regimen of MDMA. Comparable results have been described in adolescent (Aberg et al., 2007) and adult rats (Horan et al., 2000). These results are also in accordance with the finding that the acquisition of cocaine self-administration is facilitated in rats pre-exposed to MDMA (Fletcher et al., 2001). Concurring with these results, we have demonstrated that exposure to MDMA or cocaine binges during adolescence induces long-lasting changes that increase the reinforcing effects of MDMA (Daza-Losada et al., 2009b). We observed that only mice previously exposed to MDMA developed CPP after being conditioned with a sub-threshold dose of MDMA. On the other hand, although all the groups developed CPP after conditioning with 10 mg/kg of MDMA, the extinguished preference was reinstated only in animals exposed to MDMA or cocaine during adolescence, in which it also took longer for the preference to be extinguished. Extinction provides a measurement of the motivational properties of drugs, which are evident in the persistence of drug-seeking behaviour in the absence of the drug (Aguilar et al., 2009). This is a powerful means of assessing the incentive motivational properties of drug-paired stimuli or non-contingent drug administration in the reinstating response (Pulvirenti, 2003). However, when the two drugs were administered together, cocaine blocked the increases that MDMA induced in sensitivity to the MDMA-induced CPP and in vulnerability to reinstatement of the preference. Once again, as the two drugs were administered simultaneously, the competition for the same molecular target could have affected their action, leading to a weaker effect.

Most authors believe that increases in drug-induced CPP or self-administration observed in animals exposed to MDMA are due to the actions that MDMA exerts on the serotoninergic system (Horan et al. 2000; Fletcher et al. 2001). However, in many cases, it has been reported that the MDMA regimen employed did not induce dopaminergic or serotoninergic neurotoxicity, which was indeed the case in the studies mentioned above. None of the drugs, whether administered alone or together, induced significant changes in the concentration of these monoamines in the striatum, cortex or hippocampus 3 weeks later, at which time CPP was initiated (Daza-Losada et al. 2008b). Moreover, the chosen CPP schedule did not affect the concentration of monoamines (Daza-Losada et al. 2007).

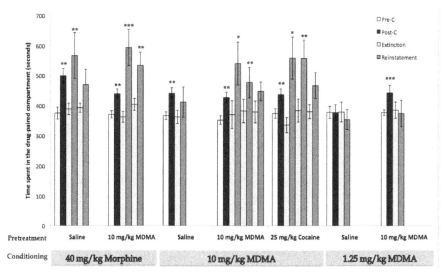

Fig. 2. Effects of MDMA or cocaine administration during adolescence on the acquisition and reinstatement of morphine or MDMA-induced CPP in adult mice. Bars represent mean (±SEM) time spent in the drug-paired compartment before conditioning session (□), after conditioning session (■), in the last extinction session (light grey), and in the reinstatement test (dark grey). During adolescence, mice were treated with six injections of physiological saline, 10 mg/kg of MDMA, or 25 mg/kg of cocaine. Three weeks later mice were conditioned with 40 mg/kg of morphine, or 10 mg/kg or 1.25 mg/kg of MDMA. After conditioning and extinction procedures, all animals received a priming injection of 50% of the drug dose administered during conditioning. In the subsequent reinstatement test, the priming doses employed were 25 and 12.5% that used during conditioning. MDMA exposure during adolescence increased the vulnerability to reinstatement of the extinguished preference induced by morphine and MDMA. This effect was also induced by administration of cocaine during adolescence. Pre-treatment with MDMA also increased its rewarding effects. * p< 0,05, **p<0.01, ***p<0.001 significant difference in time spent in Post-C or Reinstatement tests vs. Pre-C session. Modified from Daza-Losada et al 2008b, 2009b).

6.2.2 MDMA and ethanol binges

Another drug often taken by adolescents in combination with ecstasy is alcohol (Riley et al., 2001; Barrett et al., 2006). Physiological and behavioural studies in humans and rodents have demonstrated an interaction between these two drugs (Mohamed et al., 2009). In humans, ethanol enhances and prolongs the euphoria and feelings of well-being induced by MDMA

(Hernández-López et al., 2002), but moderates some of its physiological effects, such as fluid retention and hyperthermia (Dumont et al., 2010). In addition, animal models have demonstrated that the hyperpyretic effect of MDMA is modulated by Ethanol according to the moment of ethanol administration and ambient temperature (Cassel et al., 2004, 2005 and 2007).

Research has only recently begun to use animal models to evaluate ethanol–MDMA interactions. Ethanol was shown to increase MDMA concentrations not only in blood but also, and to a greater extent, in the striatum and cortex than in the hippocampus (Hamida et al. 2009). On the other hand, levels of alcohol dehydrogenase 2, which metabolizes ethanol to acetaldehyde, were found to be 35% lower in MDMA-treated rats than in controls (Upreti et al. 2009). EthOH significantly potentiates the MDMA-induced outflow of serotonin and DA in rat striatal slices (Riegert et al., 2008). EthOH also affects the neurotoxicity induced by MDMA, although discrepant results have been reported. In rats, EtOH treatment before MDMA administration enhances long-term neurotoxicity, while in mice, EtOH protects DA neurons from the toxic effects of MDMA when evaluated 72 h after the first injection (Johnson et al., 2004). At the behavioural level, EtOH administration potentiates MDMA-induced hyperlocomotion in rats (Cassel, et al. 2004; Riegert, et al. 2008), and repeated co-administration of the two drugs results in a pronounced sensitization of hyperactivity (Hamida et al., 2007, 2008). Recently, Jones and co-workers (2010) have reported CPP in rats that received MDMA plus ethOH but not in those administered just with one of these drugs. These results suggest that acute co-administration of EtOH plus MDMA potentiates the reinforcing effects of each drug alone. Moreover, administration of EtOH would appear to increase the risk of compulsive use of MDMA.

A small number of studies have evaluated chronic exposure to both ethOH and MDMA, and none have explored this interaction in adolescent animals. Employing a model of binge drinking in which animals are treated during adolescence with intermittent doses of ethOH (a total of 16 doses administered intraperitoneally; two per day for two days, followed by a two-day interval without drugs), we aimed to imitate the pattern of weekend binge drinking that is currently so common among adolescents.

Mice were injected twice per day on postnatal day 29, 30, 33, 34, 37, 38, 41, and 42 and with MDMA twice daily on postnatal day 33, 34, 41, and 42. The behavioural and neurochemical test took place three weeks after the last drug administration. Pascual and co-workers (2007) demonstrated that this pattern of ethOH administration during adolescence enhances neural cell death in several brain regions (neocortex, hippocampus, and cerebellum) and induces long-lasting neurobehavioural impairments in conditional discrimination learning as well as motor learning and discrimination between novel and familiar objects. We too have observed that exposure to ethOH during adolescence increases the anxiogenic response induced by MDMA in the elevated plus maze, with adult treated-mice spending less time in the open arms of the maze than non treated littermates. In addition, although ethOH undermines the hyperthermic response induced by MDMA, animals exposed to ethOH plus MDMA exhibit lower concentrations of DA in the striatum than those treated with MDMA only (Rodriguez-Arias et al., 2011). In the study in question, though ethanol efficiently decreased the hyperthermic response induced by MDMA, it did not protect mice treated with 20 mg/kg of MDMA and actually increased the toxic effect in those treated with 10 mg/kg of MDMA, in which a hypothermic response was observed. This effect could be the result of binge pattern ethOH administration enhancing MDMA-induced long-term neurotoxicity through a mechanism that is unrelated to changes in acute hyperthermia and which is thought to involve hydroxyl radical formation (Izco et al., 2007). All the groups that presented reduced levels of striatal DA exhibited increased levels of anxiety. We have previously observed that adolescent mice treated with a schedule of MDMA that provoked a similar decrease in DA concentration without alterations in DOPAC levels behave normally in the elevated plus maze (Daza-Losada et al. 2008b). However, in our study, the decrease in DA was accompanied by a considerable decrease in DOPAC levels, which may have been responsible for the behavioural differences observed. Dopamine plays an important role in anxiety by modulating a cortical brake that the medial prefrontal cortex exerts on the anxiogenic output of the amygdala. It also has a considerable influence on the trafficking of impulses between the basolateral and central nuclei of the amygdala. Intra-amygdaloid infusion of D1 agonists and antagonists elicits anxiogenic and anxiolytic effects, respectively, suggesting an anxiogenic role for D1 receptors in the amygdala. Analyses of the effects of D2 agonists and antagonists suggest that, depending on the model of anxiety in question, either anxiogenic or anxiolytic effects are elicited (de la Mora et al., 2010).

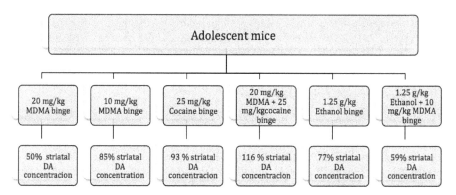

Fig. 3. Effects of MDMA, cocaine or ethanol binge administration during adolescence on the striatal DA concentration three weeks after the last drug administration. Co-administration of cocaine counteracted the neurotoxic effect of binge administration of 20 mg/kg of MDMA. However, intermittent ethanol administration increased the dopaminergic decrease induced by a non-neurotoxic dose (10 mg/kg) of MDMA. *** p<0.001 differences with respect to the saline group. Modified from Daza-Losada et al 2008a, and Rodriguez-Arias et al., 2011.

In addition to inducing long-term consequences for the rewarding effects of drugs, any manipulation or intervention during adolescence can produce other changes, such as the reactivity of the HPA axis to different stressful situations. In a series of recent reports (Ribeiro do Couto et al., 2011a, 2011b), we observed that exposure during adolescence to intermittent injections of ethOH or MDMA modify the response of mice to MDMA administration in adulthood, in addition to previous reports that pointed out long-term behavioural (an increase in anxiety) and neurochemical (a rise in MDMA-induced neurotoxicity) effects (Rodriguez-Arias et al., 2011). Pre-exposure to ethOH, MDMA or both increased the rewarding effects of an ineffective dose of MDMA (1.25 mg/kg). Although these pre-treatments did not affect acquisition of the CPP induced by higher doses, the preference was more persistent in mice pre-exposed to MDMA, ethOH or to both drugs. In addition, reinstatement of the extinguished preference was achieved with lower priming doses of MDMA in the groups pre-exposed to ethOH or MDMA (Ribeiro do Couto et al., 2011a). These effects appear to be due to the changes in the rewarding effects of MDMA rather than unspecific effects such as changes in basal motor activity or stress levels. After conditioning adults mice with an effective (but non neurotoxic) dose of MDMA (10 mg/kg), we once again observed that MDMA or ethanol exposure during adolescence increased the time required to extinguish the preference induced by MDMA and that these effects were related with an increase in either brain monoamine or corticosterone levels in response to MDMA (Ribeiro do Couto et al., 2011b). Mice treated with ethanol after the priming injection presented a significant increase in striatal DA. It is possible that this stronger neurochemical response to the priming dose of MDMA increased the efficacy of conditioning, reflected in a greater resistance to extinction. Similarly, the administration of 10 mg/kg of MDMA led to higher corticosterone values in mice exposed to MDMA during adolescence, while the response to low-mild stressors or to 5 mg/kg of MDMA did not differ, which could produce a stronger learning during conditioning.

In these series of studies, the combination of intermittent administration of ethOH+MDMA did not produce synergistic effects at either behavioural or neurochemical levels. In fact, the combination of the two drugs would seem to counteract the behavioural and hormonal effects of MDMA observed when each is administered alone. These results are in line with the previously discussed observation that adolescent exposure to MDMA exerts more powerful and longer-lasting effects on an MDMA-induced CPP than exposure to cocaine+MDMA (Daza-Losada et al., 2009). In this case, it is possible that ethanol interferes with the metabolism of MDMA and with its penetration of, and/or elimination, from the brain, and that this is responsible for the lack of effects observed after co-administration. Evidence that ethanol increases brain and blood concentrations of MDMA (Johnson et al., 2004) implies an enhanced MDMA-based neurotoxicity and an increased liability to abuse (Hamida et al., 2009). Since no neurotoxic effects were observed after any of the drug pre-treatments measured in the first reinstatement test, our results could be explained by the fact that ethanol increases the concentration of MDMA in the brain. Indeed, we found that the rewarding effects of MDMA produced an inverted U-curve in function of dose, with high doses proving to be devoid of motivational effects (Daza-Losada et al., 2007).

6.3 Cross-reinstatement and sensitization studies

This last section is dedicated to other kinds of drug interaction, cross-reinstatement and sensitization phenomena. Cross-reinstatement can be defined as the reinstatement of extinguished drug-seeking by drugs other than the previously self-administered or conditioning drug. This phenomenon has been widely demonstrated in self-administration and CPP studies. Cross-reinstatement with drugs from different classes to that of the self-administered drug has been demonstrated using the self-administration model. Cannabinoid agonists, DA agonists and re uptake inhibitors and morphine, among others, produce reinstatement of cocaine-seeking after self-administration of cocaine has ended (reviewed by Shalev et al., 2002). Similarly, amphetamine and cocaine produce reinstatement of heroin self-administration (De Vries et al., 1998). Some studies have also demonstrated cross-reinstatement using the CPP paradigm. An extinguished cocaine-induced CPP can be reinstated by a priming injection of related psychostimulants (Itzhak & Martin, 2002), and of other drugs of abuse of different pharmacological classes (Romieu et al., 2004). In the same way, we observed that a cocaine or amphetamine priming following extinction reinstated morphine-induced CPP (Ribeiro Do Couto et al., 2005). In a series of recent studies, we have also observed cross-reinstatement between cannabinoids and MDMA in adolescent animals. Extinguished MDMA-induced CPP was reinstated after a priming injection of the CB1 cannabinoid agonist WIN 55212-2, but this phenomenon only occurred in animals exposed to the cannabinoid agonist during adolescence (Rodríguez-Arias et al., 2010). However, in mice conditioned with WIN 55212-2, a priming injection of MDMA was capable of reinstating the extinguished preference without pre-exposure (Manzanedo et al., 2010). Most authors agree that the mesocorticolimbic DA system is involved in cross-reinstatement. For instance, Wang et al. (2000) suggested that opiates and psychostimulants can all activate the mesolimbic DA system to release DA, which is a mechanism underlying the relapse to drug-seeking behaviour induced by morphine, cocaine or amphetamine. It is possible that one drug cross-primes the other via this common pathway, which is involved in incentive motivation and appetitive goal-directed behaviour (Wang et al., 2000). Such evidence of cross-reinstatement between drugs of different pharmacological classes has also been found in adolescents and suggests that, in drug-abstinent individuals, exposure to an addictive drug can produce intense craving for the previously abused drug and thus lead to relapse to drug-taking and dependence.

The repeated, intermittent administration of a variety of potentially addictive drugs produces persistent increases in their incentive motivational properties (Manzanedo et al., 2004, 2005; Shippenberg & Heidbreder, 1995). Age-related differences in psychostimulant sensitization profiles have been described (Laviola et al., 1995, 1999), with adolescent rats proving to be less vulnerable to MDMA-induced sensitization, only developing this response to MDMA when administered with a high dose and within a narrow margin of time (Aberg et al., 2007). In a recent study, we have evaluated for the first time the effect of adolescent exposure to cannabinoids on the reinforcing effects of MDMA (Rodriguez-Arias et al., 2010). On postnatal day 27, animals received the first of five daily injections of the cannabinoid agonist WIN55212-2, and three days later the place conditioning procedure for MDMA was initiated. In mice pre-exposed to cannabinoids, sub-threshold doses of MDMA induced CPP and reinstatement of an extinguished preference. In the same way, delta-9-tetrahydrocannabinol administration increased hedonic reactions to sucrose and the rise of dialysate DA in the shell of the NAc (de Luca et al., in press). These results endorse the gateway hypothesis, which is sustained by numerous epidemiological studies and suggests that prior exposure to cannabinoids encourages use of other illicit drugs such as psychostimulants (Lynskey et al., 2003). Few studies have tested this hypothesis in animal models, and those that have done so do not provide firm support for it. However, the adolescent brain is particularly sensitive to external and internal variables such as drug exposure, since this phase of development is characterized by active neural changes in, for example, synapse formation and elimination, in brain areas essential for behavioural and cognitive functions (Charmandari et al., 2003; Rice & Barone, 2000). Consequently, exposure to cannabis during the adolescent period may increase vulnerability to subsequent drug abuse disorders.

Authors	Treatment employed	Specie	Age	Behaviour studied/ model employed	Drugs of abuse	Results
Diller et al 2007	acute treatment	rats	adult	MDMA- or cocaine-induced CPP	MDMA and cocaine	Both drugs induced CPP when administered alone. Co-administration produced an antagonism, except at high doses
Daza-Losada et al., 2009a	acute treatment	mice	adolescent	Anxiety (EPM) and striatal monoamine levels	MDMA and cocaine	Anxiolytic response in the elevated plus maze and increased DA turnover in the striatum only when the two drugs were administered together
Braida & Sala, 2002	acute treatment	rats	adult	Self-administration of MDMA (ICV)	MDMA and cannabinoid agonist	Cannabinoid agonists potentiated the rewarding effects of MDMA
Manzanedo et al., 2010	acute treatment	mice	adolescent	MDMA- induced CPP	MDMA and cannabinoid agonist	Low dose of the CB1 agonist increased the rewarding effects of an ineffective dose of MDMA, but higher doses of the cannabinoid agonist weakened the preference induced by effective doses of MDMA
Robledo et al (2007)	acute treatment	mice	adult	THC-induced CPP	Δ9-THC and MDMA	A sub-threshold dose of THC produced CPP in mice when combined with a non-rewarding dose of MDMA, but decreased the CPP induced by an effective dose of MDMA
Daza-Losada et al., 2008a	MDMA and cocaine binge during adolescence	mice	adolescent	Striatal monoamine levels	MDMA and cocaine	MDMA-induced long-lasting decreases in the concentration of striatal DA at high doses, but cocaine inhibited this effect
Daza-Losada et al., 2008b	MDMA binge during adolescence	mice	adolescent	Morphine-induced CPP	MDMA and morphine	Sensitivity to reinstatement of an extinguished preference was increased in morphine-induced CPP
Estelles et al., 2006	Prenatal cocaine administration	mice	adult	Morphine-induced CPP	Cocaine and morphine	Prenatal treatment with cocaine decreased the rewarding actions of morphine in adult offspring
Achat-Mendes et al., 2003	MDMA binge during adolescence	mice	adolescent	Cocaine-induced CPP	Cocaine and MDMA	A priming injection of cocaine after extinction reinstated a significantly higher CPP in mice previously exposed to MDMA during adolescence
Daza-Losada et al., 2009b	MDMA and cocaine binge during adolescence	mice	adolescent	MDMA- induced CPP	Cocaine and MDMA	Only mice previously exposed to MDMA developed CPP after conditioning with a sub-threshold dose of MDMA. The extinguished preference was reinstated only in animals exposed to MDMA or cocaine during adolescence
Jones et al (2010)	acute treatment	rats	adult	MDMA- and EtOH-induced CPP	MDMA and EtOH	CPP was detected in rats that had received MDMA plus ethanol but not in those that had been administered just one of the drugs
Rodriguez-Arias et al., 2011	MDMA and EtOH binge during adolescence	mice	adolescent	Anxiety (EPM) and striatal monoamine levels	MDMA and EtOH	An increase was observed in the anxiogenic response induced by MDMA in adult mice treated with MDMA plus EtOH. EtOH increased the neurotoxic effect of MDMA
Ribeiro do Couto et al., 2011a, 2011b	MDMA and EtOH binge during adolescence	mice	adolescent	MDMA-induced CPP	MDMA and EtOH	Pre-exposure to EtOH, MDMA or both drugs increased the rewarding effects of an ineffective dose of MDMA. Reinstatement of the extinguished preference was achieved with lower priming doses of MDMA in the groups pre-exposed to ethanol or MDMA

Table 1. Synthesis of the most relevant interactions observed in the different models explained within the text.

7. Conclusion

In conclusion, the risks associated with multi-drug exposure during adolescence are still unclear. The high frequency of the combined used of several drugs in human adolescent users demands an in-depth evaluation of their interaction. It is obvious that the developing brain is highly vulnerable to the damaging effects of drugs; effects that can be irreversible. Studies performed to date demonstrate that the combined use of drugs produces a specific neurochemical and behavioural profile which differs to that observed when each drug is administered alone. These kinds of studies are more complicated to perform than those employing only one drug and involve many more variables that need to be controlled. Nevertheless, despite their complexity and the limitations inherent in their design, each of these studies constitutes a piece of a giant jigsaw puzzle which, as it is gradually put together, provides an increasingly clearer image of the reality of drug use.

8. Acknowledgement

This work was supported by the following grants: Ministerio de Economia y Competitividad. Dirección General de Investigación (PSI2011-24762), Instituto de Salud "Carlos III" (FIS), RETICS, Red de Trastornos Adictivos (RD06/001/0016) and Generalitat Valenciana, Conselleria de Educación (PROMETEO/2009/072), Spain.

9. References

2010 Monitoring the Future (MTF) NIDA. National Institutes of Health. US Department of Health & Human Services.
       http://drugabuse.gov/drugpages/MTF.html
2010 Annual report on the state of the drugs problem in Europe. EMCDDA, Lisbon, November 2009.
       http://www.emcdda.europa.eu/attachements.cfm/att_93236_EN_EMCDDA_AR2 009_EN.pdf
Abbott, A. (2005). Physiology: an end to adolescence. Nature, Vol.433, No.7021, (January, 2005), p. 27, ISSN 0028-0836
Åberg, M.; Wade, D.; Wall, E. & Izenwasser, S. (2007). Effect of MDMA (ecstasy) on activity and cocaine conditioned place preference in adult and adolescent rats. Neurotoxicology and Teratology, Vol.29, No.1, (January-February, 2007), pp. 37–46, ISSN 0892-0362
Achat-Mendes, C.; Anderson, K.L. & Itzhak, Y. (2003). Methylphenidate and MDMA adolescent exposure in mice: long-lasting consequences on cocaine-induced reward and psychomotor stimulation in adulthood. Neuropharmacology, Vol.45, No.1, (July, 2003), pp. 106–115, ISSN 0028-3908
Adriani, W. & Laviola, G. (2003). Elevated levels of impulsivity and reduced place conditioning with d-amphetamine: two behavioral features of adolescence in mice. Behavioral Neuroscience, Vol.117, No.4, (August, 2003), pp.695–703, ISSN 0735-7044
Aggarwal, S.K.; Carter, G.T.; Sullivan, M.D.; ZumBrunnen, C.; Morrill, R. & Mayer, J.D. (2009). Medicinal use of cannabis in the United States: historical perspectives, current trends, and future directions. Journal of Opioid Management, Vol.5, No.3, (May-June, 2009), pp. 153-168. ISSN 1551-7489
Aguilar, M.A.; Rodríguez-Arias, M. & Miñarro, J. (2009). Neurobiological mechanisms of the reinstatement of drug-conditioned place preference. Brain Research Reviews, Vol.59, No.2, (March, 2009), pp. 253-277, ISSN 0165-017
Ahmed, S.H. (2010). Validation crisis in animal models of drug addiction: Beyond non-disordered drug use toward drug addiction. Neuroscience and Biobehavioral Reviews, Vol. 35, No.2, (November, 2010), pp. 172–184, ISSN 0149-7634
Allen, M.T. & Matthews, K.A. (1997). Hemodynamic responses to laboratory stressors in children and adolescents: the influences of age, race, and gender. Psychophysiology, Vol.34, No.3, (May, 1997), pp. 329-339, ISSN 0048-5772
Andersen, S.L. & Gazzara, R.A. (1993). The ontogeny of apomorphine-induced alterations of neostriatal dopamine release: effects on spontaneous release. Journal of Neurochemistry, Vol.61, No.6, (December, 1993), pp. 2247-2255, ISSN 0022-3042

Asato, M.R.; Terwilliger, R.; Woo, J. & Luna, B. (2010). White matter development in adolescence: a DTI study. Cerebral Cortex, Vol.20, No.9, (September, 2010), pp. 2122-2131, ISSN 1047-3211

Badanich, K.A.; Adler, K.J. & Kirstein, C.L. (2006). Adolescents differ from adults in cocaine conditioned place preference and cocaine-induced dopamine in the nucleus accumbens septi. European Journal of Pharmacology, Vol.550, No.1-3, (November, 2006), pp. 95-106, ISSN 0014-2999

Balogh, B.; Molnar, E.; Jakus, R.; Quate, L.; Olverman, H.J.; Kelly, P.A.; Kantor, S. & Bagdy, G. (2004). Effects of a single dose of 3,4-methylenedioxymethamphetamine on circadian patterns, motor activity and sleep in drug-naive rats and rats previously exposed to MDMA. Psychopharmacology, Vol. 173, No.3-4, (May, 2004), pp. 296–309, ISSN 0033-3158

Barrett, S.P.; Darredeau, C. & Pihl, R.O. (2006). Patterns of simultaneous polysubstance use in drug using university students. Human Psychopharmacology, Vol.21, No.4, (June, 2006), pp. 255–63. ISSN 0885-6222

Barrot, M.; Olivier, J.D.; Perrotti, L.I.; DiLeone, R.J.; Berton, O.; Eisch, A.J.; Impey, S.; Storm, D.R.; Neve, R.L.; Yin, J.C.; Zachariou, V. & Nestler, E.J. (2002). CREB activity in the nucleus accumbens shell controls gating of behavioral responses to emotional stimuli. Proceeding of the National Academy of Sciences USA, Vol.99, No.17, (August, 2002), pp. 11435–11440, ISSN 0027-8424

Baumrind, D. (1987). A developmental perspective on adolescent risk taking in contemporary America. In: Adolescent social behavior and health, Irwin Jr. CE, editor, pp. 93–125, Jossey-Bass, ISBN-10: 1555429394, San Francisco, CA.

Bauzo, R.M. & Bruijnzeel, A.W. (2012). Animal models of nicotine withdrawal: intracranial self-stimulation and somatic signs of withdrawal. Methods in Molecular Biology, Vol.829, No. 3, (2012), pp.257-268, ISSN 1064-3745

Baylen, C.A. & Rosenberg, H. (2006). A review of the acute subjective effects of MDMA/ecstasy, Addiction, Vol.101, No.7, (July, 2006) 933–947, ISSN 0965-2140

Belin, D., Besson, M., Bari, A., & Dalley, J. (2009). Multi-disciplinary investigations of impulsivity in animal models of attention-deficit hyperactivity disorder and drug addiction vulnerability. In S. Granon (Ed.), Endophenotypes of Psychiatric and Neurodegenerative Disorders in Rodent Models. New York: Oxford University Press. ISBN: 8178954028

Belin, D., Economidou, D., Pelloux, Y., & Everitt, B. J. (2010). Habit Formation and Compulsion. In M. C. Olmstead (Ed.), Animal models of drug addiction. Humana Press. ISBN-13 9781607619338

Belin, D.; Berson, N.; Balad, E.; Piazza, P.V.; Deroche-Gamonet, V. (2011) High-novelty-preference rats are predisposed to compulsive cocaine self-administration. Neuropsychopharmacology, Vol. 36, No. 3 (February, 2011), pp. 569-579 , ISSN 0893-133X

Bjork, J.M.; Smith, A.R.; Chen, G. & Hommer, D.W. (2010). Adolescents, Adults and Rewards: Comparing Motivational Neurocircuitry Recruitment Using fMRI. PLoS ONE Vol.5, No.7, (July, 2010), pp. e11440, ISSN 1932-6203

Braida, D. & Sala, M. (2002). Role of the endocannabinoid system in MDMA intracerebral self-administration in rats. British Journal of Pharmacology, Vol.136, No.8, (August, 2002), pp. 1089-1092, ISSN 0007-1188

Brenhouse, H.C. & Andersen S.L. (2011). Developmental trajectories during adolescence in males and females: A cross-species understanding of underlying brain changes Neuroscience and Biobehavioral Reviews, Vol.35, No.8, (August, 2011), pp. 1687–1703, ISSN 0149-7634

Buchanan, C.M.; Eccles, J.S. & Becker, J.B. (1992). Are adolescents the victims of raging hormones: evidence for activational effects of hormones on moods and behavior at adolescence. Psychological Bulletin, Vol.111, No.1, (January, 1992), pp. 62–107, ISSN 0033-2909

Buwalda, B.; Geerdink, M.; Vidal, J. & Koolhaas, J.M. (2011). Social behavior and social stress in adolescence: A focus on animal models. Neuroscience and Biobehavioral Reviews, Vol.35, No.8, (August, 2011), pp. 1713–1721, ISSN 0149-7634

Carlezon, W.A. Jr.; Thome, J.; Olson, V.G.; Lane-Ladd, S.B.; Brodkin, E.S.; Hiroi, N.; Duman, R.S.; Neve, R.L. & Nestler, E.J. (1998). Regulation of cocaine reward by CREB. Science, Vol.282, No.5397, (December, 1998), pp. 2272–2275, ISSN 0036-8075

Casey, B.; Jones, R.M. & Somerville, L.H. (2011). Braking and Accelerating of the Adolescent Brain. Journal of Research on Adolescence, Vol.21, No.1, (March, 2011), pp. 21-33, ISSN 1532-7795

Cassel, J.C.; Ben Hamida, S. & Jones, B.C. (2007). Attenuation of MDMA-induced hyperthermia by ethanol in rats depends on ambient temperature. European Journal of Pharmacology, Vol.571, No.2-3, (October, 2007), pp. 152–155. ISSN 0014-2999

Cassel, J.C.; Jeltsch, H.; Koenig, J. & Jones, B.C. (2004). Locomotor and pyretic effects of MDMA ethanol associations in rats. Alcohol, Vol.34, No.2-3, (October-November, 2004), pp. 285–289. ISSN 0741-8329

Cassel, J.C.; Riegert, C.; Rutz, S.; Koenig, J.; Rothmaier, K.; Cosquer, B.; Lazarus, C.; Birthelmer, A.; Jeltsch, H.; Jones, B.C. & Jackisch, R. (2005). Ethanol, 3, 4-methylenedioxymethamphetamine (ecstasy) and their combination: long-term behavioral, neurochemical and neuropharmacological effects in the rat. Neuropsychopharmacology, Vol.30, No.10, (October, 2005), pp. 1870–1882, ISSN 0893-133X

Charmandari, E.; Kino, T.; Souvatzoglou, E. & Chrousos, G.P. (2003). Pediatric stress: hormonal mediators and human development. Hormones Research, Vol.59, No.4, (2003), pp. 161–179. ISSN 0301-0163

Clemens, K.J.; Cornish, J.L.; Hunt, G.E. & McGregor, I.S. (2007). Repeated weekly exposure to MDMA, methamphetamine or their combination: long-term behavioural and neurochemical effects in rats. Drug & Alcohol Dependence, Vol.86, No.2-3, (January, 2007), pp. 183–190, ISSN 0376-8716

Colado, M.I.; O'Shea, E. & Green, A.R. (2004). Acute and long-term effects of MDMA on cerebral dopamine biochemistry and functions. Psychopharmacology, Vol.173, No.3-4, (May, 2004), pp. 249-263, ISSN 0033-3158

Colado, M.I.; Camarero, J.; Mechan, A.O.; Sanchez, V.; Esteban, B.; Elliott, J.M. & Green, A.R. (2001). A study of the mechanisms involved in the neurotoxic action of 3,4-methylenedioxymethamphetamine (MDMA, 'ecstasy') on dopamine neurones in mouse brain. British Journal of Pharmacology, Vol.134, No.8, (December, 2001), pp. 1711–1723, ISSN 1476-5381

Colado, M.I.; O'Shea, E. & Green, A.R. (2004). Acute and long-term effects of MDMA on cerebral dopamine biochemistry and function, Psychopharmacology, Vol.173, No.3-4, (May, 2004), pp. 249–263, ISSN 0033-3158

Cunningham, M.G.; Bhattacharyya, S. & Benes, F.M. (2002). Amygdalo-cortical sprouting continues into early adulthood: implications for the development of normal and abnormal function during adolescence. Journal of Comparative Neurology, Vol.453, No.2, (November, 2002), pp. 116-130, ISSN 0021-9967

Daumann, J.; Hensen, G.; Thimm, B.; Rezk, M.; Till, B. & Gouzoulis-Mayfrank, E. (2004). Self-reported psychopathological symptoms in recreational ecstasy (MDMA) users are mainly associated with regular cannabis use: further evidence from a combined cross-sectional/longitudinal investigation. Psychopharmacology, Vol.173, No.3-4, (May, 2004), pp. 398-404. ISSN 0033-3158

Daza-Losada, M.; Ribeiro Do Couto, B.; Manzanedo, C.; Aguilar, M.A.; Rodríguez-Arias, M. & Miñarro, J. (2007). Rewarding effects and reinstatement of MDMA-induced CPP in adolescent mice. Neuropsychopharmacology, Vol.32, No.8, (August, 2007), pp. 1750–1759. ISSN 0893-133X

Daza-Losada, M.; Rodríguez-Arias, M.; Maldonado, C.; Aguilar, M.A. & Miñarro, J. (2008a). Behavioural and neurotoxic long-lasting effects of MDMA plus cocaine in adolescent mice. European Journal of Pharmacology, Vol.590, No.1-3, (August, 2008), pp. 204-211. ISSN 0014-2999

Daza-Losada, M.; Rodríguez-Arias, M.; Aguilar, M.A. & Miñarro, J. (2008b). Effect of adolescent exposure to MDMA and cocaine on acquisition and reinstatement of morphine-induce CPP. Progress in Neuro-Psychopharmacology & Biological Psychiatry, Vol.32, No.3, (April, 2008), pp. 701–709, ISSN 0278-5846

Daza-Losada, M.; Rodríguez-Arias, M.; Maldonado, C.; Aguilar, M.A.; Guerri, C. & Miñarro, J. (2009a). Acute behavioural and neurotoxic effects of MDMA plus cocaine in adolescent mice. Neurotoxicology & Teratology, Vol.31, No.1, (January-February, 2009), pp. 49-59, ISSN 0892-0362

Daza-Losada, M.; Rodríguez-Arias, M.; Aguilar, M.A. & Miñarro, J. (2009b). Acquisition and reinstatement of MDMA-induced conditioned place preference in mice pre-treated with MDMA or cocaine during adolescence. Addiction Biology, Vol.14, No.4, (September, 2009), pp. 447-456. ISSN 1369-1600

de la Mora, M.P.; Gallegos-Cari, A.; Arizmendi-García, Y.; Marcellino, D.; Fuxe, K. (2010) Role of dopamine receptor mechanisms in the amygdaloid modulation of fear and anxiety: Structural and functional analysis. Proggress in Neurobiology Vol.90, No.2, (February, 2010), pp. 198-216. ISSN 0301-0082

De Luca, M.A.; Solinas, M.; Bimpisidis, Z.; Goldberg, S.R.; Di Chiara, G. (2012) Cannabinoid facilitation of behavioral and biochemical hedonic taste responses. Neuropharmacology, in press.

Deroche-Gamonet, V., Belin, D. & Piazza, P,V. (2004). Evidence for addiction-like behavior in the rat. Science, Vol. 305, No.5686, (August, 2004), pp. 1014-1017, ISSN 0036-8075

De Vries, T.J.; Schoffelmeer, A.N.; Binnekade, R.; Mulder, A.H. & Vanderschuren, L.J. (1998). Drug-induced reinstatement of heroin- and cocaine-seeking behaviour following long-term extinction is associated with expression of behavioural sensitization. European Journal of Neuroscience, Vol.10, No.11, (November, 1998), pp. 3565–71, ISSN 1460-9568

Di Giovanni, G., Esposito, E., Di Matteo, V. (2010) Role of serotonin in central dopamine dysfunction. CNS Neurosci Ther. Vol.16, No. 3, pp. 179-194, DOI: 10.1111/j.1755-5949.2010.00135.x

Diller, A.J.; Rocha, A.; Cardon, A.L.; Valles, R.; Wellman, P.J. & Nation, J.R. (2007). The effects of concurrent administration of +/−3,4-methylenedioxymethamphetamine and cocaine on conditioned place preference in the adult male rat. Pharmacology, Biochemistry & Behavior, Vol.88, No.2, (December, 2007), pp. 165–170, ISSN 0091-3057

Doremus-Fitzwater, T.L.; Elena I. Varlinskaya, E.I. & Spear, L.P. (2010). Motivational systems in adolescence: Possible implications for age differences in substance abuse and other risk-taking behaviors. Brain & Cognition, Vol.72, No.1 (February, 2010), pp. 114, ISSN 0278- 2626

Dumont, G.; Kramers, C.; Sweep, F.; Willemsen, J.; Touw, D.; Schoemaker, R.; van Gerven, J.; Buitelaar, J. & Verkes, R. (2010). Ethanol co-administration moderates 3,4-methylenedioxymethamphetamine effects on human physiology. Journal of Psychopharmacology, Vol.24, No.2, (February, 2010), pp. 165-174, ISSN 0269-8811

Eaton, D.K.; Kann, L.; Kinchen, S.; Shanklin, S.; Ross, J.; Hawkins, J.; Harris, W.A.; Lowry, R.; McManus, T.; Chyen, D.; Lim, C.; Whittle, L.; Brener, N.D. & Wechsler, H. (2010). Youth risk behavior surveillance - United States, 2009. Morbidity and Mortality Weekly Report (MMWR) Surveillance Summaries, Vol.59 No.5, (Jun, 2010), pp. 1-142, ISSN 1546-0738

Encuesta domiciliaria sobre alcohol y drogas en España (EDADES) 2009/2010. Delegación del gobierno para el plan nacional sobre drogas. Ministerio de sanidad, política social e igualdad.
http://www.pnsd.msc.es/Categoria2/observa/estudios/home.htm

Encuesta Estatal sobre Uso de Drogas en Estudiantes de Enseñanzas Secundarias (ESTUDES) (2008). Ministerio de Sanidad y Política Social, Delegación del Gobierno para el Plan Nacional sobre Drogas
http://www.pnsd.msc.es/Categoria2/observa/estudios/home.htm

Epstein, D.H.; Preston, K.L.; Stewart, J. & Shaham, Y. (2006). Toward a model of drug relapse: an assessment of the validity of the reinstatement procedure. Psychopharmacology, Vol.189, No.1, (November, 2006), pp. 1-16, ISSN 0033-3158

Erhardt, E.; Zibetti, L.C.; Godinho, J.M.; Bacchieri, B. & Barros, H.M. (2006). Behavioral changes induced by cocaine in mice are modified by a hyperlipidic diet or recombinant leptin. Brazilian Journal of Medical & Biological Research, Vol.39, No.12, (December, 2006), pp. 1625–1635, ISSN 0100-879X

Ernst, M.; Bolla, K.; Mouratidis, M.; Contoreggi, C.; Matochik, J.A.; Kurian, V.; Cadet, J.L.; Kimes, A.S. & London, E.D. (2002). Decision-making in a risk-taking task: a PET study. Neuropsychopharmacology, Vol.26, No.5, (May, 2002), pp. 682-691, ISSN 0893-133X

Ernst, M., Romeo R.D. & Andersen S.L. (2009). Neurobiology of the development of motivated behaviors in adolescence: A window into a neural systems model. Pharmacology, Biochemistry and Behavior, Vol.93, No.3, (September, 2009), pp. 199–211, ISSN 0091-3057

Estelles, J.; Rodriguez-Arias, M.; Maldonado, C.; Manzanedo, C.; Aguilar, M.A. & Minarro, J. (2006). Prenatal cocaine alters later responses to morphine in adult male mice.

Progress in Neuropsychopharmacology & Biological Psychiatry, Vol.30, No.6, (August, 2006), pp. 1073–1082, ISSN 0278-5846

Everitt, B.J.; Belin, D.; Economidou, D.; Pelloux, Y.; Dalley, J.W. & Robbins, T.W. (2008). Neural mechanisms underlying the vulnerability to develop compulsive drug-seeking habits and addiction. Philosophical Transactions of the Royal Society of London B Biological Sciences, Vol.363, No.1507, (October, 2008), pp.3125-35. ISSN 0080-4622

Faria, R.; Magalhaes, A.; Monteiro, P.R.; Gomes-Da-Silva, J.; Amelia Tavares, M. & Summavielle, T. (2006). MDMA in adolescent male rats: decreased serotonin in the amygdala and behavioral effects in the elevated plus-maze test. Annals of the New York Academy of Science, Vol.1074, (August, 2006), pp. 643–649, ISSN 0077-8923

Fisk, J.E.; Montgomery, C.; Wareing, M. & Murphy, P.N. (2006). The effects of concurrent cannabis use among ecstasy users: neuroprotective or neurotoxic? Human Psychopharmacology, Vol.21, No.6, (August, 2006), pp. 355-366, ISSN 0885-6222

Fletcher, P.J.; Robinson, S.R. & Slippoy, D.L. (2001). Pre-exposure to (+/-) 3,4-methylenedioxy-methamphetamine (MDMA) facilitates acquisition of intravenous cocaine self-administration in rats. Neuropsychopharmacology, Vol.25, No.2, (August, 2001), pp. 195–203, ISSN 0893-133X

Galici, R., Pechnick, R.N., Poland, R.E. & France, C.P. (2000). Comparison of noncontingent versus contingent cocaine administration on plasma corticosterone levels in rats. European Journal of Neuroscience, Vol.387, No.1, (January, 2000), pp. 59–62, ISSN 0953-816X

Galvan, A.; Hare, T.A.; Parra, C.E.; Penn, J.; Voss, H.; Glover, G. & Casey,B.J. (2006). Earlier development of the accumbens relative to orbitofrontal cortex might underlie risk-taking behavior in adolescents. Journal of Neuroscience, Vol.26, No.25, (June, 2006), pp. 6885–6892, ISSN 0270-6474

Gardner, E.L. & Vorel, S.R. (1998). Cannabinoid transmission and reward-related events. Neurobiology of Disease, Vol.5, No.6, (December, 1998), pp 502-533, ISSN 0969-9961

Gawin, F.H. (1991). Cocaine addiction: psychology and neurophysiology. Science, Vol.251, No.5001, (March, 1991), pp. 1580–1586, ISSN 0036-8075

Gerra, G.; Zaimovic, A.; Giucastro, G.; Maestri, D.; Monica, C.; Sartori, R.; Caccavari, R. & Delsignore, R. (1998). Serotonergic function after (+/−)3,4-methylene-dioxymethamphetamine ('Ecstasy') in humans. International Clinical Psychopharmacology, Vol.13, No.1, (January, 1998), pp. 1–9, ISSN 0271-0749

Gogtay, N.; Giedd, J.N.; Lusk, L.; Hayashi, K.M.; Greenstein, D.; Vaituzis, A.C.; Nugent 3rd, T.F.; Herman, D.H.; Clasen, L.S.; Toga, A.W.; Rapoport, J.L. & Thompson, P.M. (2004). Dynamic mapping of human cortical development during childhood through early adulthood. Proceedings of the National Academy of Sciences of the United States of America, Vol. 101, No.21, (May, 2004), pp.8174–8179, ISSN 0027-8424

Hall, B.J.; Pearson, L.S. & Buccafusco, J.J. (2010). Effect of the use-dependent, nicotinic receptor antagonist BTMPS in the forced swim test and elevated plus maze after cocaine discontinuation in rats. Neuroscience Letters, Vol.474 No.2, (April, 2010) pp. 84-87, ISSN 0304-3940

Hamida, S.B.; Plute, E.; Bach, S.; Lazarus, C.; Tracqui, A.; Kelche, C.; de Vasconcelos, A.P.; Jones, B.C. & Cassel, J.C. (2007). Ethanol-MDMA interactions in rats: the importance of interval between repeated treatments in biobehavioral tolerance and sensitization to the combination. Psychopharmacology, Vol.192, No.4, (July, 2007), pp. 555–569, ISSN 0033-3158

Hamida, S.B.; Plute, E.; Cosquer, B.; Kelche, C.; Jones, B.C. & Cassel, J.C. (2008). Interactions between ethanol and cocaine, amphetamine, or MDMA in the rat: thermoregulatory and locomotor effects. Psychopharmacology, Vol.197, No.1, (March, 2008), pp. 67–82, ISSN 0033-3158

Hamida, S.B.; Tracqui, A.; de Vasconcelos, A.P.; Szwarc, E.; Lazarus, C.; Kelche, C.; Jones, B.C. & Cassel, J.C. (2009). Ethanol increases the distribution of MDMA to the rat brain: possible implications in the ethanol-induced potentiation of the psychostimulant effects of MDMA. International Journal of Neuropsychopharmacology, Vol.12, No.6, (July, 2009), pp. 749–759, ISSN 1461-1457

Han, D.D. & Gu, H.H. (2006). Comparison of the monoamine transporters from human and mouse in their sensitivities to psychostimulant drugs. BMC Pharmacology, Vol.3, No.6, p. 6, ISSN 1471-2210

Hermann, H.; Marsicano, G. & Lutz, B. (2002). Coexpression of the cannabinoid receptor type 1 with dopamine and serotonin receptors in distinct neuronal subpopulations of the adult mouse forebrain. Neuroscience, Vol.109, No.3, (February, 2002), pp. 451-480, ISSN 0306-4522

Hernández-López, C.; Farré, M.; Roset, P.N.; Menoyo, E.; Pizarro, N.; Ortuño, J.; Torrens, M.; Camí, J. & de La Torre, R. 3, 4-Methylenedioxymethamphetamine (ecstasy) and alcohol interactions in humans: psychomotor performance, subjective effects, and pharmacokinetics. Journal of Pharmacology & Experimental Therapeutics, Vol.300, No.1, (January, 2002), pp. 236–44, ISSN 0022-3565

Heyser, C.J.; Chen, W.J.; Miller, J.; Spear, N.E. & Spear, L.P. (1990). Prenatal cocaine exposure induces deficits in Pavlovian conditioning and sensory preconditioning among infant rat pups. Behavioral Neuroscience, Vol.104, No.6, (December, 1990), pp. 955–963, ISSN 0735-7044

Hodos, W. (1961). Progressive ratio as a measure of reward strength. Science, Vol.134, No.3483, (September, 1961), pp. 943-944, ISSN 0036-8075

Horan, B.; Gardner, E.L. & Ashby, C.R. (2000). Enhancement of conditioned place preference response to cocaine in rats following subchronic administration of 3,4-methylenedioxymethamphetamine (MDMA). Synapse, Vol.35, No.2, (February, 2000), pp. 160–162, ISSN 0887-4476

Inman-Wood, S.L.; Williams, M.T.; Morford, L.L. & Vorhees, C.V. (2000). Effects of prenatal cocaine on Morris and Barnes maze tests of spatial learning and memory in the offspring of C57BL/6J mice. Neurotoxicology & Teratology, Vol.22, No.4, (July-August, 2000), pp. 547–557, ISSN 0892-0362

Insel, T.R.; Miller, L.P. & Gelhard, R.E. (1990). The ontogeny of excitatory amino acid receptors in rat forebrain: I. N-methyl-d-aspartate and quisqualate receptors. Neuroscience, Vol.35, No.1, pp. 31–43, ISNN 0306-4522

Itzhak, Y. & Martin, J.L. (2002). Effect of the neuronal nitric oxide synthase inhibitor 7-nitroindazole on methylphenidate-induced hyperlocomotion in mice. Behavioural Pharmacology, Vol.13, No.1, (February, 2002), pp. 81-86, ISSN 0091-3057

Itzhak, Y. & Ali, S.F. (2006). Role of nitrergic system in behavioral and neurotoxic effects of amphetamine analogs. Pharmacology & Therapeutics, Vol.109, No.1-2, (January, 2006), pp. 246–262, ISSN 0163-7258

Izco, M.; Marchant, I.; Escobedo, I.; Peraile, I.; Delgado, M.; Higuera-Matas, A.; Olias, O.; Ambrosio, E.; O'Shea, E. & Colado, M.I. (2007). Mice with decreased cerebral dopamine function following a neurotoxic dose ofMDMA (3, 4-methylenedioxymethamphetamine, "Ecstasy") exhibit increased ethanol consumption and preference. Journal of Pharmacology & Experimental Therapeutics, Vol. 322, No.3, (September, 2007), pp. 1003–1012, ISSN 0022-3565

Jain, R. & Balhara, Y.P. (2010). Impact of alcohol and substance abuse on adolescent brain: a preclinical perspective. Indian Journal of Physiology & Pharmacology, Vol.54, No.3, pp. 213-234, ISSN 0019-5499

Johnson, E.A.; O'Callaghan, J.P. & Miller, D.B. (2004). Brain concentrations of d-MDMA are increased after stress. Psychopharmacology, Vol.173, No.3-4, (May, 2004), pp. 278–286, ISSN 0033-3158

Jones, B.C.; Ben-Hamida, S.; de Vasconcelos, A.P.; Kelche, C.; Lazarus, C.; Jackisch, R. & Cassel, J.C. (2010). Effects of ethanol and ecstasy on conditioned place preference in the rat. Journal of Psychopharmacology, Vol.24, No.2, (February, 2010), pp. 275–279, ISSN 0269-8811

Knackstedt, L.A. & Kalivas, P.W. (2007). Extended access to cocaine self-administration enhances drug-primed reinstatement but not behavioral sensitization. Journal of Pharmacology and Experimental Therapeutics, Vol.322, No.3, (September, 2007), pp. 1103-1109. ISSN 0022-3565

Laviola, G., Adriani, W.; Terranova, M.L. & Gerra, G. (1999). Psychobiological risk factors for vulnerability to psychostimulants in human adolescents and animal models. Neuroscience & Biobehavioral Reviews, Vol.23, No.7, (November, 1999), pp. 993–1010, ISSN 0149-7634

Laviola, G.; Wood, R.D.; Kuhn, C. & Francis, R.L.P. (1995). Cocaine sensitization in periadolescent and adult rats. Journal of Pharmacology & Experimental Therapeutics, Vol.275, No.1, (October, 1995), pp. 345–357, ISSN 0022-3565

Laviola, G.; Pascucci, T. & Pieretti, S. (2001). Striatal dopamine sensitization to d-amphetamine in periadolescent but not in adult rats. Pharmacology, Biochemistry & Behavior, Vol.68, No.1, (January, 2001), pp. 115–124, ISSN 0091-3057

Lidow, M.S.; Goldman-Rakic, P.S. & Rakic, P. (1991). Synchronized overproduction of neurotransmitter receptors in diverse regions of the primate cerebral cortex. Proceedings of the National Academy of Sciences of USA, Vol.88, No.22, (November, 1991), pp. 10218–10221, ISSN 0027-8424

Luna, B.; Padmanabhan, A. & O'Hearn K. (2010) What has fMRI told us about the Development of Cognitive Control through Adolescence? Brain & Cognition, Vol. 72, No.1, (February, 2010), pp.101, ISSN 0278-2626

Lynskey, M.T.; Heath, A.C.; Bucholz, K.K.; Slutske, W.S.; Madden, P.A.; Nelson, E.C.; Statham, D.J. & Martin, N.G. (2003). Escalation of drug use in early-onset cannabis users vs co-twin controls. Journal of the American Medical Association, Vol.289, No.4, (January, 2003), pp. 427-433, ISSN 0098-7484

Maldonado, R.; Valverde, O. & Berrendero, F. (2006). Involvement of the endocannabinoid system in drug addiction. Trends in Neurosciences, Vol.29, No.4, (April, 2006), pp. 225-232, ISSN 0166-2236

Manzanedo, C.; Aguilar, M.A.; Rodríguez-Arias, M.; Navarro, M. & Miñarro, J. (2004). Cannabinoid agonist-induced sensitisation to morphine place preference in mice. NeuroReport, Vol.15, No.8, (June, 2004), pp. 1373-1377, ISSN 0959-4965

Manzanedo, C.; Aguilar, M.A.; Rodriguez-Arias, M. & Minarro, J. (2005). Sensitization to the rewarding effects of morphine depends on dopamine. NeuroReport, Vol.16, No.2, (February, 2005), pp. 201–205, ISSN 0959-4965

Manzanedo, C.; Rodríguez-Arias, M.; Daza-Losada, M.; Maldonado, C.; Aguilar, M.A. & Miñarro, J. (2010). Effect of the CB1 cannabinoid agonist WIN 55212-2 on the acquisition and reinstatement of MDMA-induced conditioned place preference in mice. Behavioral & Brain Functions, Vol.6, (March, 2010), p. 19. ISSN 1744-9081

Merola, J.L. & Liederman, J. (1985). Developmental changes in hemispheric independence. Child Development, Vol.56, No.5, (October, 1985), pp. 1184–1194, ISSN 0009-3920

Mohamed, W.M.; Hamida, S.B.; de Vasconcelos, A.P.; Cassel, J.C. & Jones, B.C. (2009). Interactions between 3, 4-methylenedioxymethamphetamine and ethanol in humans and rodents. Neuropsychobiology, Vol.60, No.3-4, pp. 188–194, ISSN 0302-282X

Morley-Fletcher, S.; Bianchi, M.; Gerra, G. & Laviola, G. (2002). Acute and carryover effects in mice of MDMA ("ecstasy") administration during periadolescence. European Journal of Pharmacology, Vol.448, No.1, (July, 2002), pp. 31–38, ISSN 0014-2999

Moser, P.; Wolinsky, T.; Duxon, M. & Porsolt, R.D. (2011). How Good Are Current Approaches to Nonclinical Evaluation of Abuse and Dependence? Journal of Pharmacology & Experimental Therapeutics, Vol.336, No.3, (March, 2011), pp. 588–595, ISSN 0022-3565

Nakazi, M.; Bauer, U.; Nickel, T.; Kathmann, M. & Schlicker, E. (2000). Inhibition of serotonin release in the mouse brain via presynaptic cannabinoid CB1 receptors. Naunyn-Schmiedeberg´s Archives of Pharmacoogy, Vol.361, No.1, (January, 2000), pp. 19-24, ISSN 0028-1298

Navarro, J.F. & Maldonado, E. (2002). Acute and subchronic effects of MDMA ("ecstasy") on anxiety in male mice tested in the elevated plus-maze, Progress in Neuropsychopharmacology & Biological Psychiatry, Vol.26, No.6, (October, 2002), pp. 1151–1154, ISSN 0278-5846

Nestler, E.J. (2004). Historical review: Molecular and cellular mechanisms of opiate and cocaine addiction. Trends in Pharmacological Sciences, Vol.25, No.4, (April, 2004), pp. 210–218, ISSN 0165-6147

O'Shea, E.; Esteban, B.; Camarero, J.; Green, A.R. & Colado, M.I. (2001). Effect of GBR 12909 and fluoxetine on the acute and long term changes induced by MDMA ('ecstasy') on the 5-HT and dopamine concentrations in mouse brain. Neuropharmacology, Vol.40, No.1, pp. 65–74, ISSN 0028-3908

Pascual, M.; Blanco, A.M.; Cauli, O.; Miñarro, J. & Guerri, C. (2007). Intermittent ethanol exposure induces inflammatory brain damage and causes long-term behavioural alterations in adolescent rats. European Journal of Neuroscience, Vol.25, No.2, (January, 2007), pp. 541–550, ISSN 0953-816X

Paus, T.; Collins, D.L.; Evans, A.C.; Leonard, G.; Pike,B. & Zijdenbos,A. (2001). Maturation of white matter in the human brain: a review of magnetic resonance studies. Brain Research Bulletin, Vol.54, No.3, (February, 2001), pp. 255–266, ISSN 0361-9230

Pazos, M.R.; Sagredo, O. & Fernández-Ruiz, J. (2008). The endocannabinoid system in Huntington's disease. Current Pharmaceutical Design, Vol.14, No.23, pp. 2317-2325, ISSN 1381-6128

Piazza, P.V. & LeMoal, M. (1998). The role of stress in drug self administration. Trends in Pharmacological Sciences, Vol.19, No.2, (February, 1998), pp. 67–74, ISSN 0165-6147

Pickles, A.; Pickering, K.; Simonoff, E.; Silberg, J.; Meyer, J. & Maes, H. (1998). Genetic clocks and soft events: A twin model for pubertal development and other recalled sequences of developmental milestones, transitions, or ages at onset. Behavior Genetics, Vol.28, No.4, (July, 1998), pp. 243–253, ISSN 0001-8244

Piomelli, D. (2005). The endocannabinoid system: A drug discovery perspective. Current Opinion on Investigational Drugs, Vol.6, No.7, (July, 2005), pp. 672-679, ISSN 1472-4472

Pulvirenti, L., (2003). Glutamate neurotransmission in the course of cocaine addiction. In: Glutamate and Addiction, Herman, B.H. (Ed.), Humana Press, New Jersey, pp. 171–181 ISBN-10: 0896038793

Ribeiro Do Couto, B.; Aguilar, M.A.; Rodríguez-Arias, M. & Miñarro, J. (2005). Cross-reinstatement by cocaine and amphetamine of morphine-induced place preference in mice. Behavioral Pharmacology, Vol.16, No.4, (July, 2005), pp. 253-259, ISSN 0955-8810

Ribeiro Do Couto, B.; Aguilar, M.A.; Manzanedo, C.; Rodríguez-Arias, M.; Armario, A. & Miñarro, J. (1996). Social stress is as effective as physical stress in reinstating morphine-induced place preference in mice. Psychopharmacology, Vol.185, No.4, (May, 2006), pp. 459-470, ISSN 0033-3158

Ribeiro Do Couto, B.; Rodríguez-Arias, M.; Fuentes, S.; Gagliano, H.; Armario, A.; Miñarro, J. & Aguilar, MA. (2011). Adolescent pre-exposure to ethanol or MDMA prolongs the conditioned rewarding effects of MDMA. Physiology & Behavior, Vol.103, No.5, (July, 2011), pp.585-593, ISSN 0031-9384

Ribeiro Do Couto, B.; Daza-Losada, M.; Rodríguez-Arias, M.; Nadal, R.; Guerri, C.; Summavielle, T.; Miñarro, J. & Aguilar, M.A. (2011). Adolescent pre-exposure to ethanol and MDMA increases conditioned rewarding effects of MDMA and drug-induced reinstatement. Addiction Biology, in press, ISSN 1369-1600

Rice, D. & Barone, S. Jr. (2000). Critical periods of vulnerability for the developing nervous system: evidence from humans and animal models. Environment Health Perspectives, Vol.108, No.3, (June, 2000), pp. 511–533, ISSN 0091-6765

Riegert, C.; Wedekind, F.; Hamida, S.B.; Rutz, S.; Rothmaier, A.K.; Jones, B.C.; Cassel, J.C. & Jackisch, R. (2008). Effects of ethanol and 3, 4-methylenedioxymethamphetamine (MDMA) alone or in combination on spontaneous and evoked overflow of dopamine, serotonin and acetylcholine in striatal slices of the rat brain. International Journal of Neuropsychopharmacology, Vol.11, No.6, (September, 2008) pp. 743–763, ISSN 1461-1457

Riley, S.C.; James, C.; Gregory, D.; Dingle, H. & Cadger, M. (2001). Patterns of recreational drug use at dance events in Edinburgh, Scotland. Addiction, Vol.96, No.7, (July, 2001), pp. 1035–1047, ISSN 0965-2140

Rivers, S.E.; Reyna, V.F. & Mills, B. (2008). Risk taking under the influence: a fuzzy-trace theory of emotion in adolescence. Developmental Review, Vol.28, No.1, (March, 2008), pp. 107–144, ISSN 0273-2297

Robinson, T.E. & Berridge, K.C. (2008). Review. The incentive sensitization theory of addiction: some current issues. Philosophical Transactions of the Royal Society B: Biological Sciences, Vol.363, No.1507, (October, 2008), pp. 3137–3146, ISSN 0080-4622

Robledo, P.; Trigo, J.M.; Panayi, F.; de la Torre, R. & Maldonado, R. (2007). Behavioural and neurochemical effects of combined MDMA and THC administration in mice. Psychopharmacology, Vol.195, No.2, (December, 2007), pp. 255-264, ISSN 0033-3158

Rodríguez-Arias, M.; Manzanedo, C.; Roger-Sánchez, C.; Do Couto, B.R.; Aguilar, M.A. & Miñarro, J. (2010). Effect of adolescent exposure to WIN 55212-2 on the acquisition and reinstatement of MDMA-induced conditioned place preference. Progress in Neuropsychopharmacology & Biological Psychiatry, Vol.34, No.1, (February, 2010), pp. 166-171, ISSN 0278-5846

Rodríguez-Arias, M.; Maldonado, C.; Vidal-Infer, A.; Guerri, C.; Aguilar, M.A. & Miñarro, J. (2011). Intermittent ethanol exposure increases long-lasting behavioral and neurochemical effects of MDMA in adolescent mice. Psychopharmacology, May 10. DOI: 10.1007/s00213-011-2329-x, ISSN 0033-3158

Rodrıguez de Fonseca, F.; Ramos, J.A.; Bonnin, A. & Fernandez-Ruiz, J.J. (1993). Presence of cannabinoid binding sites in the brain from early postnatal ages. NeuroReport, Vol.4, No., (mes, 1993), pp. 135–138, ISSN 0959-4965

Romieu, P.; Meunier, J.; Garcia, D.; Zozime, N.; Martın-Fardon, R.; Bowen, W.D. & Maurice, T. (2004). The sigma1 ($\square$1) receptor activation is a key step for the reactivation of cocaine conditioned place preference by drug priming. Psychopharmacology, Vol.175, No.2, (September, 2004), pp. 154–162, ISSN 0033-3158

Rubovitch, V.; Gafni, M. & Sarne, Y. (2002). The cannabinoid agonist DALN positively modulates L-type voltage-dependent calcium channels in N18TG2 neuroblastoma cells. Molecular Brain Research, Vol.101, No.1-2, (May, 2002), pp. 93-102, ISSN 0169-328X

Sanchis-Segura, C. & Spanagel, R. (2006). Behavioural assessment of drug reinforcement and addictive features in rodents: an overview. Addiction Biology, Vol.11, No.1, (March, 2006), pp. 2-38, ISSN 1369-1600

Sarne, Y. & Keren, O. (2004). Are cannabinoid drugs neurotoxic or neuroprotective? Medical Hypotheses, Vol.63, No.2, pp. 187-192, ISSN 0306-9877

Schensul, J.J.; Convey, M. & Burkholder, G. (2005) Challenges in measuring concurrency, agency and intentionality in polydrug research. Addictive Behaviours, Vol.30, No.3, (March, 2005), pp. 571-574, ISSN 0306-4603

Schramm-Sapyta, N.L.; Walker, Q.D.; Caster, J.M.; Levin, E.D. & Kuhn, C.M. (2009). Are adolescents more vulnerable to drug addiction than adults? Evidence from animal models. Psychopharmacology, Vol.206, No.1, (September, 2009), pp. 1-21, ISSN 0033-3158

Seeman, P.; Bzowej, N.H.; Guan, H-C; Bergeron, C.; Becker, L.E.; Reynolds, G.P.; Bird, E.D.; Riederer, P.; Jellinger, K.; Watanabe, S. & Tourtellotte, W.W. (1987). Human brain dopamine receptors in children and aging adults. Synapse, Vol.1, No.5, pp. 399–404, ISSN 0887-4476

Segal, D.S. & Kuczenski, R. (1997). An escalating dose "binge" model of amphetamine psychosis: behavioral and neurochemical characteristics. Journal of Neuroscience, Vol.17, No.7, (April, 1997), pp. 2551–2566, ISSN -0270-6474

Shalev, U.; Grimm, J.W. & Shaham, Y (2002). Neurobiology of relapse to heroin and cocaine seeking: a review. Vol. Pharmacological Reviews, Vol.54, No.1, (March, 2002), pp. 1–42, ISSN 0031-6997

Shippenberg, T.S. & Heidbreder, C. (1995). Sensitization to the conditioned rewarding effects of cocaine: pharmacological and temporal characteristics. Journal of Pharmacology & Experimental Therapeutics, Vol.273, No.2, (May, 1995), pp. 808–815, ISSN 0022-3565

Shippenberg, T.S. & Koob (2002) Recent Advances in Animal Models of Drug Addiction, In: Neuropsychopharmacology: The Fifth Generation of Progress, Kenneth L. Davis, Dennis Charney, Joseph T. Coyle, and Charles Nemeroff (Eds), pp.1381-1397, American College of Neuropsychopharmacology, ISBN-10: 0781728371, Nashville, TN.

Shippenberg, T.S.; LeFevour, A. & Thompson, A.C. (1998). Sensitization to the conditioned rewarding effects of morphine and cocaine: differential effects of the kappa opioid receptor agonist U69593. European Journal of Pharmacology, Vol.345, No.1, (March, 1998), pp. 27–34, ISSN 0014-2999

Shippenberg, T.S.; Zapata, A.; Chefer, V.I. (2007) Dynorphin and the pathophysiology of drug addiction. Pharmacology and Therapeutics, Vol. 116, No. 2 (November, 2007) pp. 306-321, ISSN 0163-7258

Sowell, E.R.; Trauner, D.A.; Gamst, A. & Jernigan, T.L. (2002). Development of cortical and subcortical brain structures in childhood and adolescence: a structural MRI study. Developmental Medicine & Child Neurology, Vol.44, No.1, (January, 2002), pp. 4–16, ISSN 0012-1622

Spear, L.P. (2000). The adolescent brain and age-related behavioral manifestations. Neuroscience & Biobehavioral Reviews, Vol.24, No.4, (June, 2000), pp. 417-463, ISSN 0149-7634

Spear, L.P. (2011a). Rewards, aversions and affect in adolescence: Emerging convergences across laboratory animal and human data. In: Developmental Cognitive Neuroscience, Ron Dahl and Louk Vanderschuren (Eds), Vol. 1, No.4, pp.390-403. ISSN: 1878-9293.

Spear, L.P. (2011b). Adolescent neurobehavioral characteristics, alcohol sensitivities, and intake: Setting the stage for alcohol use disorders?. In: Child Development Perspectives, Vol.5, No.4, pp.231-238. ISSN 1750-8606.

Sprague, J.E. & Nichols, D.E. (2005). Neurotoxicity of MDMA (ecstasy): beyond metabolism. Trends in Pharmacological Sciences, Vol. 26, No.2, (February, 2005), pp. 59–60, ISSN 0165-6147

Steketee, J.D. & Kalivas, P.W. (2011). Drug Wanting: Behavioral Sensitization and Relapse to Drug-Seeking Behavior. Pharmacological Reviews, Vol.63, No.2, (June, 2011) pp. 348–365, ISSN 0031-6997

Stone, E.A. & Quartermain, D. (1998). Greater behavioral effects of stress in immature as compared to mature male mice. Physiology & Behavior, Vol.63, No.1, (December, 1998), pp. 143–145, ISSN 0031-9384

Sturman, D.A. & Moghaddam, B. (2011). The neurobiology of adolescence: Changes in brain architecture, functional dynamics, and behavioral tendencies. Neuroscience & Biobehavioral Reviews, Vol.35, No.8, (August, 2011), pp. 1704-1712, ISSN 0149-7634

Teicher, M.H.; Andersen, S.L. & Hostetter, J.C. Jr. (1995). Evidence for dopamine receptor pruning between adolescence and adulthood in striatum but not nucleus accumbens. Developmental Brain Research, Vol.89, No.2, (November, 1995), pp. 167–172, ISSN 0165-3806

Tzschentke, T.M. (1998). Measuring reward with the conditioned place preference paradigm: a comprehensive review of drug effects, recent progress and new issues. Progress in Neurobiology, Vol.56, No.6, (December, 1998), pp. 613–672, ISSN 0301-0082

Upreti, V.V.; Eddington, N.D.; Moon, K.H.; Song, B.J. & Lee, I.J. (2009). Drug interaction between ethanol and 3,4-methylenedioxymethamphetamine ("ecstasy"). Toxicology Letters, Vol.188, No.2, (July, 2009), pp. 167–172, ISSN 0378-4274

Vázquez, D.M. (1998). Stress and the developing limbic–hypothalamic– pituitary–adrenal axis. Psychoneuroendocrinology, Vol.23, No.7, (October, 1998), pp. 663–700, ISSN 0306-4530

Vigil, P.; Orellana, R.F.; Cortes, M.E.; Molina, C.T.; Switzer, B.E. & Klaus, H. (2011). Endocrine Modulation of the Adolescent Brain: A Review. Journal of Pediatric and Adolescent Gynecology, (April 20), doi:10.1016/j.jpag.2011.01.061 ISSN 1083-3188

von Sydow, K.; Lieb, R.; Pfister, H.; Hofler, M. & Wittchen, H.U. (2002). Use, abuse and dependence of ecstasy and related drugs in adolescents and young adults – a transient phenomenon? Results from a longitudinal community study. Drug & Alcohol Dependence, Vol.66, No.2, (April, 2002), pp. 147–159, ISSN 0376-8716

Wagner, E.F., Myers, M.G. & McIninch. J.L. (1999). Stress-coping and temptation-coping as predictors of adolescent substance use. Addictive Behaviors, Vol.24, No.6, (November-December, 1999), pp. 769-779, ISSN 0306-4603

Walters, C.L.; Kuo, Y.C. & Blendy, J.A. (2003). Differential distribution of CREB in the mesolimbic dopamine reward pathway. Journal of Neurochemistry, Vol.87, No.5, (December, 2003), pp. 1237–1244, ISSN 0022-3042

Wang, B.; Luo, F.; Zhang, W.T. & Han, J.S. (2000). Stress or drug priming induces reinstatement of extinguished conditioned place preference. NeuroReport, Vol.11, No.12, (August, 2000), pp. 2781–2784, ISSN 0959-4965

Weiss, F. (2010). Advances in Animal Models of Relapse for Addiction Research. In: Advances in the Neuroscience of Addiction. Kuhn CM, Koob GF, (Eds). CRC Press, Frontiers in Neuroscience. ISBN-10: 0849373913 Boca Raton (FL)

Wolfer, D.P. & Lipp, H-P. (1995). Evidence for physiological growth of hippocampal mossy fiber collaterals in the guinea pig during puberty and adulthood. Hippocampus, Vol.5, No.4, pp. 329–340, ISSN 1098-1063

Therapeutic Strategies –
Behavioural, Social and Analytical Approaches

Proposals for the Treatment of Users of Alcohol and Other Drugs: A Psychoanalytic Reading

Cynara Teixeira Ribeiro[1,2,3] and Andréa Hortélio Fernandes[4,5]
[1]Pontifícia Universidade Católica de São Paulo (PUC/SP)
[2]Universidade Federal da Bahia (UFBA)
[3]Universidade Federal Rural do Semi-Arido (UFERSA)
[4]Université de Paris VII
[5]Universidade Federal da Bahia
[4]France
[1,2,3,5]Brazil

1. Introduction

Currently, the harmful use of alcohol and other drugs is recognized as a serious public health problem in many countries (WHO, 2002). However, it has not always been so. The reason is because, for quite a long time, the prevention and treatment related to the use of psychoactive substances were neglected in the context of public health policies, and delegated to other institutions such as justice and public safety. This fact gave rise to initiatives of total character attention[1] and to therapeutic practices that aimed mainly at the abstention from psychoactive consumption. Hence, traditionally, the great majority of treatments offered to users of alcohol and other drugs was based on the abstinence proposal (Marlatt; Larimer & Witkiewitz, 2012).

Nevertheless, a worldwide discussion about the difficulties that alcohol and other drug addicts have to drastically stop consuming such substances identified the need for the development of other treatment models as an alternative to the abstinence proposal (Brasil, 2005; Paes, 2006). As a consequence, many countries all over the world adopted the approach of harm reduction as the official strategy for prevention, treatment and education of people who use psychoactive substances in a harmful way (Brasil, 2001).

Another existing perspective in the treatment of alcohol and other drug users is the psychoanalysis proposal (Director, 2005; Laxenaire, 2010; Loose, 2000; Valentine & Fraser, 2008). Its main specificity lies in recognizing the different ways in which the subject relates to the toxic substances and consequently, understanding that drug use is anchored in the subjective dimension. Besides, psychoanalysis points to the fact that certain types of relationship to drugs can provide a kind of paradoxical and deadly satisfaction, called

---

[1] The term "initiatives of total character attention" is a mention to the term "total institutions", coined by Erving Goffmann (1985/2001).

jouissance (enjoyment)[2] (Lacan, 1969/1992; Laxenaire, 2010; Melman, 2000; Olievenstein, 2002), which is articulated to the unconscious and the death drive.

Thus, taking into consideration the abstinence proposal, the damage reduction proposal and the psychoanalytic proposal, this chapter will discuss the particular features of each one of these treatment models. Besides, it will also analyze the controversial and convergent points that exist among them, paying special attention to the debate between psychoanalysis and harm reduction. Finally, the chapter will briefly consider how the treatments of drug users can be optimized, as the result of the 'approximation' between these proposals.

2. The treatment proposals of drug use

In order to start a discussion on the treatments offered to users of alcohol and other drugs, first it is necessary to emphasize the historical character of the phenomenon of psychoactive substance use. As several authors have pointed out, the human practice of drug consumption is universal and ancient. In fact, in nearly all civilizations and human societies, the consumption of drugs capable to promote changes in what are considered as the human beings' states of consciousness has been a resource of great social and subjective importance (Mcrae, 2001; Seibel & Toscano Jr., 2001; Carneiro, 2006).

Although this consumption was historically widespread, it is important to highlight that, until a certain moment in history, it was restricted to small groups and happened in connection to collective ceremonies and sacred rituals, according to socially shared norms and conventions, which gave a predominantly symbolic value to the use of these substances. For instance, some ancient people believed that the consumption of certain substances made it possible for the spiritual representatives of certain groups to incorporate supposedly supernatural powers. This association between psychoactive substances consumption and religion lasted for quite a long time, including the medieval period, when the use of drugs was condemned because it was considered a hedonistic and sinful behavior.

However, this conception was strongly challenged from the seventeenth century on, with the development of medical studies, when certain vegetal products that have psychoactive effect started to be valued as a source of energy, stamina, humor and temper balance. As examples, we can mention the opium, originated from the poppy, which was for a long time prescribed as a painkiller, antitussive and antidiarrheal medication, and the marijuana, prescribed as a general sedative, for the specific treatment of rheumatism, neurosis, insomnia, headaches, diarrhea, seizures and anorexia as well as in the therapy of tetanus and cholera (Carneiro, 2006).

Furthermore, with the isolation of the active principles of the psychoactive substances in the eighteenth century, trade was established and certain products started to be available to the general population. Simultaneously, there was the weakening of the socio-cultural regulation strategies for the use of these substances, as well as the rise of a number of social issues that contributed to the large dissemination of drugs consumption, both for therapeutic and recreational ends. This dissemination, in turn, revealed the capacity of these substances to cause physical and psychological dependence in some users.

---

[2] 'Jouissance' means 'pleasure' or 'enjoyment', but the terms in English lack the sexual connotation that the word has in French. Hence, in consonance with the majority of the English translations of Lacan's works, the original term was adopted in this text.

Thereafter, the phenomenon of drug use was regarded both as a social and health problem, leading many scholars to devote themselves to the systematic investigation of the several types of addiction originated from the consumption of psychoactive substances. Consequently, especially from the nineteenth century on, the use of drugs has become the object of study in the field of psychiatry and started to be considered a psychopathology, and as such, it needed to be treated (Conte, 2000). This was the context in which several treatments for drug dependence appeared, which, in a first moment, focused mainly on the detoxification and/or the isolation of drug users.

In a review of the existing treatments, it is noticeable that the field of drug addiction presents a great variety of offers. These offers can be classified as: medicamental treatments, with or without internment (especially through pharmacological interventions aimed at detoxification); non-medicamental treatments with internment (in therapeutic communities, recovery program farms, etc); non-medicamental treatments through the engagement in mutual help groups (such as Alcoholics Anonymous and Narcotics Anonymous, based on the Minnesota Method, also known as the Twelve-Step Model); cognitive-behavioral therapies (with emphasis on counseling techniques, motivational interviewing, relapse prevention and skill training); psychoanalysis (through individual and/or group psychotherapy care) and more recently, harm reduction (which provides services of drop-in, needle exchange, target delivery of healthcare, outreach and drug consumption rooms) (Stevens, Hallam & Trace, 2006).

According to Queiroz (2001), except for psychoanalysis and harm reduction, the other treatments are predominantely grounded in the principle of abstinence. Hence, as previously mentioned, in the scope of drug addiction treatments at least three different proposals can be identified: abstinence, harm reduction and psychoanalysis.

3. The proposal of treatments that aim at abstinence

Considering that drug abuse treatments appeared mainly due to the recognition of drug addiction as a psychopathology by the psychiatry field, it is not difficult to understand why these treatments have been developed based on assumptions originated from psychiatry. Being a branch of medicine, initially psychiatry incorporated the hegemonic biomedical model and its strong emphasis on the organic and biological aspects of both physical and mental diseases (Pratta & Santos, 2009; Rothshild, 2010). Thus, due to the strong influence of the biomedical model on the psychiatry field, especially during the nineteenth and twentieth century, in many countries the treatments for drug use were led to adopt the same logic implemented in the therapies of other psychopathologies.

Therefore, traditionally, these treatments had as their main feature the hospitalocentric model, with predominantly pharmacological therapies aiming at healing, which in general, in the case of psychoactive substance users, was considered equivalent to the abstention of drug use (Faria & Schneider, 2009; Rothschild, 2010; Valentine & Fraser, 2008). Although this fact was more evident in some countries, such as the USA, who have lived under the aegis of a real 'war on drugs', in a way it did have, and still has, effects upon how certain organizations around the world deal with the drug addiction phenomenon[3] (Marlatt,

---

[3] An example of the influence of the prohibitionist concept on worldwide agencies were the three International Conventions organized by the UN Commission of Narcotic Drugs, that aimed at

Larimer & Witkiewitz, 2012). The concept underlying this type of this viewpoint about drug use was that drug addiction would be a neurochemical dysfunction caused by the use of drugs (Freda, 1989/1993; Khantzian, 1995; Olievenstein, 2002).

In the mid-nineteenth century, a moral model of religious or spiritualist origin was added to this classic psychiatric view of psychopathology and treatment (Marlatt & Witkiewitz, 2010). This model proposed that drug use was the result of character deviation, and rehabilitation, correlated to abstinence, was of divine nature (Faria & Schneider, 2009; Stevens, Hallam & Trace, 2006). This moral model is still adopted by some therapeutic communities and by a great part of the self-help groups, which propose that chemical dependence is an incurable physical, mental and spiritual disease.

In fact, according to Bastos (2009), there are still remaining practices of these ideas of morality in current treatment for drug users. Such practices determine that drug use treatments inserted into this logic take the strand of reward and punishment, to mould the drug users' behavior into the one desired by the public health service, that usually is the abstinent behavior. This way, it is noticeable that both treatments, the one originated from the classic psychiatry and the one originated from the moral model, have as their common objective to make the user abandon the use of drugs and reach the goal of abstinence.

In this sense, one may say that abstinence consists of a treatment proposal that is influenced by these two models, in that both establish the total abstention of consumption as the easiest way to avoid drug users to lose control in face of psychoactive substances. As a consequence, many countries that adopt abstinence based treatments (for examples, USA, Japan, Singapore, Malaysia, and others) favoring the therapeutic models based on the isolation of users (Alves, 2009; Pratta & Santos, 2009). It is worth mentioning that this preference for treatments with internment reveals the influence of the asylum model in mental health, which has been sharply questioned by the anti-psychiatry movement[4] (Marchant, 2010).

Among other reasons, this preference comes from the belief that inpatient care allows for better surveillance and control of the users, which would assure the abstention of drug consumption, at least while under treatment. However, one of the main criticisms to treatments in closed institutions lies in the fact that the patient's isolation from society creates an artificial environment which characteristics cannot be reproduced outside the institution's walls. Hence, once the treatment ends, the patient's reintegration to the family and social environment tends to be disturbing, favoring the occurrence of numerous relapses (Alves, 2009; Brasil, 2005; Marlatt; Larimer & Witkiewitz, 2012; Rothschild, 2010).

This idea of making users' access to psychoactive substances difficult is justified by the basic assumption that grounds the abstinence treatment proposal, which is that the drug makes the drug addict (Freda, 1989/1993). According to this viewpoint, drugs are seen as having a

---

implementing a common program to combat drugs in all its member states (Alves, 2009). In 1998, this same Organization devised an action plan, ratified in 2003, whose title was "A drug free world: We can do it," establishing the year 2008 as the deadline to reach this goal in several countries.

[4] It is important to emphasize that, in some countries such as France and Switzerland, due to the influence of psychoanalysis, historically the psychiatric treatments were not so subordinated to the biomedical model. However, a steady increase of an organicist perspective in mental health has been perceived lately, even in these countries (Decker, 2008).

supposedly intrinsic power of getting subjects addicted to them. Thus, the idea conveyed is that anyone who uses drugs will compulsorily become, sooner or later, a drug addict. This is considered especially true in regard to those drugs viewed as more powerful, such as cocaine, heroin and crack. But in a way, this is a belief that is extended to the remaining psychoactive substances – mainly in cases in which the consumption of these drugs goes beyond the socially established standards. However, this viewpoint ends up favoring the pharmacological aspect of drugs, and ignoring the individual, subjective, social and cultural aspects implied by the phenomenon of drug abuse and addiction.

Thus, in the perspective of treatments that aim uniquely and exclusively at abstinence, drug abuse is generally considered as a problem that concerns the disease, not the subject (Dufour, 2004; Olievenstein, 2002; Passos & Souza, 2011). By doing this, it is not taken into consideration the possibility that the use of drugs represents a way the subject found to deal with his/her conflicts and with the pain of existing, that is, the discontent that, in some measure, affects all human begins (Freud, 1930/1996)[5].

Therefore, in the abstinence proposal, it is assumed that the only means to prevent or treat drug addiction would be the non-use of drugs. This is one of the reasons why many drug addicts that are treated by the abstinence proposal say that they are permanently in recovery, regardless how long ago the last drug use was, and affirm that they are 'clean just for today'. The explanation for this type of discourse is based on the fact that relapses are seen as a great threat in the horizon of those who undergo this model of treatment. And since relapses are considered the total treatment failure, abstinence is thus placed as the objective to be pursued daily and for the whole life.

This conception favors the idea that once a drug addict, forever a drug addict. As a consequence, the abstinence proposal ends up promoting an imaginary collage of drug users to the signifiers 'addict', 'toxicomaniac', 'sick', etc. In turn, this collage makes it difficult for the user to get out of the subjective position of dependence on psychoactive substances. This is because the former user who structures his/her life around the abstinence from drugs continues to delegate to the drug a central role in his/her life, and to live under the aegis of an imperative: it is as if he/she had simply replaced the statement "I have to consume" for "I have to *not* consume", thus remaining in the same subjective position of being subjected to toxic substances. In this case, the patient, whether using drugs or not, continues to use the resource to the toxic as a subterfuge to avoid confronting his/her psychic issues, so that his/her submission to the external imperative of abstinence ends up exempting him/her from the need to make his/her own choices and be responsible for them (Rothschild, 2010).

Another criticism to drug treatments that aim exclusively at abstinence is the fact that they don't generally consider the different modalities of drug use and consequently, the fact that

---

[5] The concept that drug use is tied to a subjective need of the user was strongly advocated by Khantzian (1995), who, from the perspective of ego psychology, proposed that the intoxication practices were a type of self-medication which the subject used in an attempt to better deal with his torments. However, the association between the use of certain substances and the existence of specific psychological problems, proposed by this author, did not resist empirical tests and clinical experience. On the other hand, the hypothesis of self-medication ended up contributing to the spread of the adoption of the psychoanalytical approach in the treatment of drug users, which will be explained in more detail in following sessions.

not every drug user becomes what is considered a drug addict. This view ignores that most users of drugs do so for recreational or occasional purposes, but never come to a dependency relationship with them (Araújo, 2007; Nery Filho & Torres, 2002; Rezende, 2000; Stevens, Hallam & Trace, 2006)[6].

Nevertheless, the differences among the types of drug consumption are acknowledged in several fields of knowledge. In this respect, the UNESCO, for example, distinguishes four types of drug users: the experimenter, who tries one or several types of drugs, but limits this contact to the first experience; the occasional user, who occasionally uses one or several drugs, but is not a drug dependent; the habitual user, that frequently uses drugs, but still functions socially; and the dependent user (also called a drug addict or toxicomaniac), who lives by and for the drugs, and has his/her social bonds severely hampered or even broken by them (Rezende, 2000). Hence, the definition of drug addiction does not include the modalities of drug use in which the subject, although he/she uses the drug, does not place it at the center and as a destructive element in his/her life, and manages to preserve the social ties.

As a result of the various criticisms to the abstinence proposal, many authors have considered that, given the impossibility or great difficulty to maintain abstinence and eradicate drugs, the most interesting posture to be adopted is to try to manage the effects of drug use and minimize the damage caused by it, as proposed by the harm reduction strategy (Rezende, 1999; Queiroz, 2001; Pratta & Santos, 2009). And in fact, although the zero-tolerance policy to drug use still prevails in some countries, many other, especially in the European Union, adopt the harm reduction approach in the prevention and treatment of drug addiction as well as in the problem arising from it (Marlatt & Witkiewitz, 2010; OEDT, 2011).

4. The proposal of the harm reduction strategy

Harm reduction[7] is currently defined as a public health strategy that targets at reducing the damage caused to the individuals' health and controlling the possible adverse consequences that result from the adoption of risk practices (Marlatt; Larimer & Witkiewitz, 2012). In the specific context of alcohol and other drugs, harm reduction implies a set of interventions with the purpose of preventing the negative consequences of the consumption of psychoactive substances, without the requirement of immediate and automatic abstinence.

Among these interventions, it is worth of notice the distribution of syringes, needles and pipes, the presentation of educational lectures and the referral of users that are outside the health services to specialized institutions. Besides, the harm reduction approach is also dedicated to teach the patient the supposedly most efficient way to deal with the variety of risk factors that lead to the abuse of psychoactive substances, in order to help the patient to reach the goal he/she established for him/her, be it the total abstinence or moderate consumption. Hence, harm reduction presents an alternative perspective to treatments based on the abstinence logic, when it considers possible to prevent the negative effects of drug addiction without its compulsory interruption.

---

[6] According to the report published by the UM in 2007, approximately 200 million people use drugs worldwide, and only one-eighth of these have dependence problems. The remaining are occasional users (Araújo, 2007).

[7] In some places, the term harm reduction is replaced by risk reduction, and these two terms are often used as synonymous, although they are not.

The harm reduction approach, as a general guideline for action, was originated in England in 1926, through the development of the Rolleston Report (Stevens, Hallam & Trace, 2006). A ministerial committee chaired by the UK Ministry of Health established that the most adequate treatment for certain patients would be the maintenance of the use of certain substances, thereby regulating the right of British doctors to prescribe opiates to addicts of this type of drug. In the same Report, it was established that the criterion adopted for this prescription should be the need, after several failed attempts at abstinence, to manage the syndrome caused by the abstention of certain substances, besides the observation that the patient would not be able to lead a normal and productive life without a minimal dose of the drug administered regularly (Brasil, 2001).

This procedure was known as substitution treatment, and until today is one of the harm reduction strategies used (Marlatt & Witkiewitz, 2010; Stevens, Hallam & Trace, 2006). It consists of changing the substance which the user is dependent on for another substance that will offer lower risk. The most common strategy is the substitution of heroin by methadone, a synthetic opioid agonist with long half-life, which is consumed orally, helps to relieve some of the heroin withdrawal symptoms, causes less organic and psychological damage and is considered a substance with lower addictive power. Although this model of treatment appeared in a context different from the current, it is still in use in several countries such as England, Holland, Croatia and Norway, among others, especially in the European Union (Alves, 2009; OEDT, 2011).

Thus, the initial objectives of the harm reduction approach were to make it possible for users who were psychoactive dependents to lead a more stable and useful life, and to minimize the harmful health effects of drug use. However, after the 1980's, with the spread of the HIV/AIDS virus due to the large contamination originated from the sharing of needles, the harm reduction strategies also aimed at preventing this contamination among the users of injectable drugs.

As a consequence, due to some positive results obtained in the prevention of contamination in several countries such as Belgium, Australia, Germany, Switzerland, France and others (Brasil, 2001; Paes, 2006), many harm reduction programs appeared as public health strategies. Brazil was one of the countries that has most recently adopted this approach, when in 1994 the harm reduction model was embraced as the official policy by the Health Ministry (Brasil, 2005), resulting from the recognition of the harmful use of alcohol and other drugs as a serious public health problem. In addition, the observation that the majority of drug users are not capable or do not want to stop consuming such substances weighed heavily on this decision[8]. However, it is important to point out that despite all the incentives created by the Brazilian government, there has not yet been a significant adherence to this strategy that would allow for the institutionalization of the harm reduction policy in the entire public health system (Passos & Souza, 2011).

From a public health perspective, the adoption of harm reduction as a strategy for the treatment of addiction to psychoactive substances aims to recover the users' self-regulating

---

[8] One of the reasons why drug users do not want and/or do not manage to interrupt the consumption is the fact that they have already incorporated the drugs they use to their personal and relationships routine (Rothschield, 2010). Besides, in most cases, such substances are a source of jouissance, which they are not willing to do without (Laxenaire, 2010; Olievenstein, 2002).

role and citizenship, while stimulating their inclusion and mobilization in the society, through the expansion of their social relationships and the increase of the chances within the society in which they live. Theoretically, the objectives of the harm reduction proposal can be reached through the adoption of certain strategies of action, namely those that seek to reach users who, due to their socio-economic characteristics (lack of permanent housing, close relationship with illegal practices, lack of health concerns, etc), are generally excluded from health services (Marlatt & Witkiewitz, 2010; Pinheiro, 2002; Stevens, Hallam & Trace, 2006). Furthermore, there are other strategies that intend to promote drug users' moderation of consumption, such as drug consumption rooms and target delivery of healthcare.

As a consequence, the harm reduction proposes that, with the implementation of this new treatment model, users of alcohol and other drugs can receive counseling and adequate treatment in order to avoid the most serious consequences of drug abuse, such as deaths by overdose, organic damages and virus contamination. This way, there is the hope of contributing to a safer drug use and a global and less prejudicial understanding of this phenomenon.

In fact, many authors argue that the treatment of drug users with the harm reduction approach is not only more efficient but also less costly, when compared to the abstinence model policies of drug use combat, because it contributes to decrease the number of deaths and illnesses associated to the use of drugs and to improve the social functioning of psychoactive substances users (Marlatt & Witkiewitz, 2010; OEDT, 2011; Stevens, Hallam & Trade, 2006). Nonetheless, this effectiveness is difficult to be supported by statistical data, partly because, although abstinence and harm reduction are grounded in apparently opposite philosophies, many drug users that start treatment with the objective of achieving abstinence end up redefining their goals during the process and begin to seek moderation in consumption (Neale, Nettleton & Pickering, 2010). From this perspective, in a number of health services, abstinence and harm reduction become part of the same treatment strategy, and can actually be used together (McKeganey, 2011). Besides, because studies on efficacy, effectiveness, and cost-effectiveness of the varied types of treatment have often employed methods and research designs of varied quality (such randomized controlled trials, clinical trials, case series, reviews, meta-analysis, etc), it is difficult to make a direct comparison of the different interventions. These are the reasons why there is a growing need for the development of more research focusing on these issues (CIAR, 2008).

In spite of this, it is possible to state that, because it places lower demands, the harm reduction proposal seems more attractive to many users, and decreases the number of patients that give up treatment (Alves, 2009; Rothschild, 2010). In addition, some authors defend that the rampant increase in the consumption of illicit drugs and the growth of the progression from the use of least to most powerful drugs are less frequent in countries and areas that adopt the harm reduction perspective (Alves, 2006; OEDT, 2011).

Especially because of these reasons, harm reduction is considered an "ethical landmark" in the field of prevention and treatment of disorders associated with the use of alcohol and other drugs. From this perspective, the proponents of harm reduction programs defend that this approach "recognizes each user in his/her *singularities*, designing with him/her the strategies to defend his/her life" (Brasil, 2005, p.42)[9].

---

[9] All the translations from the Portuguese original versions were made by the author.

However, it is worth debating whether the ethic that the harm reduction strategy deals with actually takes into account the subjectivity of each user. Regarding this aspect, it is important to highlight that, in mental health practices based on harm reduction, the place occupied by the subjective aspects of the one who resorts to intoxication remains open to questioning. In this respect, it is valid to inquire whether this approach considers the dimension of *jouissance* coupled with the intoxication practices[10].

This issue deserves a thorough, deep discussion, to avoid falling in the empty promise of change, which will lead us to trade a practice that just considers the use of drugs as a disease, either physical or spiritual, for another practice that takes the drug use in its exclusively social dimension. Hence, it is important to note that drug addiction is a complex and multifaceted phenomenon. Thus, it is not possible to adopt a reductionist position, be it biological, moral, social or psychological, in relationship to it. This reservation derives from the assumption, advocated by some authors, that social inclusion and citizenship recovery in mental health, though important, tends to neglect the subjective nature entailed by the psychic suffering and the mode of *jouissance* of each subject (Kyrillos Neto, 2007; Rinaldi, Cabral & Castro, 2008).

The request for the inclusion of the singularities and the listening of the patient in mental health practices is strongly considered by some psychoanalysts (Figueiredo & Tenório, 2002; Valentine & Fraser, 2008), who, although recognizing the advances obtained by psychosocial rehabilitation, highlight that the emphasis on the citizen of rights can lead the current mental health practices to a new kind of subjective dismissal (Fernandes & Freitas, 2009). This is because there is a contemporary perspective in psychoanalysis that adverts that any rehabilitation proposal can only succeed if it follows the subject's discourse, since the rehabilitation that denies the clinic will inevitably fall into the trap of re-education (Viganó, 1999).

In this way, to psychoanalysis, the emphasis is placed on the subject, which makes the psychoanalytical practice different from the other approaches that are centered on the social determinants of the phenomena considered psychopathological, in spite of the agency and subjective choices (Valentine & Fraser, 2008). Thus, the psychoanalytical treatment focuses attention on what the patient says about him/herself, since the meaning of the symptoms, and consequently, the production of what Freud (1905/1996) called 'talking cure', will only be possible to emerge from the elements that the subject him/herself brings. Hence, the importance of psychoanalysis lies in the fact that this approach opens a space in which the patient's talking can be listened to, interpreted and analyzed.

5. The psychoanalysis proposal

Thus, psychoanalysis also presents a specific proposal for treating users of alcohol and other drugs. This psychoanalytical proposal for the understanding and treatment of drug addictions was outlined along psychoanalysis' own history. For, in this field, it was Freud who first became interested in this phenomenon, laying the conceptual foundations that

---

[10] It is important to emphasize that, from the psychoanalytical perspective, every type of drug use provides some kind of jouissance. However, in the case of drug addiction, the jouissance provided invades and dominates the user, in such a way that the subject remains subjected to the psychoactive substances.

made possible the subsequent development of psychoanalytical-based propositions on drug use such as the ones developed by Abraham (1908), Rado (1933), Krystal (1975), Lacan (1976), McDougall (1978), Wurmser (1995), Khantzian (1995), among others. Although all the theories formulated by these authors refer to the conceptual field of psychoanalysis, they are very different. Explaining each one of them is beyond the scope of this chapter, so the following considerations are embedded in the framework of Lacanian psychoanalysis, which stands out for having remained faithful to the Freudian doctrine and for being the only one that can explain why, in the use of drugs, pleasure and harm are inexorably interwoven (Loose, 2000).

Nevertheless, it is important to highlight that, despite the existence of so many psychoanalytical readings on drug use, "the association between psychoanalysis and drug addiction is not common" (Laxenaire, 2010, p. 524). One reason is the fact that there is currently a strong demand for evidences of cost-effectiveness of the several existing treatments. And psychoanalysis is usually assessed as a long-term treatment, which proofs of efficacy are still insufficient (CIAR, 2008; Harrison et al, 2003). One of the main explanations for this assessment is the fact that psychoanalysis does not work on the same efficacy parameters that are adopted by other fields. Because the therapeutic efficacy is always related to a certain conception of cure and the psychoanalytical view of cure differs from the other fields, since psychoanalysis recognizes the existence of something incurable in the subject, and hence, is warned that it is not possible to ensure a full state of well-being, for suffering, to some extent, is at the core of human existence (Freud, 1930/1996; Lacan, 1966/1998; Loose, 2000). Even so, many psychoanalysts have published works that demonstrate promising effects of the psychoanalytical treatment for drug addiction through the reports of clinical cases[11] (Rothschield, 2010; Loose, 2000; Marlo & Kalinian, 2002).

To start discussing the treatment proposal oriented by psychoanalysis, it is crucial to highlight that the psychoanalytical treatment operates under a view that is radically different from the therapeutic proposal originated in the medical-psychiatric field and from the one derived from the moral field as well (Silva, 2010). This is because psychoanalysis works with the notion of the subject of the unconscious, conceived as being beyond the individual and beyond the illness.

The psychoanalytical concept of the unconscious refers to a psychic system that runs parallel to the conscious system, and that operates in a determined way, having an order and structure of its own (Fink, 1995). But, unlike the conscious system, the unconscious can only appear as a stumble, just in the gaps of the conscious manifestations, in what Lacan (1957/1999) coined as the formations of the unconscious: dreams, lapses, faulty actions (Freudian slips), jokes and symptoms, which reveal a meaning that so far had been hidden to the subject him/herself. By doing this, the unconscious indicates to the self the existence of an instance which is, at the same time, inside and conflicting with it.

Whereas the consciousness operates in articulation with the reality principle, the unconscious operates in articulation with the pleasure principle, and, most importantly,

---

[11] This method of demonstration of results is justified because, as psychoanalysis emphasizes the singularity and the subject, it would be absolutely incoherent to expect that its efficiency could be demonstrated by statistical evidence. Hence, what can be expected from further research in this field are meta-analysis based studies that provide within-subject measures related to drug consumption, demonstrating the improvement of drug users that have undergone psychoanalytical treatment.

with the beyond pleasure principle. Whereas the reality principle, because it is articulated to the material reality, makes detours and delays in search of satisfaction, the pleasure principle seeks satisfaction in the shortest and most direct way (Freud, 1911/1996). The beyond pleasure principle, in turn, is articulated to the death drive, which Freud (1920/1996) defined as a certain tendency, inherent to all living beings, to seek the pacification of all the tensions – which ultimately can only be achieved with death.

This is why, in psychoanalysis, the resource to intoxication is understood as a choice of the subject who, moved by the unconscious laws, searches actively for a *jouissance* that is extended towards death. To psychoanalysis, this search does not happen despite the subject, as other psychotherapeutic approaches propose. Yet, it is a choice[12] made by the subject him/herself, but a choice that does not come from rational and logic elements alone, but also results from desires that many times escape rationality, since they resort to the unconscious and are articulated to the death drive.

In fact, according to Laxenaire (2010), the unconscious search for death is well evidenced in drug addiction. Thus, one of the main particularities of the psychoanalytical proposal in comparison to the other treatment modalities lies on the emphasis given to the subjective structure at the expense of the pathological phenomenon. This is so much true that, while the medical-psychiatric diagnosis is most of the times phenomenological and based on a set of previously defined signs, the psychoanalytic diagnosis is structural and is from this structural diagnosis that the psychoanalytical treatment will develop.

The structural diagnosis refers to the differentiation of the three clinical structures: neurosis, psychosis and perversion, which concern the mode of the resolution of the Oedipus Complex. This diagnosis results from the evaluation of the position assumed by the subject before the Other (Figueiredo & Tenório, 2002). This is explained by the fact that, to psychoanalysis, what marks out the structuring of the human psychism is the relationship with the Other, understood not as another person, but as the whole symbolic universe to which the individual finds him/herself referred to (the discourses, rituals, codes, beliefs, etc). Although this symbolic universe is initially transmitted by one primordial other (such as the mother or the one who is in charge of the child's insertion in the world of language), in the Lacanian theory the Other represents the entire culture, and is considered an indispensable element for the human subject constitution, in that it makes it possible for the individual not to be a mere biological representative of the human species, but to become a being provided with thoughts and feelings, and inserted into social bonds (Lacan, 1939/1985). From this perspective, every human subject is dependent on the Other, since no subject can engender him/herself on his/her own (Laxenaire, 2010).

From this viewpoint, addiction would be a posterior dependence, but anchored exactly in the mode of relationship the subject established with the world around him/her (Laxenaire,

---

[12] The term choice is used by psychoanalysis not in the sense of a pondered decision, but as something that is chosen because it relates to what is most intimate to the subject, his/her unconscious. Hence, to psychoanalysis the choices are overdetermined by his/her psychic reality. In other words, psychoanalysis refers to choices that are not always rational, such as for example, the choice of abusive intoxication that many times threatens the subject. However, despite the sometimes hazardous effects caused by the subjective choices, psychoanalysis emphasizes how important it is for health professionals who work with drug addiction issues to keep alert to the fact that, in some way, users make the choice of intoxication.

2010). This is why the structural diagnosis is of paramount importance in the psychoanalytical treatment of drug addiction, keeping in sight that it will enlighten the reasons why the inexorable dependence on the Other was transmuted into the dependence on a fixed object, which may give access to a kind of *jouissance* that is steady and repetitive, and to which the subject, from a certain moment on, becomes subordinated.

Thus, psychoanalysis defends that if, in the beginning, the consumption of drugs has basically a recreational function, it is during its use that the drug, for some users, turns into a product that acquires a vital and indispensable role, configuring thereby an addiction. Several reasons converge to explain why addiction happens only in a subgroup of drug users. Among them are individual, social, economic, cultural and family factors. However, the psychoanalytical treatment emphasizes the subject that resorts to drugs, and consequently, to the particular function that drugs have in the psychism of each drug user and/or addict, and also highlights the importance of a diagnosis that differentiates between drug consumption and drug addiction.

Hence, from a psychoanalytical perspective, "it is necessary to differentiate the simple uses of stupefiers from the imperative of treatment of the organism by a toxic drug, when this becomes the only means to shelter, on a daily basis, the body from an intolerable pain" (Kaufmann, 1996, p. 542). Thus, to psychoanalysis, drug addiction is defined as an "intense and exclusive relationship, in which the use of drugs has already been established as a function in the subject's psychic life" (Conte, 2000, p. 11).

For this reason, from a psychoanalytical viewpoint, the drug is not a problem in itself, since what can become problematic is certain types of drug use that some subjects make, which can turn into a form of the subject's own destruction. This means that, in the psychoanalytical treatment of drug addiction, it is a matter of removing the biological characteristic from the drug (although not denying its existence), to give value to something else, converting it in something other than a simple object that produces psychological or physiological effects, which, by the way, can only be apprehended by the signifier, by what the patient reports. In this sense, if the treatment modalities based on abstinence claim that the drug makes the addict, to the extent that drugs are considered as having the supposedly intrinsic power to get the subjects addicted, psychoanalysis states that the drug addict makes the drug (Freda, 1989/1993), because it understands that this is a private relationship between the subject and the object, that grants to the latter the power to become a source of satisfaction which the subject himself cannot do without.

From a psychoanalytical point of view, then, the addictions and the symptom have similar forming mechanisms, insofar as they both are a solution to an underlying conflict, but a solution that is not perfect, since it does not solve everything. But even being imperfect, it is a repeated solution, because there is something in it that the subject is not willing to give up, despite all the suffering that it brings (Loose, 2000). Hence, in the psychoanalytical treatment for drug addiction, it is understood that the subject's choice to use drugs, the relapses and the excessive use of the psychoactive substance will only stop being an escape for the subject when the treatment enables him/her to find other forms of symbolization that allow him/her to abstain from drugs, in cases when this outcome is possible – for there are cases in which, due to a extremely unstable psychic configuration, the addiction is simply the one and only way the subject finds to manage to continue living.

Thus, in the psychoanalytical treatment, it is necessary to take into account the function and the meaning of the drug use to each subject, in order to make possible the identification of the relationship established between the subject and the drug. And to psychoanalysis, this identification is only viable when it comes from the knowledge produced by the subject him/herself during the treatment. According to this perspective, the role of the psychoanalyst in toxicomania treatments is to conduct a quality listening of the subject, enabling the emergence of the unsaid, of what is not obvious, of what is beyond the pleasure principle, which, by nature, point at the subject of the unconscious. In other words, if addictions result from the choice for a *jouissance* in the body, a *jouissance* that does not express itself through language, so the psychoanalytic treatment objective is to enable the subject to make a movement "from ad-diction to diction" (Loose, 2000, p. 80).

According to Loose (2000), drugs and alcohol can only exert massive and extreme effects on the subject because they work pushing him/her out or against the language domain. In this sense, re-inserting him/her in the symbolic chain, in the diction domain, means going exactly in the opposite direction of the drug effects. Thus, the main difference from the psychoanalytical treatment is due to the ethic that guides psychoanalysis, which is radically different from any moralizing perspective. This is because, similarly to the medical-psychiatric treatments, the treatments originated from the moral model assume to know, *a priori*, about the subject and what is supposed to be the best for him/her. This characteristic results from the fact that the moral model aims at responding to a social demand of standardization and adaptation of deviant behaviors, rather than fulfilling the users' needs. Hence, the treatments based on this model end up promoting the subject's orthopedic framing or re-education, to the extent that they intend to teach him/her what is considered as the adequate behavior, which is, in this case, the social ideology of sobriety and aims at a certain preservation of the other citizens' life.

Still in regard to the moral model of treatment, psychoanalysis advises that, when the professional embodies the position of knowing about the subject, there is no room for the subject to produce any knowledge about him/herself (Bastos, 2009). And in a context in which the subject is not given the means to produce his/her own knowledge, it is very likely that he/she will remain at the mercy of the professionals or institutions, being unable to make his/her own choices and/or to be responsible for them. Consequently, instead of becoming responsible, the subject under treatment remains in a state of tutelage, in which there is an attempt to remove all of his/her possible responses that do not conform to the expectations of the health professionals and institutions. In sum, the great contribution that psychoanalysis offers to the treatments of drug abuse and addiction is to call the attention to the fact that, if the subject choses his/her addiction as a solution that makes him/her suffer and at the same time brings him/her *jouissance*, then, only the subject him/herself is able to, through treatment, choose what to do with what affects his/her body and life so radically.

6. Psychoanalysis and harm reduction: controversies and convergences

Reviewing the literature, it is possible to confirm the extent to which psychoanalysis, while a specific field of knowledge, has long adopted a critical position with regard to the existing drug use treatments based on the mandatory abstinence (Conte, 2004; Melman, 2000; Queiroz, 2001; Rothschield, 2010). For this reason, in the first instance, it would be possible to identify an approximation between psychoanalysis and harm reduction proposals, insofar as they both problematize the model of treatment guided by the logic of abstinence.

In fact, according to Paes (2006), "the literature on drugs that has psychoanalytical basis has often been used by technicians who work on the training of harm reducers" (p. 129). Since the 1970s, there has been an increase in the number of professionals with a psychoanalytical focus, who offer chemical dependents a different kind of treatment and express serious criticism to the existent models of treatment (Paes, 2006). One of the main psychoanalysts that represent this viewpoint is the psychiatrist Claude Olievenstein, who, in the 1970s, founded the Centre Médical Marmottan, an institution for the treatment of drug addicts in Paris that became a benchmark and was inspirational for many treatment centers worldwide (Freda, 1989/1993; Marchant, 2010).

Queiroz (2001) also believes that it is possible to consider an approximation between the psychoanalytical assumptions and the harm reduction approach, insofar as the programs that adopt the latter introduce the "dimension of the particularity of the subject" (p. 3) and therefore, acknowledges "drug users as particular subjects and citizens, who have the right to health and to a treatment that is in fact effective and produces meaning" (Queiroz, 2001). In this case, the production of meaning refers to the fact that both the harm reduction policies and the psychoanalytical approach grant drug users the right to use drugs, which makes possible for them to build significations for this use without necessarily having to interrupt it (Marchant, 2010; Rotschild, 2010).

Adopting a similar perspective, Conte (2004) states that not only the harm reduction approach but also the advances achieved by the psychosocial rehabilitation paradigm do come close to psychoanalysis. According to the author, in both of them "there is the common refusal to flatten the subject to a passiveness that asks for social assistance or to a subject-body condition (organic and biologic) that asks for a "medicamental solution" (Conte, 2004, p.26).

On the other hand, Conte (2004) warns that the principles that underlie the harm reduction proposals are not the same that guide psychoanalysis, and in this respect, adverts that "the differences are due to *the ethic*, the objectives of the interventions and those who they turn to" (p. 27). Hence, this proposal of conciliation between the singularity dimension, represented by the subject's clinic and grounded in psychoanalysis, and the universal dimension, represented by the perspective of social rehabilitation and consequently, harm reduction, is not consensual.

In this respect, Dufour (2004) presents a more critical position regarding the social emphasis given by some mental health policies, and advocates that "it is not about encouraging carelessness – as one is soon blamed when one shows the slightest reservation about the humanitarian conduct – but observing the effects, opposed to the desired ones, caused by the coercive kindness" (p.37). Therefore, the author indicates the existence of a certain amount of coercion in the psychosocial rehabilitation practices in mental health, and makes sure to explicitly include the harm reduction proposal under this view.

When referring to the movement that he coined as "to limit the damage" or "reduce the harm", Dufour (2004) states that:

the surprising fact in this type of proposal is that it does not take into consideration the opinion of the ones involved. It searches for their happiness and health, regardless of them. Some rebel against it. For example, a patient who lived with an HIV-positive woman used to say about precautions: 'you know, for me, making plastified love is not my business' (p.37).

It is important to pinpoint that, as previously mentioned, because it is a public health strategy, harm reduction is inserted in the psychosocial rehabilitation logic. Then, the harm reduction objectives are to reduce the damage caused by the use of psychoactive substances, and promote the bio-psychosocial well being of the health service users, having for main focus of attention the citizen of universal rights. Therefore, harm reduction aims to provide a treatment for everyone, and is thus based on the principle of equal rights and connected to the universal dimension. This universalizing perspective in public health and in harm reduction may bring a number of complicating factors in regard to the possibility of approximation with psychoanalysis, which points to the singularity of each subject's treatment.

Henceforth, although psychoanalysis and harm reduction may initially come close, because they both oppose the abstinence model, the possibilities of convergence between these two fields need to be more deeply investigated. Whereas psychoanalysis adopts an ethic that foregrounds the subjective position and the modality of *jouissance* achieved by the intoxication practices, the harm reduction approach, being a public health strategy, advocates in its principles the bio-psychosocial well being of the health service users.

7. Final considerations

In the mental health field, it is possible to outline the existence of at least three prevalent models: the exclusively biomedical or pharmacological, the exclusively sociological and the subjective (Rigter at al, 2004; Kyrillos Neto, 2007). The exclusively organicist model has as its object the mental disorders, taken as a "biologizing degradation of nosology", that ignores the subjective, political and social aspects of the psychic suffering, and has the purpose of treating them exclusively through the psychopharmaceutical sovereignty. In the specific context of alcohol and drug abuse, it would be possible to state that this model guides its treatments by abstinence, insofar as they do not consider the subjective and social issues that the use of psychoactive substances imply, and seem to give importance only to the neurochemical effects caused by toxic drugs.

On the other hand, the exclusively sociological model takes as its object the man in his suffering existence, and is guided by the notion of individual originated from the liberal ideology and the human rights advocated by the constitution of the democratic regime. This model draws attention to the need for development and empowerment of individuals and communities so that, thereafter, they become able to have democratic participation in the actions devised to protect and promote their own health (Duggan, Cooper & Foster, 2002). It is possible to approximate this sociological model to some proposals derived from the psychosocial rehabilitation perspective, insofar as these place the emphasis on the citizen of universal rights and on the socio-political dimension. Thus, in the realm of the treatments offered to drug users, we can assume that this exclusively sociological model would be represented by the harm reduction approach.

Finally, the subjective model has as its object the "subject of desire", defined by Lacan (1969/1992) as constituted from its position before the Other. Among the existing proposals for the treatment of drug abuse, this subjective model is almost exclusively represented by psychoanalysis.

According to Kyrillos Neto (2007), it is noticeable that, unfortunately, these three models are considered mutually exclusive in most health mental services. However, it is important to highlight that overcoming the impasses that arise daily in these services depends on an approach that does not rely only on the exclusive considerations of the social determinations nor on a purely clinical focus, but rather on the articulation of these important factors.

Consequently, it is necessary that the harm reduction strategies, when proposed as a mental health policy, be able to reach these multiple sides that outline the complexity of the phenomenon of drug abuse and addiction. In this respect, psychoanalysis has great contributions to offer, since the psychoanalytical treatment aims at promoting the articulation between the universal aspect of the structure and the singular nature of the psychic reality of each individual, allowing the treatment of the universal (the structure) through the singular (the subject).

Hence, despite the recognized need for more research in the field of treatments offered to drug users, it is important to ponder that any proposed treatment cannot leave out the consideration for the psychic aspects involved in the phenomenon of drug addiction (OEDT, 2011). This is why current reports have demanded more studies analyzing the effects generated by the several types of existing psychological interventions, considering that, until now, the collected data are not sufficient to show evidence of the compared efficacy of each intervention. However, many studies suggest that such interventions are fundamental to act upon both the causes and the psychological consequences associated to drug use, especially when combined with other treatments, such as, for instance, the substitution treatments (CIAR, 2008; Marlatt; Larimer & Witkiewitz, 2012). And it is precisely in this context that psychoanalysis becomes a treatment proposal that, for placing the subject as the focus of any therapeutic action, presents itself as extremely promising.

8. References

Abraham, K. (1908/1927). The psychological relations between sexuality and alcoholism. *Selected Papers on Psychoanalysis*. London: Karnac.

Alves, V. S. (2009). Modelos de atenção à saúde de usuários de álcool e outras drogas: discursos políticos, saberes e práticas. *Cadernos de saúde pública*, 25 (11), p. 2309-2319.

Araújo, T. (2007). Drogas: proibir é legal? *Revista Superinteressante*, 244, p. 62-71. São Paulo: Ed. Abril.

Bastos, A. (2009). *Considerações sobre a clínica psicanalítica na instituição pública destinada ao atendimento de usuários de álcool e/ou drogas*. (MA Dissertation). Universidade do Estado do Rio de Janeiro, Rio de Janeiro, RJ.

Brasil (2001). *Manual de Redução de Danos*. Brasília: Ministry of Health.

Brasil (2005). *Reforma Psiquiátrica e Política de Saúde Mental no Brasil.* Brasília: Ministry of Health.

Carneiro, H. (2006). As drogas no Brasil: entre o delírio e o perigo. *Revista Nossa História, 33,* p. 12-26. São Paulo: Ed. Vera Cruz.

Conte, M. (2000). *A clínica psicanalítica com toxicômanos: o corte & costura no enquadre institucional.* (PhD Thesis). Pontifícia Universidade Católica de São Paulo, São Paulo, SP.

Conte, M. (2004). Psicanálise e redução de danos: articulações possíveis. *Revista da Associação Psicanalítica de Porto Alegre, 26,* p. 23-33.

Decker, S. H. (2008). *Drug Smugglers on Drug Smuggling: lessons from the inside.* Philadelphia: Temple University Press.

Director, L. (2005). Encounters with omnipotence in the psychoanalysis of substance users. *Dialogues,* 15 (4), p. 567-584.

Dufour, A. (2004). Opiacidade. *Revista da Associação Psicanalítica de Porto Alegre, 26,* p. 34-57.

Duggan, M.; Cooper, A. & Foster, J. (2002). *Modernising the social model in mental health: a discussion paper.* England: SPN by Topss.

Faria, J. G. & Schneider, D. R. (2009). O perfil dos usuários do CAPS ad-Blumenal e as políticas públicas em saúde mental. *Psicologia e Sociedade, n. 21,* vol. 3, pp. 324-333.

Fernandes, A. & Freitas, L. (2009). Tempos de reforma psiquiátrica: a clínica da recepção e a direção do tratamento no Hospital Juliano Moreira de Salvador – Bahia. *Psicologia: Teoria e Prática, n. 11,* vol. 1, 2009, p. 97-109.

Figueiredo, A. C. & Tenório, F. (2002). O diagnóstico em psiquiatria e psicanálise. *Revista Latinoamericana de Psicopatologia Fundamental, vol. 5,* n. 1, p. 29-43, mar/2002.

Fink, B. (1995). *The Lacanian Subject: between language and jouissance.* Princeton: Princeton University Press.

Freda, H. (1989/1993). Quem lhe disse isso? *Coletânea de textos sobre toxicomania e alcoolismo do Centro Mineiro de Toxicomania* (p. 1-13). Belo Horizonte: Centro Mineiro de Toxicomania.

Freud, S. (1905/1996). Fragmento da análise de um caso de histeria. In: *Edição Estandard Brasileira das Obras Psicológicas Completas* (Vol. VII.). Rio de Janeiro: Imago.

Freud, S. (1911/1996). Dois princípios do funcionamento psíquico. In: *Edição Estandard Brasileira das Obras Psicológicas Completas* (Vol. XII.). Rio de Janeiro: Imago.

Freud, S. (1920/1996). Além do princípio do prazer. In: *Edição Estandard Brasileira das Obras Psicológicas Completas* (Vol. XVIII.). Rio de Janeiro: Imago.

Freud, S. (1930/1996). O Mal-estar na Civilização. In: *Edição Estandard Brasileira das Obras Psicológicas Completas* (Vol. XXI.). Rio de Janeiro: Imago.

Goffmann, E. (1985/2001). *A representação do eu na vida cotidiana.* Petrópolis, RJ: Vozes.

Harrison, L.; Cappello, R.; Alaszewski, A.; Appleton, S. & Cooke, G. (2003). *The effectiveness of treatment for substance dependence within the prison system in England: a review.* Canterbury, Kent: Centre for Health Services Studies.

Kaufmann, P. (1996). *Dicionário Enciclopédico de Psicanálise.* Rio de Janeiro: Jorge Zahar Ed.

Khantzian, E. (1995). Self-regulation vulnerabilities in substance abusers: treatment implications. In: Dowling, S. (Ed.). *The psychology and treatment of addictive behavior,* Madison, CT: International Universities Press.

Krystal, H. (1975). Affect tolerance. *Annual of Psychoanalysis,* 3, p. 179-219.

Kyrillos Neto, F. (2007). *Efeitos de circulação do discurso em serviços substitutivos de saúde mental.* (PhD Thesis). Pontifícia Universidade Católica de São Paulo, São Paulo, SP.

Lacan, J. (1939/1985). *Os complexos familiares na formação do indivíduo.* Rio de Janeiro: Jorge Zahar Ed.

Lacan, J. (1957/1999). *O Seminário, Livro V: As formações do inconsciente.* Rio de Janeiro: Jorge Zahar Ed.

Lacan, J. (1966/1998). A ciência e a verdade. *Escritos.* Rio de Janeiro: Jorge Zahar Ed.

Lacan, J. (1969/1992). *O Seminário, Livro XVII: o avesso da psicanálise.* Rio de Janeiro: Jorge Zahar Ed.

Lacan, J. (1976). Journées des cartels de l'École Freudienne de Paris. *Lettres de l'École Freudienne,* Paris, 18, p. 263-270.

Laxenaire, M. (2010). Psychanalyse et addictions sans substances. *Annales Médico-Psychologiques,* 168, p. 524-527.

Loose, R. (2000). The addicted subject caught between the ego and drive: the post-freudian reduction and simplification of a complex clinical problem. *Psychoanalytische Perspectieven,* 41/42.

Marchant, A. (2010). Answering drug epidemic at the beginning of the 1970s: experimenting new patterns, creating new practices, building standardization in matters of help care policy. *Conference Standardizing and Marketing the Drugs in the XXth Century.* History of Medicine University La Charité: Berlin (Allemagne), 7-8th October, 2010.

Marlatt, G. A. & Witkiewitz, K. (2010). Update on Harm-Reduction Policy and Intervention Research. *Annual Revue Psychology,* 6, p. 591-606.

Marlatt; G. A.; Larimer, M. E. & Witkiewitz, K. (2012). *Harm reduction: pragmatic strategies for managing high-risks behaviors.* New York: The Guilford Press.

Marlo, H. & Kalinian, H. (2002). Utilizing psychoanalytic psychotherapy in the treatment of substance abusers. *Clinical Psychology and Psychotherapy,* 9, p. 211-223.

McDougall, J. (1978). *Plea for a measure of abnormality.* New York: International Universities Press.

McKeganey, N. (2011). Abstinence and harm reduction: can they work together? *International Journal of Drug Policy,* doi: 10.1016/j.drugpo.2011.04.001.

Mcrae, E. (2001). Antropologia: aspectos sociais, culturais e ritualísticos. In: Seibel, S. & Toscano JR., A. (Eds.). *Dependência de drogas.* São Paulo: Atheneu.

Melman, C. (2000). *Alcoolismo, delinqüência e toxicomania – uma outra forma de gozar.* São Paulo: Escuta.

Nery Filho, A. & Torres, I. M. A. (Eds.) (2002). *Drogas: isso lhe interessa? Confira aqui.* Salvador: CETAD/UFBA/CPTT/PMV.

OEDT (2011). *Relatório anual 2011: a evolução do fenômeno da droga na Europa.* Luxemburgo: Serviço das Publicações da União Européia.

Paes, P. (2006). *Ensino e aprendizagem na prática da Redução de Danos.* (PhD Thesis). Universidade Federal de São Carlos, São Carlos, SP.

Passos, E. H. & Souza, T. P. (2011). Redução de danos e saúde pública: construções alternativas à política global de "guerra às drogas". *Psicologia & Sociedade,* 23 (1), p. 154-162.

Pinheiro, R. (2006). Redução de Danos e psicanálise aplicadas à toxicomania. In: Cirino, O. & Medeiros, R. (Eds.). *Álcool e outras drogas: escolhas, impasses e saídas possíveis.* Belo Horizonte: Autêntica.

Pratta, E. M. M. & Santos, M. A. (2009). O processo saúde-doença e a dependência química: interfaces e evolução. *Psicologia: Teoria e Pesquisa, n. 2,* vol. 25, p. 203-211.

Queiroz, I. (2001). Os programas de redução de danos como espaços de exercício da cidadania dos usuários de drogas. *Psicologia: ciência e profissão, 21,* 4, dez/ 2001.

Rado, S. (1933/1984). The Psychoanalysis of Pharmacothymia. *Journal of Substance Abuse Treatment,* I, p. 59-68.

Rezende, M. (1999). *Tratamento com dependentes de drogas: diálogos com profissionais da área de saúde mental.* (PhD Thesis). Universidade Estadual de Campinas, Campinas, SP.

Rezende, M. (2000). Uso, abuso e dependência de drogas: delimitações sociais e científicas. *Revista Psicologia & Sociedade, 12,* 144-155.

Rigter, H.; Van Gageldonk, A.; Ketelaars, T. & Van Laar, M. (2004). *Treatment of problematic use of drugs. State of the art for evidence based treatments and other interventions.* Utrecht (Niederlande): Trimbos Institute.

Rinaldi, D.; Cabral, L. & Castro, G. (2008). Psicanálise e reabilitação psicossocial: limites e possibilidades de articulação. *Revista Estudos e Pesquisas em Psicologia, vol. 8,* n. 1, jan./abr. 2008.

Rothschild, D. (2010). Partners in treatment: relational psychoanalysis and harm reduction therapy. *Journal of Clinical Psychology: In Session,* 66 (2), p. 136-149.

Seibel, S. & Toscano Jr., A. (Eds.). *Dependência de drogas.* São Paulo: Atheneu.

Schulte, B.; Thane, K.; Rehm, J.; Uchtenhagen, A; Stöver, H.; Degkwitz, P & Reimer, C. (2008). *Review of the efficacy of drug treatment interventions in Europe.* Hamburg: Centre for Interdisciplinary Adicction Research (CIAR).

Silva, J. R. (2010). *A clínica psicanalítica das toxicomanias.* (MA Dissertation). Universidade do Estado do Rio de Janeiro, Rio de Janeiro, RJ.

Stevens, A.; Hallam, C. & Trace, M. (2006). *Treatment for dependent drug use: a guide for policymakers.* Beckley: The Beckley Foundation Drug Policy Programme.

Viganó, C. (1999). A construção do caso clínico em saúde mental. *Curinga – Psicanálise e Saúde Mental, n. 13,* set./1999.

Valentine, K. & Fraser, S. (2008). Trauma, damage and pleasure: rethinking problematic drug use. *International Journal of Drug Policy,* 19, p. 410-416.

WHO (2004). *Neurociências: consumo e dependência de substâncias psicoativas.* Genebra: WHO
    Library Cataloguing-in Publication Data.
Wurmser, L. (1995). *The hidden dimension: psychodynamics of compulsive drug use.* New Jersey:
    Jason Aronson Inc.

5

Research and Intervention for Drug-Addicted Mothers and Their Children: New Perspectives

Paolo Stocco[1], Alessandra Simonelli[2],
Nicoletta Capra[3] and Francesca De Palo[2]
[1]*Therapeutic Community "Villa Renata", Venice,*
[2]*Department of Developmental and Social Psychology, Padua University,*
[3]*Mother-Child Therapeutic Community "Casa Aurora e Villa Emma," Venice,*
Italy

1. Introduction

According to research carried out by the EMCDDA, drug-addicted women in Europe account for at least one quarter of the total European population consuming illicit substances (Emcdda, 2006a). A specific research platform entitled "Women and Drugs" was created within the context of the second European project "Democracies, Cities and Drugs." This platform is focused on what characterizes and distinguishes female substance addiction from male substance addiction: its manifestation, its attributes, and the interventions or services which can be put into effect while devoting special attention and offering specialized care to this phenomenon. Our findings confirm that women substance users are exposed to a great number of risks such as medical, social, economic, familial and psychopathological risks requiring intervention through specific tools and aimed responses (see Brentari, Hernandez, Tripodi, 2011). The investigated factors included pregnancy, parenthood and the well-being as well as development of the child, while taking into account institutional and ethical reflections regarding this complex theme.

The substance abuse phenomenon indeed affects a high number of fertile women. When drugs are consumed during pregnancy, they can have serious, direct and indirect effects on the postpartum development with subsequent effects on the child (OTIS, 2010). Substance abusing mothers represent an at-risk parenting situation which, in turn, profoundly influences the quality of the mother-child relationship. The awareness of these at-risk situations for children along with the widely accepted notion that ideally, children should always be raised by their mothers led to the introduction of residential treatment in Italy. These services deal with maternal pathologies and provide care and assistance for children; in fact, these therapeutic communities accommodate addicted mothers as well as their children.

Up until recently, therapies for children (particularly medical ones) were administered by institutions outside of the community, while no therapeutic treatment was mandated for minors. The first therapeutic communities for drug addicted mothers and their children appeared in Europe in the early nineties. These institutions must provide assistance to children and assure them the greatest possible social, psychological and physical well-being. In addition to the funds available for each mother, funds for each individual minor are made available on a daily basis. Our project: "Research and intervention on minors in communities for addicted mothers and their children: from at-risk parenting to child well-being" was promoted within this specific intervention framework. The project aims to secure child well-being by assessing maternal parenting as well as by carrying out direct and indirect observations of the child, his/her caregivers and the caregiver-child relationship. At the same time, the most suitable intervention for each single subject is put into effect.

2. Female substance addiction, pregnancy and parenthood

As stated above, there is an ever increasing interest towards defining characteristics which are specifically related to substance abuse in the female population, with specific reference to the following two crucial aspects.

a. general differences, in terms of individual and relational characteristics, life history and family history which single out addicted women as subjects with experiences of trauma, abandonment or neglect, from either a physical or psychological standpoint (Parsec Association, 2004; Stocco et Al., 2000, 2002; Studio VEdeTTE, 2007). These subjects suffer also for their specific medical problems (HIV, sexually transmitted pathologies, etc.), for their social situation (prostitution, access to the job market, etc.) and institutional difficulties (organization and access to services). From this point of view, the interest is to detect and realize any available data projections referring to female substance addiction and feasible interventions from the legislative and health perspective (Home Ministry Government, 2010).

b. specific issues related to pregnancy and parenthood in substance abusing women from the medical-gynecological perspective, including all psychological aspects which might have an impact on the subsequent relationship with a child.

2.1 Substance abuse

All international data confirm a commonly shared view according to which male drug users outnumber women drug users by far (UNODC, 2004). However, recent research suggests that the gender gap may be narrowing, at least with reference to some types of drugs (EMCDDA 2006a). For example, for cannabis use and binge drinking, differences in drug use between men and women have substantially narrowed, at times showing an almost equal consumption between the genders. Another trend indicated a higher percentage of female rather than male students using tranquilizers or sedatives which are bought without prescription. Patterns of drug use based on gender differences are illustrated by the percentage of patients entering treatment services in Europe. The percentage of female patients is around 20% (EMCDDA 2005): among those receiving drug treatment, problems relating to amphetamine-type stimulant drugs (ATS) are most common among young people (under 20 years old), whereas problems relating to the use of sedatives or pharmaceutical drugs are most widespread among older patients (over 39 years old) (EMCDDA 2005).

With reference to intravenous drug use (IDU), the WHO reported a rapid increase in the rate of female IDUs in recent years, especially in Eastern Europe and Asia (Pinkham and Malinowska-Sempruch, 2007). According to available epidemiological data, women are more likely than men to abuse and become dependent on substances such as tranquilizers and sedatives when used without prescription (Simoni-Wastila et. al, 2004). It has also been shown that women typically become dependent on substances more quickly than men: this holds good for cannabis, cocaine and other stimulants, as well as opioids, inhalants and hallucinogens (UNODC, 2004).

With respect to "binge drinking"[1], an EMCDDA gender perspective report underlines that male predominance in general is lower in those countries where the prevalence of binge drinking is highest. Gender correlation with respect to cannabis use and binge drinking increases proportionally according to the increased use of those substances (EMCDDA, 2006a). Other studies show that in recent years, risky alcohol consumption has increased among young girls and adolescents (Anderson, Baumberg, 2006; O.N.Da, 2008).

Several studies suggest that women are more likely to use and abuse prescribed psychoactive drugs such as painkillers, sleeping pills and tranquillizers (EMCDDA, 2006a). This remark applies especially to opioids and depressants of the central nervous system. Sleeping-pill and anti-anxiety drug abuse is less visible than other, more common forms of addiction among women (PNS, 2008; Stocco, 2000). Actually, this seems related to the high incidence of depression or anxiety disorders in women (WHO, 2000). It is important to note that a lifetime prevalence of benzodiazepine use (for sleep or anxiety problems) without medical prescription among school students between the ages of 15 and 16 is significantly higher in females than in males (EMCDDA, 2006a).

2.2 Mental health and dual diagnosis

A high percentage of women substance users suffer from mental disorders. This specific type of diagnostic comorbidity, called *dual diagnosis*[2] was defined as the co-existence, in one

---

[1] Binge drinking is defined as a dangerous practice of consuming large quantities of alcoholic beverages in a single session. More specifically, experts agree that binge drinking occurs when one consumes 5 or more alcoholic drinks within a couple of hours.

[2] The term "comorbidity" was introduced by Feinstein and further specified by Klerman (1990) who used it to denote two or more disorders occurring at the same time or in the life course of one and the same subject. Cloninger (1990) stated that comorbidity implied the likeliness for a subject with a specific index disorder to develop a second disorder. Finally, Golberg (1996) very interestingly pointed out that it was only possible to talk of comorbidity when the assessed disorders were clearly distinct entities: symptoms of interrelated domains should not be classified as comorbidity. This clarification must be kept in mind since comorbidity only occurs when two different disorder categories can be recognized and described: however, it cannot be considered irrelevant that a "disorder" should be accompanied by symptoms or clusters of symptoms belonging to domains that are to a greater or lesser extent interrelated with the psychopathological domain of the index disorder. Rather, this reveals a "specific vulnerability" for a psychopathological development of the interrelated domain to reach disorder level and, therefore, comorbid condition (Di Sciascio, Nardini, 2005).

and the same subject, of a disorder related to psychoactive substance abuse and another psychiatric disorder (World Health Organization, WHO, 1995). As far as addiction is concerned, co-morbidity refers to the co-presence of a serious mental disorder and a disorder caused by substance abuse/dependence when such causality can be demonstrated (De Leon, 1989; Buckley, Brady, Hermann, 2010; Bobes, Casas, Szerman, 2009).

Dual diagnosis is more frequent among women than among men, particularly with regard to affective and anxiety disorders. Affective disorders (especially depression, moodiness and low self-esteem, loss of interest or pleasure in enjoyable activities) and anxiety disorders (excessive anxiety with physical and emotional effects such as apprehension, nervousness or fear) are common and serious pathologies to be treated in addicted women. A recent comprehensive study in United States confirmed that feelings of depression, hopelessness, sadness and suicidal ideation are more frequent in high school girls than in boys and that these feelings are more likely associated with a high risk for drinking and other drug use in girls (CASA 2003, cit. in Brady, Back, Greenfield, 2009). Also personality disorders (mostly Cluster B), posttraumatic stress disorders, suicide attempts and eating behavior disorders have to be treated in addict women. Schizophrenia and other psychotic symptoms are also frequent in women (Stocco et al., 2000, Instituto de la Mujer, 2007).

Particularly, exposure to trauma is a very frequent condition in drug-addicted women and it is the environmental basis for a posttraumatic stress disorder: sexual assault is the most frequent type of trauma experienced by women, but all different kinds of abuse are suffered by women before or during drug addiction. All in all, women are four times more likely to develop this disorder than men after exposure to traumatic events (Ciechanowski, 2010; Instituto de la Mujer, 2007)

Moreover, a lifetime prevalence of eating disorders (such as anorexia and bulimia) was found in women misusing substances: these disorders are thought to be behavioural patterns stemming from emotional conflicts that need to be solved so that the patient can develop a healthy relationship with food (Charles & Pull, 2004). Among psychiatric disorders, these are serious mental illnesses with a high incidence of co-morbidity and also with a high mortality rate (Ibidem).

Causes for high co-morbidity between substance misuse and mental health issues are not known and prevalence varies among different populations. Etiological theories in dual diagnosis include factors that are common to both disorders: a substance use disorder secondary to mental illness; a mental illness secondary to substance use, as well as bidirectional models. Women have more difficulties than men when treated for dual pathologies: these difficulties are related to drug addiction and mental illness. Drug addiction damage in a woman's body occurs earlier and more intensely than in men. Women seek treatment later than men, and addiction treatments do not often include a suitable program for dual diagnosis cases. In addition to this, women with mental illness usually suffer from some degree of impaired cognition. This makes them feel embarrassed, and contributes to a lack of compliance and difficulties when confronted with the need to change their lifestyle. Moreover, these women don't seek specific services: on the contrary, they usually prefer to see general practitioners. Women typically don't ask for mental or addiction treatments nor for social help. As a result, doctors that are unprepared to treat these cases may delay assistance (Instituto de la Mujer, 2007).

Finally, reference should be made to the co-dependence phenomenon (also called bi-dependence): more often than not, drug-addicted women experience problematic relationships with multi-problematic partners who also have drug- or alcohol-addiction problems (Moral Jiménez & Sirvent Ruiz, 2007).

2.3 Medical implications

Drug use, particularly intravenous drug use (IDU) remains one of the major risk factors for acquiring blood-borne infections for both men and women. With reference to the risk of infections related to sharing needles and other drug paraphernalia, it has been demonstrated that a significant number of women begin using drugs in the context of a sexual relationship (Unodc, 2004; Price & Simmel, 2002). Women are also more likely than men to borrow or share injection equipment, particularly with their sexual partners. They also often rely on men to acquire and inject them with drugs (Doherty et al. 2000; Vidal-Trecan at al, 1998, Pinkham et al. 2007). Women share needles with more people in their social network than men do (Sherman et al. 2001). This leads to an increased risk for acquiring blood-borne infections, particularly HIV and hepatitis C, which is generally very high among intravenous drug users.

Biological and social factors contribute to the increase of women drug users' risks for HIV. The overall data available for 25 European countries in 2005 showed that 35% of newly diagnosed cases of HIV were among women, reaching 41% in Eastern Europe, where the epidemic was mainly concentrated among IV drug users (Euro-HIV, 2007). Studies in nine EU countries showed that the average HIV prevalence was more than 50 percent higher among women IV drug users than among their male counterparts (EMCDDA, 2006). The correlation of IV drug use, sex work and unsafe sexual practices led to a significantly increased risk of HIV infection among women (UNODC, 2004).

Risk behaviour for infections needs to be considered not only with reference to HIV, but also to other blood-borne diseases such as Hepatitis C and B. Hepatitis C is the most common infectious disease among IV drug users, since it is transmitted through the sharing of needles, syringes and, unlike HIV, other injection-related equipment (Eurasian Harm Reduction Network (2007b). In 2006, the EMCDDA reported that median sero-prevalence of hepatitis C virus (HCV) is quite similar in male and female IV drug users: 58.1 % in males and 56.4 % in females. It is generally understood that it is more difficult to acquire HCV through sexual transmission than it is to acquire HIV. Infection among IV drug users will therefore be almost exclusively the result of sharing syringes and other injecting paraphernalia (EMCDDA, 2006).

2.4 Gender violence and social conditions

Neglect and abuse in childhood are common trends in the personal backgrounds of many female substance users.

European data estimates that one in five women experiences some form of physical or sexual violence (European Women's Lobby, 2001; Stocco, Llopis et al., 2000). In England and Wales alone, there were over 1 million female victims of domestic violence between 2009-2010. In the same area, every year over 300,000 women are sexually assaulted and 60,000 women are raped. Overall in the UK, more than one in four women experience domestic abuse during their lifetime (Home Minister Government, 2010)[3].

These women tend to define their substance use as the best coping mechanism available to them. Parental negligence and lack of attention in addition to the trauma of physical or sexual abuse make women more vulnerable to developing problems with substance abuse. In the absence of adequate support, such conditions can become a descending spiral (EMCDDA, 2009).

The link between substance use and gender violence/domestic abuse is complex. There is no reliable evidence of a cause-effect link between the two. However, where problems with substance use exist, domestic abuse is often present as well. Physical or sexual abuse on women is often perpetrated by a male partner or other male family members. Studies show that women with substance use problems are more likely than men to have experienced physical and/or sexual abuse (UNODC, 2004). A history of violence can have an impact on a woman's experience with substance abuse and mental health problems. Women who use substances are also more likely to live in environments where violence or sexual abuse is a common pattern: a study by Vogt (1998) and Zenken et Al. (2003) found that a significant background variable for female drug addiction are past experiences of violence, especially sexual exploitation. In line with this view, some Italian research studies have shown that about 50 % of young female drug users with anti-social behaviour and one-third of female psychiatric patients were victims of untreated sexual abuse during childhood (Gelinas, 1983; Malacrea, 2006).

Social, physical and psychological deprivations expose women to the influence and exploitation of male partners. Substance use can also drive women into sex work as a source of income (EMCDDA, 2009).

2.5 Pregnancy and parenthood

Women drug users who become pregnant form an additional sub-group requiring specific attention and care, both for them and for their babies (EMCDDA, 2006a). Drug use is associated with direct and indirect complications throughout pregnancy, postnatal morbidity and developmental delays (Hunter and Powis 1996): for instance, within the groups studied by Aronica et al. (1987) and by Palmieri (1991), 50% of the subjects were pregnant women with one or more children. Alleged reproduction difficulties in this population were attributed both to neuroendocrine alterations induced by substances such as heroin and opioids and to an irregular and inconstant lifestyle, alimentary deficits and poor hygienic, sanitary habits (Genazzani, 1987). However, neither of the two classes of factors seem to significantly reduce the chances for these subjects to bear children (Ibidem).

These women usually report deep feelings of anguish and dismay which build up their inner world, always suspended between impotence and manipulative, boundless omnipotence. Actually, addicted women often wish to get pregnant and bear a child as a form of vital defense or a redemption experience, even though this idealized view does not prevent the emergence of phases of anguish which are tied to the clashing of evidence against the ever incumbent denial of the event (Tempesta, et al., 1987). Evidence of this

---

[3] Figures from 2009/10 British Crime Survey data http://rds.homeoffice.gov.uk/rds/

denial can be found in the failed acknowledgement of a delayed period as a "sign" of pregnancy, the delay with which they finally resolve to taking a pregnancy test and, later on, their carelessness towards the fetus' needs (Tempesta et al., 1987). Moreover, these women often keep on using drugs during pregnancy while keeping their lifestyle unchanged for as long as possible, in homage to drug addiction homeostasis (Di Cagno et al., 1985). Even when drug consumption is discontinued during pregnancy, it is often resumed after delivery or during the postpartum period in an attempt to feel up to the new task and soothe the sense of guilt and failure.

In fact, for an addicted woman, delivery may imply having to cruelly realize what she was not able to do for her child and her negligence towards him/her: when real life needs become too hard, either because of the child's or the mother's difficulties or else for lack of a support network, the dream embodied in the fetus/child is shattered and heavy, depressive feelings may ensue which, up to that point, had been kept at bay by a megalomaniac investment on the child and on an idealized maternal image (De Zordo, 1997; Tempesta, et al., 1987).

No matter whether these women remain abstinent or else resume drug consumption, their difficulties in carrying out parenting functions emerge fairly early. Generally speaking, these mothers seem to find it difficult to build and maintain gratifying interpersonal relationships (with their partners and their families of origin), they tend to adopt a lifestyle leading to isolation and, above all, they have trouble in recognizing and satisfying their children's needs (Fiks, Johnson, Rosen, 1985). Their more or less conscious inadequacy in performing the parenting function has been suggested to derives from their early feelings and experiences: affective deprivation, losses, separations, lack of affective continuity in their families of origin (Johnson, Cohen, Brown, et al., 1999; Ravndal, Lauritzen, Frank, Jansson, Larsson, 2001). This inadequacy seems to be at the root of their educational style which is often characterized by an authoritarian overinvolment of the child: any external influence is rejected with a tendency to isolation, while the child is urged to become independent as quickly as possible and communication is controlled and avoided (Wellisch, Steinberg, 1980). Moreover, ambivalence seems to be a complex and typical feature of the relationships these mothers build with their children: they often expect them to take their mothers' expectations and wishes on themselves and consequently, they induce a role reversal and a process whereby these children are forced to think and act like adults, something they also experimented during their infantile past (Malagoli Togliatti, Mazzoni, 1993).

Finally, becoming a mother to a newborn does not coincide with a renewed motivation to seek counselling and/or treatment, rather, it strictly depends on a wide range of variables (McMahon, Luthar, 2000): according to the data available in the literature, mothers seem to be more prone to entering a detoxification and drug treatment when they are in young age, have more than one child, have got financial and legal problems, have suffered physical mistreatment and, above all, when they join advanced therapeutic programs (Grella et Al., 2006).

3. Children of drug-addicted mothers

It is indisputable that the development of children born from drug-addicted parents is highly at risk already before their birth, because the interaction of personal, relational and social factors does not support the individual's adjustment to his/her environment (see Nicolais, 2010). In this respect, Cicchetti and Rizley (1981) identify two categories of developmental risk factors: endogenous risk factors, such as physical or behavioral anomalies and psychological disorders, which make it difficult for the parent to take care of the child; exogenous risk factors, related to the environmental context in which the child is raised, such as features of his/her parents' personal histories, their psychological characteristics as well as ecological aspects of his life context or the one of the whole family. Both categories have become the subject of interest in several studies on this special children population.

3.1 Endogenous risk factors

Many research studies on children of addicted mothers, originally from US, focused on the harmful effects on the fetus following exposure to psychotropic substances, since recent data indicate that around 5% of all pregnant women aged between 15 and 44 years use substances (Substance Abuse and Mental Health Service Administration, 2005) which leads to the birth of approx. 375,000 babies with withdrawal symptoms every year.

In fact, psychoactive substances can have various harmful perinatal effects. Among others, the authors listed: rupture of the placenta and premature birth, low weight at birth and APGAR[4] scores below normal, low cranial circumference, the occurrence of perinatal stroke, congenital deformities and neurobehavioral disorders in newborns who had been exposed to cocaine and heroin during pregnancy (Lutinger, Graham, Einarson, Karen, 1991; Mayes, Granger, Bornstein, Zuckermann, 1992; Zuckerman, Bresnahan, 1991; Zuckerman et al., 1989). Moreover, the fetus can develop a dependency to the substances used by the mother: after delivery, when drug intake is abruptly discontinued, the baby runs the risk of undergoing real withdrawal crises (Foetal Drug Syndrome, FDS) which intensity may vary according to the used substance and its intake method (Finnegan, 1986; Zacchello, Giaquinto, 1997; Zuckerman, Brown, 1993).

Finally, it must be pointed out that many of these children test HIV-positive at birth: in most cases, remission occurs during the first months of life but for some of them, it is indicative of infection. Similar data are reported also for other infective pathologies such as hepatitis, syphilis, toxoplasmosis, cytomegalovirus (Zacchello, Giaquinto, 1997).

Later on, some studies report rhythm irregularities in the sleep-awake state and in food intake, as well as a tendency to hyperactivity (Zuckerman, 1994) already in early infancy. Learning difficulties, low attentive capacities and a higher degree of aggressiveness in

---

[4] Apgar: Abbreviation for the Apgar score, a practical method of evaluating the physical condition of a newborn infant shortly after birth. The Apgar score is a number arrived at by scoring the heart rate, respiratory effort, muscle tone, skin color, and response to a catheter in the nostril. Each of these signs can receive 0, 1, or 2 points. A perfect Apgar score of 10 means an infant is in the best possible condition. An infant with an Apgar score of 0-3 needs immediate intensive care. The Apgar score is measured routinely 60 seconds after delivery and then it is repeated after 5 minutes. In the event of a difficult resuscitation, the Apgar score may be done again at 10, 15, and 20 minutes. An Apgar score of 0-3 at 20 minutes of age is predictive of high morbidity (disease) and mortality (death). <http://www.medterms.com/script/main/art.asp?articlekey=2302>

preschool and school age (Cavazzuti, Frigieri, Finelli, 1987; Fundaro, Salvataggio, 1987; Oloffson, Buckley, 1983; Sanderegger, Zimmermann, 1978; Wilson, McCreary, Kean, Baxter, 1979) are also reported in these children, even if, compared to controls, neither differences in IQ levels nor alterations of intellectual functions are to be found (Azuma, Chasnoff, 1993). In this respect, Lester and Tronick (1994) offer an outlook on the effects of prenatal drug exposure which takes into consideration functional difficulties in the "4A" childhood areas (attention, arousal, affectivity and action). However, we should also remember the results of a research by Alessandri, Bendersky and Lewis (1998) revealing a correlation between the severity of the child's developmental deficit and the amount of substance (in their specific research, heroin) consumed by the mother during pregnancy. The neurobehavioral vulnerability which is typical of children who were exposed to drugs *in utero* must, therefore, be considered within a wider context including relational and environmental aspects too, two factors which also have an influence upon child development immediately after birth.

The clinical presentation of the "addicted babies" depends on the type of substances used by the mother during pregnancy, by value, frequency and time since last use / abuse. Substances commonly used by drug addicts are Alcohol, Nicotine, Marijuana, Tranquilizers, Cocaine and opioids in general, as well as 'heroin and methadone (Johnson & Kate, 2000; Lester & Barry, 2000). It was found that if the mother has made extensive use of drugs such as alcohol, hypnotics, or heroin–that could be considered "not exciting" the nervous system– the infant will manifest respiratory depression problems immediately after birth. Expressions of neonatal abstinence syndrome could be constant irritability, tremors and stiffness of muscle tone. Other possible symptoms include: irritability of the nervous system, gastrointestinal disorders, vomiting, diarrhea, hysterical crying, sleep disturbances, rapid breathing.

When we consider the effects of the substance exposure on the development of the child, the researches reveal that the global development is slowed and more in deficit at the cognitive level but not completely destroyed. In general, the child exposition to heroin and methadone during intrauterine development, is already evident after 48 hours of birth, while the exposure to the Alcohol leave marks immediate developing a real withdrawal syndrome. With reference to the specific symptoms related to different substances, many studies are interested to the exposure to Cocaine, that is a stimulant causing the blood vessels : this substance decreases the oxygen supply to the fetus and, consequently, the infant is at risk of suffocation. Also, the infants exposed to cocaine in the last gestational period reveal a state of reduced alertness and reduced responsiveness to external stimulation, when compared with controls.

In the table below are classified as such direct effects, distinguishing them according to the type of substance used by the mother (Wright & Walker, 2001).

3.2 Environmental factors: the attachment contribution

In addition to the various aspects highlighted in the studies mentioned above, we should not forget the multiple postnatal factors which contribute to determine the developmental outcomes of children who were born from drug-addicted parents.

The effect of drugs on mother and baby				
Drug	Antepartum	Intrapartum	Post-partum	Long term
Smoking	Growth restriction	Fetal Distress	Increases in Infant deaths	
Alcohol	Fetal Alcohol Syndrome		Maternal withdrawal symptoms	Fetal Alcohol syndrome Mental Impairment
Heroin / Opiates	Preterm Labor Growth restriction	Problem with analgesis	Neonatal abstinence syndrome	Probably not
Cocaine	Placental Pathology Growth Restriction Impaired brain development Abruption	Placental Pathology Low birth weight Fetal distress	Prolonged fetal withdrawal (3 days – 3 weeks) Chaotic lifestyle	Aggressive children Neurodevelopme ntal delay
Amphetamine	Growth restriction Maternal hypertension Antisocial behavior	Maternal cardiovascular disturbances	Chaotic lifestyle	
Ecstasy	Congenital defects			
Benzodiazepines	Cleft lip and palate			Neurodevelopme ntal delay

Table 1. The effect of drugs on mother and baby. Source: Wright & Walker, 2001

A large part of research in this domain have focused interest on the role of the quality of the proximal environmental factors on child development and well being; one of the most important factors that have an impact on child's early development is the quality of interactions and relations between child and the significant adults who play a protective role for him (the mother and/or other caregivers). In this perspective, the "Attachment theory" (Bowlby, 1969-1980) has provided useful theoretical and methodological tools to study the affective-relational development during the first years of life both in normal as well as in "at-risk" populations, in order to study the role of the quality of early interactions on the child well being and adaptation to the context.

According to this theoretical model, feeling safe and secure is the first and most important, early developmental task during the child's first year of life and one major protection factor in the process of adjusting himself/herself to the environment. Various research studies investigated the parent and child role and how they influenced the quality of the attachment bond: however, the contribution of each of the two parties is still not clear.

Van IJzendoorn, Goldberg, Kroonenberg, and Frenkel (1992) carried out a meta-analytical work on the influence of the child's and/or the parents' problems on the development of attachment during the first year of life. Attachment was assessed using the Strange Situation

Procedure[5] (Ainsworth, Blehar, Waters, Wall, 1978): researchers found a lower percentage of Secure attachment (B) and an increase in the Disorganized/Disoriented (D) category among samples of mother-child dyads at risk which differentiated them from the distributions observed in the general population. Moreover, a prevalent influence of maternal problems and difficulties rather than of children's endogenous risk factors came to light affecting the quality of infant-mother attachment. In fact, attachment distributions within groups of children of mistreating mothers (Carlson, Cicchetti, Barnett, Braunwald, 1989, Crittenden, 1985; Schneider-Rosen, Braunwald, Carlson, Cicchetti, 1985), mentally disturbed mothers or drug addicted mothers (Rodnig, Beckwith, Howard, 1989) revealed high divergence when compared to normative samples, more so than in case of problems coming from the child's side only. In fact, the child's problems did not seem to jeopardize the process of creating a secure attachment bond with the mother (van JIzendoorn et al., 1992).

Research studies with groups of parents suffering from psychiatric disorders, behavioral disorders or else mistreating their children seem to proceed along the same direction: once again, they reveal a high percentage of insecure attachment and, more specifically, entangled attachment (E) and unresolved attachment (U) tied to experiences of trauma and bereavement. These subjects seem to have difficulties in working through life experiences which they went through during childhood while their caregivers only proved to be scarcely adequate and supportive (van IJzendoorn, Bakermans-Kranenburg, 1996). Therefore, parents belonging to clinical populations do not seem to be emotionally secure, which represents a potential risk factor for their children, because of the process of intergenerational transmission of attachment, according to which the mother's representational world has got a fundamental role in the co-construction of a bond with the

---

[5] The Strange Situation is a standardized observation procedure (Ainsworth et al., 1978; Ainsworth, Wittig, 1969) which aims at activating and intensifying the child's attachment behavior towards his/her parent by exposing the child to a moderately, yet increasingly stressful situation. In fact, the Strange Situation takes place within a context – an observation laboratory – which is not familiar to the child: it foresees the presence of an unfamiliar adult and a series of two separations and reunions with the mother (or any other adult figure we might be interested in studying the child's attachment relationship with). This procedure is applicable to children between 12 and 24 months of age: between two subsequent administrations, a time interval of at least 6 months must be respected, so that the child can forget the situation and the stressful feelings tied with it (Ainsworth, 1985; Ainsworth, Bell, Stayton, 1971). The procedure is subdivided into eight short episodes, each of them lasting approximately three minutes and following one another according to a fixed order and a clearly stated consignment.
The SSP coding is based on the observation of the overall organization of a child's attachment behavior and foresees two assessment levels: the first one is based on graduated ordinal scales on a 7-point Likert scale (range 1 – 7), which refer to specific behavioral sequences the child can display in the various episodes. They can be applied to each procedure episode at 15-second intervals. The second level leads to the assignment of an attachment pattern according to four categories. It is based on the observation of the way in which the behavioral systems of attachment and exploration are organized during the whole procedure both towards the caregiver, as well as the stranger, while various stress elements are introduced, one after the other. The four categories are (Scheme 3): secure attachment (B) – research studies referring to "non-clinical" United States children show that between 54.9% and 67% of the population fall into this category; avoidant attachment (A) is observed in an average range of 20.5% - 22.9% of the population. Resistant attachment (C) is less frequent among the population (7.5% -12.5%), while disorganized/disoriented attachment (D) is observed in 14.7% of the children (van IJzendoorn, Goldberg, Kroonenberg, Frenkel, 1992).

child (Benoit, Parker, 1994; Fonagy, Steele, Steele, 1991; Ward, Carlson, 1995; van IJzendoorn, Bakermans-Kranenburg, 1997; Zeanah, 1992).

4. Therapeutic communities and the intervention model in Italy: an overview

In Europe, during the past years, referral to Juvenile Court was the most commonly applied procedure to drug-addicted mothers (Pomodoro, 1993, 1996). More often than not, these cases resulted in the suspension or revocation of parental rights, until the mother or both parents passed examinations which were required by the Court and administered by services in charge of evaluating and following the case. In case of substance addiction, a common solution during evaluation period was to separate the child from the mother (or both parents) and relocate him/her elsewhere, that is, for instance, at the grandparents' home, or else, at other out-patients services'. The first TC for mothers and children were founded in Switzerland, Germany and Italy in the early 1990s, then also in Spain and Portugal. Further solutions included admitting the child to family crisis intervention homes or placing the child in an extra-familial home or elsewhere, depending on the resources available in the territory. As for Italy, the juvenile judges' reluctance to place children in therapeutic communities – even though this would guarantee the presence of their mothers at their side – was justified by the fact that this environment – although run by professionals – did not seem to guarantee adequate attention to the child, nor did community workers seem to possess adequate training and the right methodological tools to operate for the well-being of the child and the mother-child couple. Therefore, more often than not, judges would take steps towards a separation of the mother-child dyad. These measures clearly indicated a lack of alternative possibilities within the enlarged network of fostering services but also un underlying prejudice towards drug-addicted parents who were considered "irredeemable" with regard to their capability to offer adequate care and protection to their children, especially in the very first years of their lives (Pomodoro, 1993, 1996). Confiding the child to his/her grandparents in foster care has become the most frequently adopted measure when one or both parents are drug-addict, even though this measure is still considered controversial as for its outcomes (Cirillo, 1996; Ghezzi, 1996). More specifically, criticism is raised towards its generalized and almost automatic use: if it is true, on the one hand, that it can provide an answer to the child's immediate need for protection, on the other hand it can turn into a very heavy obstacle against a possible recovery of the child's parents (Cirillo et Al., 1996). For this reason – as well as many others - the need has arisen for new intervention paths to be sought and experimented.

4.1 Therapeutic communities for drug-addicted women and their children

Over the past twenty years, the Veneto region has radically modified the functions of therapeutic communities for addicted mothers and their children, rethinking assessment and intervention measures in case of female drug addiction while paying special attention to children's well-being and to the results obtained in the short and long run. Communities for drug-addicted women and their children offer residential care to the mother-child dyad (sometimes to the father too) and provide a comprehensive rehabilitation program which takes place during a two-year stay. Many of these facilities are now present on the whole national territory: they greatly differ from each other in terms of constituent aspects which have now been included into a complex and articulated regulation that also leaves room for autonomous regional organization and definition (available places, internal arrangement, monthly fee etc.). These facilities can accommodate up to 10-12 dyads: as for the children's age, the range spans from few-months-old babies (but more and more often, pregnant women are admitted too) up to school age children. In the first place, communities give hospitality to drug-addicted women (already detoxified or on methadone therapy and followed by the "Ser.T.", territorial services), who are offered a comprehensive rehabilitation path

One further aspect of paramount importance is that, within a mother-child therapeutic community, addicted mothers are offered parenting support. Admitting the mother-child dyad into the community means guaranteeing an adequate intervention for the adult, while providing a protective environment for the child. Indeed, many of the problems associated with child development when a mother suffers from addiction can be addressed more easily and eventually solved once these children are offered an appropriate and stable relational context (Chasnoff, 1992). Moreover, a direct admittance of the mother-child dyad satisfies the need to overcome barriers between generations, since both the addicted woman's and her partner's families of origin are often not willing to help looking after the child. Moreover, it has been demonstrated how implementing assistance tools for children and families with a family-based approach prevents treatment dropouts (McComish, et al., 2000; Grella, et al., 2000). In fact, a droupout risk exists from the very first moment addicted mothers enter a therapeutic community, which is for them a very difficult step to take. These mothers fear that they might be labeled as incapable of caring for their children and consequently, that they have to be separated from them (National Institute on Drug Abuse, 1996; Stevens, et al., 1989).

As for the intervention methods, a combined treatment (that is, for the parent and the child together) is carried out on an intensive basis (the dyads are in residential care): in other words, it is typical of these communities to offer a therapeutic rehabilitation program which is centered on the family-parent-child system taken as a whole (Meisels, Dichtelmiller, Fong-Ruey Liaw, 1993). Usually, the mother is the primary focus of the intervention: however, special attention is given to the mother-child relationship too in all facilities offering support to the dyad. An intervention on the child is carried out only when it becomes clear that there is a need for it: in fact, in most cases, these children are physically and psychologically healthy but their caregiving environment reveals a symptomatology which must be tackled and solved. However, in recent times, greater and greater attention has been paid to ensuring the well-being of children living in therapeutic communities, since having a drug-addicted parent is indeed considered as a sort of risk factor in relation to the child's evolutionary path (Capra, 2011). The length of time mothers have to devote to their rehabilitation program actually affects children too. At a very early stage in their lives, when many new experiences should be made and new things should be learnt, they spend a long time at a therapeutic community's. Actually, already during the gestation period, they were exposed to the drugs consumed by the mother and often had to endure their mother's irregular alimentation and burdensome life rhythms. Even when delivery and the post partum period went well and without complications, during the first months of life most of these children experienced multiple separations from their mothers or closest caregivers, who were often scarcely respectful of their rhythms and needs. Others had to confront themselves with new people and environments: for instance, with specialized health care services, or else they had to meet social workers, psychologists or community workers.

Finally, some of them had to endure sudden changes in their daily life and moved to another house or a different town etc. Because of all this, one of the primary interventions in favor of children residing at a community's is to offer them stable life conditions, deep affective experiences as well as sound routine practices. With reference to the last mentioned aspect, communities seem to work as a place of physical and psychological attachment within which it becomes possible to create new and adequate affective relationships: all this is made possible thanks to the "holding" function supplied by the community as a context of early caregiving and a guarantee of protection from danger, as well as a secure base for the exploration of the environment. This concept of community allows us to consider it, all in all, as a parenting environment where the a growth towards motherhood can be followed and supported, where mothers are no longer blamed or punished for their inadequacy and difficulties but rather are offered a very important chance to experience regression to the role of daughters and children in need (who are taken care of by community workers, psychologists etc.). The chance to experience mixed feelings towards their institutional "parents" seems to make it possible for these women to trace down the relational and representational bonds which were cut short during their infancy and adolescence favoring a review of their own past which is very beneficial to the relationship with their children.

5. A research and intervention project on minors in therapeutic communities for addicted mothers and children

Until a few years ago, in Italy, communities for drug-addicted mothers and their children provided treatments to disintoxicate mothers and favour their rehabilitation into society, while also ensuring overall medical and social support for their children's development, for whom no specialized health treatment was foreseen (in case of need, treatment would be carried out by facilities outside of the community). However, in the last few years, a radical and much needed-for reorganization has come into effect in the field of residential and semi-residential services for drug-addicts and alcohol-addicts. More specifically, during the years 2006-2007 in North-Eastern Italy, new service units have been defined for addiction treatment, among others: swift admission services, semi-residential services, residential services (type A – B – C), type C1 (for drug-addicted mothers with minor children) and C2 (for drug-addicted minors). Moreover, requirements and standards authorizing socio-sanitary and social facilities to offer assistance have been redefined so as to bestow them recognition at institutional level. Over the years, especially in the Veneto region, it became clear that it was necessary to better define professional competences together with the methodological and organizational pre-requisites which are at the root of the intervention procedures in these specialized services. Treatment paths and management procedures within these services were redefined, whereby treatment must include a parallel series of medical-pharmacological, psychological and socio-educational interventions which are offered not only to the mother, but to the child too. Therefore, since 2008, the mother-child dyad and the quality of the caregiving relationship which develops between the two in the course of time have acquired prominent focus in the assessments and interventions by professionals who work in this specific field. The combination of all these assessment procedures is extremely important in order to arrange the best therapeutic and rehabilitation path for the mother who, up to that point, had been considered the sole subject to be taken therapeutic charge of in the community.

However, when minors are sent to therapeutic communities together with their mothers, this usually happens following a decree by a tutelary judge of the juvenile court so as to make sure that they receive protection and their psycho-physical health condition is assessed. For this reason, it was necessary to reconsider all areas of competence within direct and indirect interventions in favour of minors. Following this path, as of 2010, new socio-sanitary services for children in therapeutic communities type C1 have received official recognition. They are conducted by health professionals and technicians and foresee individualized interventions (individual psychological support, psychomotility , pet therapy), group psychomotility, clinical observation and assessment of the father-child and mother-child relationship, neuropsychiatric observation and assessment, mother-child relationship supervision and relational psychotherapy. Therefore, nowadays, not only are mothers but also their children officially considered clients of a community, where they are offered specific interventions of socio-psycho-physical health care.

It is not easy to combine clinical and rehabilitation activities with research. The authors have striven to set innovative research projects in motion which methodological principles are going to be described in the following pages. In so doing, we hope to stimulate cultural growth while improving care giving practices. The first, preliminary results are presented in this chapter.

The project "Research and intervention on minors in communities for drug-addicted mothers and their children: from at-risk parenting to child wellbeing" is the result of joint work carried out by the Psychology Department of the University of Padua and two therapeutic communities for addicted mothers and their children, *Villa Emma* and *Casa Aurora,* located in Venice and its mainland (Mestre) and run by the social cooperative *Villa Renata.*

The project provides a multi-method evaluation through a longitudinal approach aimed at programming and monitoring the interventions performed by parents while following the development of children living in therapeutic communities. Developmental risk factors and/or clinically relevant, real life symptoms are identified as they emerge. Our theoretical and methodological points of reference are based on the study of parenting and development according to the current, dynamic, multi-factor models of influence (Belsky, 1984; Gabble, Belsky, Crnic 1992; De Palo, 2010).

The setting of the project is the therapeutic community and its complex caregiving system. The focus of the assessment is set on three areas, each of which is investigated at different levels: (a) evaluation of the mother's psychic condition, in terms of personality and individual characteristics, assessed through interviews (such as the Adult Attachment Interview[6], SCID-II[7]), questionnaires and dynamic tests (Rorchach[8]); (b) evaluation of the

---

[6] **The Adult Attachment Interview** (AAI) developed by George, Kaplan and Main (1985) is a semi-structured interview assessing attachment in adolescence and adult age. The interview includes a series of questions through which a subject is asked to recall his/her attachment history and attachment experiences with his/her caregivers during infancy. The AAI coding scheme foresees two distinct phases: a first phase during which text content and form are analyzed through Evaluation Scales (Scales of Subjective Experience and Scales of the State of Mind) and a second phase during which the interview is analyzed as a whole in order to formulate a categorical classification of the subject's attachment.

mother's parenting capabilities as well as those of the father's (if present), through the observation of their interactions with the child both in daily routine exchanges and/or in structured settings (Attachment Q-Sort[9], Lausanne Trilogue Play[10], Emotional Availability Scales[11]); (c) evaluation of the child's development and adjustment through assessment measures for the developmental age (Vineland Scales[12], Child Behavior Check List[13], Attachment Story Completion Task[14]), aimed at identifying a developmental diagnosis according to the indications of the current 0-3 classification system for early infancy; (d) a comprehensive analysis of the progressive and current context of relations between caregiver and child, exploring limits and points of strength; (e) data obtained at various observational levels are shared by a professional team striving to achieve data integration so as to guarantee a very careful and comprehensive evaluation. Thanks to these organized data, it is possible to acquire a deeper knowledge and a better understanding of the

---

[7] **The Structured Clinical Interview for DSM-III-R** . The SCID-II (First, Gibbon, Spitzer, Williams, & Benjamin, 1997) allows diagnostic evaluations of a potential personality disorder such as the ones included on Axis II of DSM-IV, passive-aggressive and depressive disorders (Appendix B of DSM-IV) and unspecified personality disorder (UPD). The Italian version of the SCID for DSM-IV was published in 2003.

[8] **The Rorschach Test** (Rorschach, 1921) is a perception, projective, psycho-diagnostic instrument. It is composed of 10 standardized cards out of 23 (5 black and grey, 2 red and grey and 3 multi-coloured), each of them carrying a symmetric ink-blot. With this test, it is possible to observe both stable personality traits as well as a possible psychopathology or possible affective disorders. Moreover, this test offers very valuable information on the subject's intelligence and cognitive processes. As for data analysis and interpretation, they are carried out both at quantitative and at qualitative level.

[9] **The Attachment Q-Sort** (Waters, & Deane, 1985) allows repeated data acquisition over one single week, so as to compare the attachment bonds created by the child with his/her caregivers, as well as a measurement of children's attachment over a longer period of time (from 1 to 5 years). The AQS comprises 90 items which describe a child's attachment behaviours in his/her natural, everyday home environment.

[10] **The Lausanne Trilogue Play** (LTP, Fivaz-Depeursinge, Corboz-Warnery, 1999) is a semi-standardized, laboratory, play procedure during which mother, father and child interact. This procedure allows observation and evaluation of the quality of interactions within the mother-father-child family system during a play interaction where all three partners are involved at the same time. The coding scheme of the LTP procedure is made up of 10 scales, each of them defining an observation variable (Lavanchy, Cunnet, Favez, 2006). They are graduated on a 5-point Likert Scale (range 1 – 5) and coded for each of the four parts of the procedure.

[11] **Emotional Availability Scales** (EAS, Biringen Robison Emde, 1998) Interactive adult-child video-recordings are observed and evaluated according to the adult's sensitivity, his/her capacity to frame the environment, his/her non-intrusiveness and non-hostility. The child's involvement and his/her replies to the adult are evaluated too.

[12] **The Vineland scales** allow measurement – by means of a semi-structured interview –of 4 main dimensions (scales) and 11 sub-dimensions (subscales). They can find application in various clinical, educational and research settings: they are particularly useful to observe adaptive behaviours and to investigate to what degree a disability, if present, can have an impact on the subject's everyday performances.

[13] **Child Behavior Check List Achenbach CBCL** (1991, 1992) This scale allows to investigate social competencies and behavioural problems in children aged 18 months - 18 years. Its items favour a description of the child's behavioural and emotional repertoire through the narratives supplied by parents, teachers and/or educators supporting the evaluation of a potentially problematic conduct as listed in the behavioural scales.

[14] The **Attachment Story Completion Task** (ASCT; Bretherton, Ridgeway, Cassidy, 1990) was designed to assess attachment style in preschool and school age. Five story stems referring to attachment-relevant family themes are presented to the child who is asked to complete them freely using a set of dolls and props.

1st PHASE	Assessment of mother's parental capabilities		
OBJECTIVE	Investigate mother's personality characteristics and her attachment history since these are indexes of her parental competence.		
INVESTIGATED AREAS	Personality ↓	Pathology self-perception ↓	Attachment ↓
MEASURES	Rorschach Test	SCID II (Structured Clinical Interview for DSM-IV)	AAI (Adult Attachment Interview)
2nd PHASE	a) Indirect assessment of the child (through mothers/educators)		
OBJECTIVE	1) Evaluation of the child's relational and developmental competencies and psychopathological aspects 2)Give mothers a chance to compare and share their perceptions of their children with those of the educators, so as to find a common language on the main topics referring to the children		
INVESTIGATED AREAS	Development ↓	Symptomatology ↓	Attachment relationship ↓
MEASURES	VABS (Vineland Adaptive Behavior Scales)	CBCL (Child Behavior Checklist)	AQS (Attachment Q-Sort)
	b) Assessment of adult-child relationships		
OBJECTIVE	1) Observation and evaluation of the mother-child dyadic relationship (if possible, the father-child relationship too) then comparison with the educator-child dyadic relationship 2) If possible, observation and evaluation of the mother -father -child triadic relationship		
OBSERVED RELATIONSHIPS	Mother-Child Educator-Child Father-Child		Mother-Father-Child
MEASURES	EAS (Emotional Availability Scales)		LTP (Lausanne Trilogue Play).
3rd PHASE	Direct assessment of the child		
	This investigation is only carried out on children who show dysfunctional or pathological characteristics during screening phase 2		

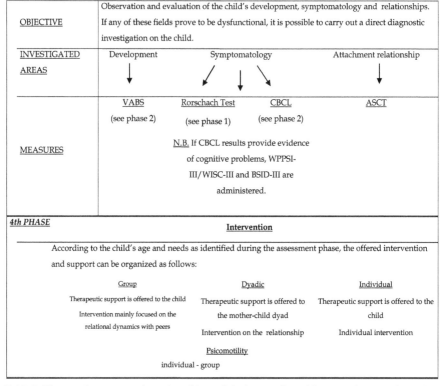

OBJECTIVE	Observation and evaluation of the child's development, symptomatology and relationships. If any of these fields prove to be dysfunctional, it is possible to carry out a direct diagnostic investigation on the child.		
INVESTIGATED AREAS	Development	Symptomatology	Attachment relationship
MEASURES	VABS (see phase 2)	Rorschach Test (see phase 1) CBCL (see phase 2) N.B. If CBCL results provide evidence of cognitive problems, WPPSI-III/WISC-III and BSID-III are administered.	ASCT

4th PHASE	**Intervention**	
	According to the child's age and needs as identified during the assessment phase, the offered intervention and support can be organized as follows:	
Group	Dyadic	Individual
Therapeutic support is offered to the child	Therapeutic support is offered to the mother-child dyad	Therapeutic support is offered to the child
Intervention mainly focused on the relational dynamics with peers	Intervention on the relationship	Individual intervention
	Psicomotility individual - group	

Table 2. Phases of our research project: "A model of research and intervention on minors in communities for drug-addicted mothers and their children: from at-risk parenting to child wellbeing".

caregiver, the child and their relationship: these data also help professionals to more clearly identify the therapeutic and pedagogical objectives to be suggested to the dyad, which can then be supported and monitored over time. These objectives can be modified and re-elaborated according to each individual project but also to the changes observed during the intervention. In fact, the same evaluation procedure is administered at different times during the mother-child residential period. It aims at monitoring the interventions and any possible change as well as identifying eventual aspects of danger and/or increased risk that may require the use of further community facilities. A continuous assessment of the intervention is a powerful instrument to reflect, both clinically and ethically, on the opportunity to go on providing care to mother-child pairs featuring elements of danger and pathology. This assessment also examines the presence of prejudicial clinical manifestations of the child and any developmental difficulties related to inadequate maternal care which can arise in spite of the protective and rehabilitative intervention provided by the community and its comprehensive setting. In 2010, we started gathering data which are presently being processed and which will be described in depth in this chapter.

6. Conclusions

Our project started in 2009: the following, preliminary results are now available (De Palo, Simonelli, Capra, 2010). Twenty-four mothers took part to the program: they were evaluated according to the 1st phase protocol. The reported data refer to the first twelve of them, whom data have already been processed for. Generally speaking, 31 is their mean age: they entered the community at different times from 2007 to 2010. Most of them started consuming substances during pre-adolescence/adolescence (12-19 years).

The first aspect refers to personality diagnosis: 10 subjects were diagnosed a structure of personality with borderline features (polydrug use of psychotropic substances with heroin as the main substance of abuse). This characteristic shows a clinically significant association with some other investigated aspects, particularly, with an insecure attachment style which is prevalent within the group and which seems to be rooted in experiences of traumatic and/or doleful events during these women's infancy, especially physical and sexual abuse which most of them experienced in intra-familial environments. Moreover, their attachment style, which developed on the basis of their infantile experiences with their caregivers, is associated to disorganization characteristics and a difficulty to work through early experiences of loss or trauma. The educational style they experienced in their families of origin was predominantly coercive. To sum up, at exploratory level we can say that, in the mothers accommodated at the community, we notice associations between early traumatic events (coercive educational style and abuse) experienced within their families of origin, an insecure working-through of their own attachment history and borderline personality features. These results urge us towards a reflection on feasible intervention methods for patients presenting similar clinical pictures where drug-addiction almost seems just a symptom of a more complex pathology. At the same time, this reflection seems of paramount importance to globally re-think interventions in favor of minors living in the community: in fact, shouldn't the fact of being born to mothers with similar characteristics be considered in itself a vulnerability factor which shall issue to psychopathology?

We believe that a possible answer can be found within the described project, since the main objective of our research and intervention model is to observe the child's level of development and the risk and protective factors characterizing his/her growth so as to plan taylor-made interventions to satisfy each single minor client's needs and support each single mother-child relationship. Therefore, within the model we presented in this paper, attention is focused on the well-being of minors who were born to drug-addicted mothers. Reason for this choice is the unavoidable need to carefully and realistically consider the condition of these children: their drug-addicted mothers present an at-risk parenting function and are therefore supported by educators who play the role of more adequate, alternative caregivers. The "adolescent" aspect of drug-addicted women can be a major risk factor against the assumption of their parental role: these mothers are often envious of the therapeutic support which is given to the child and which develops in a situation of conflict between mother and child. Moreover, these patients often have great difficulties in acknowledging limits, even physical ones, between their child and themselves: these mothers often find it hard to distinguish themselves from their child, especially if it is a female child, and they mix up their thoughts, actions and feelings with those of their daughters. When they have a male child, they find it difficult to differentiate their sons from their own fathers or partners. Therefore, by choosing to set up a project on minors' health, all research objectives are focused on the viable, most adequate actions to be taken in order to achieve the set goal, that is, the well-being of children born to adults with parenting function at risk.

To this extent, a parallel administration of evaluation measures both to the mother and to the educator makes it possible to investigate what is the latter's (and the community's) image of the child. Carefully monitoring the idea the community has of a child makes it possible to create a univocal perception of him/her which otherwise gets lost in the various circumstances characterizing the community environment. The attention educators continuously devote to the child is shared with the mother, with whom they strive to create a univocal, shared image of the minor. Actually, within a community for drug-addicted mothers and their children, both educators and the very treating team perform the function of secure base which neither the mother nor the child have found elsewhere: they offer an alternative and vicarious relational model both to women and their children. Since educators possess characteristics that are typical of early caregivers (closeness, continuous presence, responsiveness etc.), they often find themselves emotionally involved in the relationship with the child: for this reason, their continuous training and supervision aim at helping them to stick to their professional role, without wanting to replace the mother's role.

7. References

Achenbach, T.M. (1991). Manual for the Child Behavior Check List/4-18 and 1991 Profile. Burlington: University of Vermont.

Achenbach, T.M. (1992). Manual for the Child Behavior Check List/2-3 and 1992 Profile. Burlington: University of Vermont.

Ainsworth, M. D. S. (1985). Patterns of infant-mother attachment: antecedents and effects on development. Bulletin of the New York Academy of Medicine, 61, 771-791

Ainsworth, M. D. S, Wittig B. A. (1969). Attachment and exploratory behavior of one-year-olds in a strange-situation. In B. M. Foss (Eds), Determinants of infant behavior IV, Methuen, London, 113-136.

Ainsworth, M. D. S., Bell, S. M., Stayton, D. J. (1971). Infant-mother attachment and social development: socialization as a product of reciprocal responsiveness to signals. In M. P. M. Richards (Eds) (1971). The integration of a child into a social world, Cambridge University Press, London, 99-135

Ainsworth, M. D. S., Blehar, M. C., Waters, E., & Wall, S. (1978). Patterns of attachment: A psychological study of the strange situation. Hillsdale, NJ: Erlbaum.

Alessandri S. M., Bendersky, M., Lewis, M. (1998). Cognitive functioning in 8- to 18-month-old drug-exposed infants, Dev Psychol. 1998 May;34(3):565-73. Retrieved from <http://www.ncbi.nlm.nih.gov/pmc/articles/PMC1531636/?tool=pubmed>

Anderson, P., & Baumberg, B. (2006). Alcohol in Europe. A public health perspective. Analysis for the European Commission. Institute of Alcohol Studies, UK. Retrieved from <http://ec.europa.eu/health/ph_determinants/life_style/alcohol/documents/alcohol_europe.pdf >

Aronica E. et Al. (1987). Il rapporto tra donna e droga. Alla ricerca di possibili differenze e specificità. Atti del Convegno "La donna e l'eroina". Torino: CIC Ed. Internaz.

Associazione Parsec (2004, April, 16). In-Dipendenza Donna: Workshop su Tossicodipendenza e Maternità, Paper presented at meeting of Istituto Superiore di Sanità, Roma.

Azuma, C.D., & Chasnoff, I. J. (1993). Outcome of children prenatally exposed to cocaine and other drugs: A path analysis of three-year data. Pediatrics, 92(3), 396-402.

Belsky, J. (1984). The Determinants of Parenting: A Process Model. Child Development, 55, 83-96

Benoit, D., & Parker, K.C.H. (1994). Stability and Transmission of Attachment across Three Generations. Child Devolopment, 65, 1444-1456.

Biringen, Z., Robinson, J., & Emde, R.N. (1998). The emotional availability scales (3rd ed.). Unpublished manuscript, Department of Human Development & Family Studies, Colorado State University, Fort Collins, CO.

Bobes J., Casas M., Szerman N. et al. (2009). "Manejo clínico del paciente con patología dual. Recomendaciones de expertos". In Socidrogalcohol. Valencia. Retrieved from <www.socidrogalcohol.org>

Bowlby, J. (1969). Attachment: Attachment and Loss (Vol. 1). New York: Basic Books (trad. it. Attaccamento e perdita (Vol. 1): L'attaccamento alla madre, Boringhieri, Torino 1972.)

Bowlby, J. (1973). Separation: Anxiety & Anger: Attachment and Loss (Vol. 2). London: Hogarth Press (trad. it. Attaccamento e perdita (Vol. 2): La separazione dalla madre, Boringhieri, Torino, 1975).

Bowlby, J. (1980). Loss: Sadness & Depression: Attachment and Loss (Vol. 3). London: Hogarth Press (trad. it. Attaccamento e perdita (Vol. 3): La perdita della madre, Boringhieri, Torino, 1983.)

Brentari, C., Herrera Hernandez, B., Tripodi, S. (2011, in press). Attention to Women Drug Users in Europe, Guidelines of the "Democracy, Cities and Drugs II" Project. A Public Health Executive Agency project. Retrieved from <www.democitydrug.org>

Bretherton, I., Ridgeway, D., & Cassidy, J. (1990). Assessing internal working models of the attachment relationships: An Attachment Story Completion Task for 3-year-olds. In M.T. Greenberg, D. Cicchetti, & E.M. Cummings (Eds.), Attachment in the preschool years: Theory, research, and intervention (pp. 273-308). Chicago: University of Chicago Press.

Buckley, P., Brady, K., & Hermann, R.. (2010). Dual diagnosis: Severe mental illness and substance use disorders. UpToDate, Inc. MA. Online 18.2:, Retrieved from <www.uptodate.com>

Capra, N. (2011). Presentazione del progetto terapeutico di presa in carico residenziale in comunità per madri tossicodipendenti e i loro figli. Paper presented at International conference "L'esposizione dei minori alle droghe: dalla vita prenatale all'adolescenza", February 24-26 2011 Padova, Italy.

Carlson, V., Cicchetti, D., Barnett, D., & Braunwald, K. (1989). Disorganized/disoriented attachment relationships in maltreated infants. Developmental Psychology, 25, 525-531.

Cavazzuti, G.B., Frigieri, G., & Finelli, P. (1987). Il follow up del bambino nato da madre farmacodipendente. Bollettino per le farmacodipendenze e l'Alcolismo, 10(6), 20-28.

Charles Pull, C.B., (2004). Binge Eating Disorder. Current Opinion in Psychiatry, 17(1), 43-48.

Chasnoff, I.J. (1992). Cocaine, pregnancy, and the growing child. Current Problems in Pediatrics, 22, 302–321.

Cicchetti, D., & Rizley, R. (1981). Developmental perspective on the etiology,Intergenerational trasmission and Sequelae un Child Abuse and Neglect. Journal of American Accademy of Child Adolescent Psychiatry, 34, 541-565.

Ciechanowski, P., Katon W., Stein, B.M., & Hermann R. (2010), Post-traumatic stress disorder: Epidemiology, pathophysiology, clinical manifestations, and diagnosis, UpToDate, Inc. MA. Retrieved from <www.uptodate.com>

Cirillo S. et Al., (1996), La famiglia del tossicodipendente, Cortina, Milano

Cloninger, C. (1990). The empirical structure of psychiatric comorbidity and its theoretical significance. US: American Psychiatric Association.

Crittenden, P.M. (1985). Maltreated infants: Vulnerability and resilience. Journal of Child Psychology and Psychiatry, 26, 85-96.

De Leon, G. (1989). Psychopathology and substance abuse and psychiatric disorders: what is being learned from research in therapeutic community. Journal of psychoactive drugs, 21, 177/188.

De Palo, F. (2010). The trasmission gap: quali influenze familiari e contestuali nel passaggio tra rappresentazioni dell'adulto e comportamenti di attaccamento del bambino. Ph.D. Thesis. Milan University

De Palo, F., Simonelli, A., & Capra, N. (2010). Madri tossicodipendenti: attaccamento personalità e trattamenti possibili. Paper presented at "Congresso Nazionale dell'Associazione Italiana di Psicologia (AIP) – Sezione di psicologia clinica" September 24-26 2010. Università degli Studi di Torino.

De Zordo, M.R. (1997). Genitori e bambini: genitori-bambini. In G. Fava Vizziello & P. Stocco (Eds.), Tra genitori e figli la tossicodipendenza (pp. 103-120). Milano: Masson.

Di Cagno, L., et al. (1985). Distorsione della relazione oggettuale e persistente della tossicodipendenza. Giornale di Neuropsichiatria dell'Età Evolutiva, 5,(2) 133-138.

Di Sciascio, G., & Nardini, M. (2005). Comorbidità fra disturbi mentali e dipendenze patologiche: il problema della cosiddetta "Doppia Diagnosi". DITE-Edizioni Scientifiche.

Doherty, M.C., Garfein, R.S., Monterroso, E., Latkin, C., & Vlahov, D. (2000). Gender difference in the initiation of injecting drug use among young adults. Journal of Urban Health, 77(3), 397

Eurasian Harm Reduction Network. (2007). Hepatitis C among Injecting Drug Users in the New EU Member States and Neighboring Countries. Situation, Guidelines and Recommendations. Vilnius: Eurasian Harm Reduction Network.

EuroHIV. (2007). HIV / AIDS Surveillance in Europe, Mid-year report 2006, No. 74. French Institute for Public Health Surveillance, Saint-Maurice.

European Monitoring Centre for Drugs and Drug Addiction (EMCDDA). (2005). Differences in patterns of drug use between women and men. Paper presented at meeting of European Drug Situation, Lisbon. Retrieved September 10, 2010 from <http://www.emcdda.europa.eu/html.cfm/index34278EN.html>

European Monitoring Centre for Drugs and Drug Addiction (EMCDDA) (2006). The state of the drugs problem in Europe. Annual report. EMCDDA. Luxembourg: Publications Office of the European Union.

European Monitoring Centre for Drugs and Drug Addiction (EMCDDA) (2006a). A gender perspective on drug use and responding to drug problems. Paper presented at meeting of European Drug Situation, Lisbon.

EMCDDA (European Monitoring Center for Drugs and Drug Addiction) (2009). The State of the Drugs Problems in Europe. Annual Report. Luxembourg: Publications Office of the European Union, 2009 — ISBN 978-92-9168-384-0

European Women's Lobby (2001), Young Women's Guide to Equality between Women and Men in Europe, EWL- LEF, Brussels, Retrieved from
<http://www.womenlobby.org>

Ficks, K.B., Johnson, H.L., & Rosen, T.S. (1985) Methadone-Mantained Mothers: Three-Year Follow-up of Parental Functioning. The international journal of the addiction, 20(5), 45-57.

Finnegan, 1986. Neonatal Abstinence Syndrome (NAS) Clinical Presentation and Management.

First, M.B., Gibbon, M., Spitzer, R.L., Williams, J.B.W., & Benjamin, L.S. (1997). Structured Clinical Interview for DSM-IV Axis II Personality Disorders, (SCID-II). Washington: American Psychiatric Press.

Fivaz-Depeursinge, E., & Corboz-Warnery, A. (1999). The Primary Triangle: A develompmental system view of fathers, mothers and infants. New York: Basic Books. (Trad. it. Il triangolo primario: Le prime interazioni triadiche tra padre, madre e bambino, Cortina, Milano, 2002).

Fonagy, P., Steele, M., & Steele, H. 1991, Maternal representation of attachment during pregnancy predict the organisation of infant-mother attachment at one year of age. Child Development, 62, 891-905.

Fundaro, C. & Salvataggio, E. 1987, Lo sviluppo del bambino di madre tossicodipendente. Bollettino per le Farmacodipendenze e l'Alcolismo, X, 6.

Gable, S., Belsky, J., & Crnic, K. (1992). Marriage, Parenting, and Child Development: Progress and Prospects. Journal of Family Psychology, 5, 276-294.

Ghezzi, D., & Vadilonga, F.1996, (Eds.) La tutela del minore. Milano: Raffaello Cortina Editore.

Gelinas, D. (1983). "The persisting negative effects of incest". Psychiatry, 46, p. 312-332

George, C., Kaplan, N., & Main, M. (1985). Adult Attachment Interview. Unpublished manuscript, Department of Psychology, University of California, Berkeley.

Genazzani, A.R., Santoro, V., Carino, M., Golinelli, S., Maietta Latessa, A., & Volpe, A. (1987). Riproduzione e farmacodipendenza. Bollettino Farmacologico e Alcol, 6, 609-615.

Goldberg, D. (1996), A dimensional model for common mental disorders, British Journal of Psychiatry, Vol 168 (Suppl 30), Jul 1996, 44-49.

Grella, C.E., Joshi, V., & Hser, Y.I. (2000). Program variation in treatment outcomes among women in residential drug treatment. Evaluation Review, 24(4), 364-383.

Grella, C.E., Hser, Y,I., Huang, Y.C. (2006). Mothers in substance abuse treatment: differences in characteristics based on involvement with child welfare services, Child Abuse Neglect, Jan; 30(1), 55-73.

Home Ministry Government (2010). Call to End Violence against Women and Girls, ISBN: 978-1-84987-377-2, London, Retrieved from <http://www.homeoffice.gov.uk/publications/crime/call-end-violence-women-girls/vawg-paper?view=Binary>

Hunter G and Powis B., (1996). Women drug users: barriers to service use, and service needs. The Centre for Research on Drugs and Health Behaviour: Executive Summary, 47, 1996

Instituto de la Mujer. (2007). Ministerio de Trabajo y Asuntos Sociales. Intervención en drogodependencias con enfoque de género. Nipo: 207-07-132-8. Madrid. Retrieved from <http://www.mtas.es/mujer>

Ijzendoorn M. H. Van, Goldberg S., Kroonenberg P. M., Frenkel O. J. (1992). The relative effects of maternal and child problems on the quality of attachment: a meta-analysis of attachment in clinical samples, Child Development , 63, 840-858

Johnson, J., G., Cohen, P., Brown, J., et al. (1999). Childhood maltreatment increases risk for personality disorders during early adulthood. Archives of General Psychiatry, 56, 600-606.

Johnson, K. (2000). Prenatal Cigarette, Cocaine Exposure Tied to Language Problems. OB GYN News, 35, 13.

Klerman, G.L. (1990). Approaches to the phenomena of comorbidity. American Psychiatric Association, US

Lavancy, C., Cuennet & Favez, N. (2006). Coding manual for Family Alliance Assessment Scale (Evaluation grid of the Lausanne Triadic Play). Fourth version. Manoscritto non pubblicato. Centre d'Etude de la Famille (CEF). Lausanne.

Lester, B. M. & Tronick, E. Z. 1994, The effects of prenatal cocaine exposure and child outcome. Infant Mentaal Health Journal, 15(2), 107-120.

Lester, Barry. (2000). Drug-addicted Mothers Need Treatment, Not Punishment. Alcoholism & Drug Abuse Weekly, 12, 5.

Malacrea, M., (2006). Caratteristiche, dinamiche ed effetti della violenza su bambini e bambine", In: Bianchi, D., Moretti, E., (2006). Vite in bilico. Indagine retrospettiva su maltrattamenti e abusi in età infantile. Ministero della Solidarietà Sociale, Centro Nazionale Documentazione e Analisi per l'Infanzia e l'Adolescenza. Retrieved from <http://ems.cilea.it/archive/00000763/01/Vite_in_bilico_Q40.pdf>

Malagoli Togliatti, M., Mazzoni, S. (1993). Maternità e tossicodipendenza. Milano: Giuffrè

Mayes, L. C., Granger, R. H., Bornstein, M. H., & Zuckerman, B. 1992, The problem of prenatal cocaine exposure: A rush to judgment. Journal of the American Medical Association, 267, 406-408

McComish, J.F., Greenberg, R., Ager, J., Chruscial, H., & Laken, M. (2000). Survival analysis of three treatment modalities in a residential substance abuse program for women and their children. Outcomes Management for Nursing Practice, 4(2), 71-77.

McMahon, T.J., Luthar, S.S. (2000). "Women in Treatment: Within-Gender Differences in the Clinical Presentation of Opioid-Dependent Women", In Journal of Nervous & Mental Disease: October 2000 - Volume 188 - Issue 10 - pp 679-687

Meisels, S. J., Dichtelmiller, M., & Fong-Ruey L. (1993). Un'analisi multidimansionale dei programmi di intervento per la prima infanzia. In C.H. Zeanah (Ed.), Manuale di salute mentale infantile (pp.317-339). Milano: Masson.

Ministero della Salute (2010). Rilevazione attività nel settore tossicodipendenze: Anno 2008. Retrieved October 3, 2010, Retrieved from <http://www.salute.gov.it/imgs/C_17_pubblicazioni_1306_allegato.pdf>

Moral Jiménez, M., Sirvent Ruiz, C. (2007). Codependence and Gender: exploratory analysis in differences in tds- 100 symptomatic factors. 8° Congreso Vrtual de Psiquiatría. Interpsiquis Febrero 2007. Psiquiatria.com, Retrieved from <http://www.fispiral.com/wp/wp-content/uploads/2012/01/21.pdf>

National Institute on Drug Abuse (NIDA) (1996). National pregnancy and health survey: Drug Use Among Women Delivering Livebirths. Rockville, MD: National Institutes of Health Publications.

NSW Department for Women, Young Women's health: depression and risk taking behavior. Retrieved from <www.women.nsw.gov.au/pdf/young_womens_health>

Oloffson, M. & Buckley,W. (1983). Investigation of 85 children born by drug-addicted mothers. II Follow up 1-10 years after birth. Acta Pediatr. Scand., 72, 407-413.

O.N.Da. (Osservatorio Nazionale sulla salute della Donna). (2008). La Salute della Donna. Proposte, strategie, provvedimenti per migliorarla. Libro verde, FrancoAngeli Milano

OTIS (Organization of Teratology Information Specialists) (2010), O.T.I.S. Fact Sheets ©. Retrieved from <http://www.otispregnancy.org/otis-fact-sheets-s13037#6>

Palmieri, V. (1991). Osservazione e analisi del tossicodipendente detenuto. Progetto carcere: Quaderni della Fondazione Villa Maraini, 1, Roma.

Pinkham S., Malinowska-Sempruch K. (2007). Women, Harm Reduction, and HIV. New York: International Harm Reduction Development Program of the Open Society Institute. Retrieved from <http://www.idpc.net/sites/default/files/library/IHRD_WomenHRHIV_EN.pdf>

Pomodoro, L. (1993). Aspetti giuridici. In M. Malagoli Togliatti & S. Mazzoni (Eds.), Maternità e tossicodipendenza (pp.13-24). Milano: Giuffrè.

Pomodoro, L. (1996). Introduzione. In D. Ghezzi & F. Vadilonga (Eds.), La tutela del minore (pp.1-13). Milano: Raffaello Cortina Editore.

PNS: Ministerio del Interior (Delegación del Gobierno para el Plan Nacional sobre Drogas) (2000 – 2008). Estrategia Nacional Sobre Drogas. España. NIPO: 126-99-041-3.

Price A. and Simmel C. (2002). Partners' Influence on Women's Addiction and Recovery: the Connection Between Substance Abuse, Trauma and Intimate Relationships (Berkeley, California, National Abandoned Infants Assistance Resource Center, School of Social Welfare, University of California at Berkeley, 2002). Retrieved from <http://aia.berkeley.edu/media/pdf/partners.pdf>

Ravndal, E., Lauritzen, G., Frank,O., Jansson, I., Larsson, J. (2001). "Childhood maltreatment among Norwegian drug abusers in treatment". In International Journal of Social Welfare, 10, 142-147.

Rorschach, H. [1921] (1932). W. Morgenthaler (Ed.), Psychodiagnostik (2nd ed.). Bern-Berlin: Hans Huber (trad. it. Psicodiagnostica, Kappa, Roma, 1981).

Rodning, C., Beckwith, L., & Howard, J. (1989). Characteristics of attachment organization and play organization in prenatally drug-exposed toddlers. Development and Psychopathology, 1, 277-289.

Sanderegger,T. & Zimmermann, E. 1978, Adult behavior and adrenocortical function following neonatal morphine treatment in rats. Psychopharm., 56, 103-109.

Schneider-Rosen, K., Braunwald, K. G., Carlson,V., & Cicchetti, D. (1985). Current perspectives in attachment theory: Illustration from the study of maltreated infants. In I. Bretherton & E. Waters (Eds.), Growing points of attachment theory and research. Monographs of the society for research in child development, 50(209), 194-210.

Sherman, S. G., Latkin, C. A., & Gielen, A.C. Social factors related to syringe sharing among injecting partners: a focus on gender, Substance Use and Misuse, vol. 36, No. 14 (2001), pp. 2113-2136.

Simoni-Wastila, L., Ritter, G., & Strickler, G. (2004). Gender and other factors associated with the nonmedical use of abusable prescription drug. Substance Use and Misuse, 39(1), 1-23.

Stevens, S., Arbiter, N., & Glider, P. (1989). Women residents: Expanding their role to increase treatment effectiveness in substance abuse programs. International Journal of the Addictions, 24, 425-434.

Stocco, P., Llopis Llacer, J.J., De Fazio, L., Calafat, A., & Mendes, F. (2000). Women drug abuse in Europe: Gender identity. Palma de Mallorca: European Institute of Studies on Prevention (IREFREA). Retrieved April 8, 2010 from <http://www.irefrea.org/uploads/PDF/Stocco%20et%20al_2000_Women%20Dru g%20Abuse.pdf>

Stocco, P., Llopis Llacer, J.J., de Fazio, L., Facy, F., Mariani, E., Legl, T., et al. (2002). Women and opiate addiction: A European Perspective. Palma de Mallorca: European Institute of Studies on Prevention (IREFREA). Retrieved April 08, 2010 from <http://www.irefrea.org/uploads/PDF/Stocco%20et%20al_2002_Women%20Opi ate.pdf>

Studio VEdeTTE (2007). Monografia n. 7: Differenze di genere nello studio VEdeTTE. Spoleto (PG): Litografia Spoletina-Del Gallo.

Substance Abuse and Mental Health Services Administration (2005), Overview of Findings from the 2004 National Survey on Drug Use and Health, Office of Applied Studies, NSDUH Series H-27, DHHS Publication No. SMA 05-4061. Rockville, MD.

Tempesta, E., et al. 1987, Storia psichica della gravida tossicodipendente. Bollettino delle Farmacodipendenze e Alcoolismo, 6, X, 602-607.

United Nations Office on Drug and Crime (2004, August). Substance abuse treatment and care for women: Case studies and lessons learned. Wien. Retrieved September 11, 2010 Retrieved from <http://www.unodc.org/pdf/india/womens_corner/sustance_abuse_treat_care. pdf>

van IJzendoorn, Bakermans-Kranenburg, (1996). Attachment representations in mother, fathers, adolescents, and clinical groups: a meta-analytic search for normative data. Journal of Counseling and clinical psychology, 64.

van IJzendoorn, M. H. & Bakermans-Kranenburg, M. J. (1997). Intergenerational transmission of attachment: A move to the contextual level. In L. Atkinson, & K. J. Zuckerman (Eds.), Attachment and psychopathology (pp. 135-170). New York: Guilford Press.

van IJzendoorn, M. H., Kroonenberg, P. M., & Frenkel, O. J. (1992). The relative effects of maternal and child problems on the quality of attachment: A meta analysis of attachment in the clinical samples. Child Development, 63, 840-858.

Vidal-Trécan, G, Coste, J, Coeuret, M, Delamare, N, Varescon-Pousson, I, Boissonnas, A (1998). Risk behaviors of intravenous drug users: are females taking more risks of HIV and HCV transmission? Rev Epidemiolo Sante Publique; 46(3):193-204

Vogt, I., Gender and drug treatment systems. In Klingemann H, Hunt G (eds), Drug Treatment Systems in an International Perspective: Drugs, Demons and Delinquents. Sage, London, 1998

Ward, M. J. & Carlson, E. A. 1995, Association among adult attachment representations, maternal sensibility, and infant-mother attachment in a sample of adolescent mothers. Child Development, 66, 69-79.

Waters, E., & Deane, K. E. (1985). Defining and assessing individual differences in attachment relationships: Q-methodology and the organization of behavior in infancy and early childhood. In I. Bretherton & E. Waters (Eds.), Growing points of attachment theory and research. Monographs of the Society for Research in Child Development, 50(1-2), 41-65.

Wellish, D.H. & Steinberg, M.R. 1980, Parenting Attitudes of Addicts Mothers. The International Journal of Addictions, 15, 6.

WHO (1995). The World Health Report 1995. Bridging the gaps, Geneva, World Health Organization, Retrieved from <http://www.who.int/whr/1995/en/whr95_en.pdf>

WHO (2000). Women's Mental Health: An Evidence Based Review, WHO, Geneva.

WHO (2007a), Interventions to address HIV in prisons: HIV care, treatment and support. Geneva, World Health Organization (Evidence for Action Technical Papers; Retrieved from <http://www.who.int/hiv/pub/advocacy/idupolicybriefs/en>

Wilson, G. S., McCreary, R., Kean, J., & Baxter, J. C. 1979, The developmental of preschool children of heroinaddicted mothers: A controlled study. Pediatrics, 63(1), 135-141.

Wright A., Walker J. (2001). Drugs of abuse in pregnancy. Best Practices Res Clin Obstet Gynaeco, 1, pp. 987-998.

Zacchello, F. & Giaquinto, M. (1997). Figlio di madre tossicodipendente. Problemi clinici e assistenziali. In G.M. Fava Vizziello & P. Stocco (Eds.), Tra genitori e figli la tossicodipendenza (pp.161-168). Milano: Masson.

Zeanah, C.H. (1992). L'esperienza soggettiva nella relazione di attaccamento: la prospettiva di ricerca. In M. Ammaniti & D. N. Stern (Eds.), Attaccamento e psicoanalisi, Roma: Laterza.

Zenker ,C., Bammann, K.and Jahn, I., (2003). Genese und Typologisierung der Abhängigkeitserkrankungen bei Frauen. Baden-Baden, Schriftenreihe des Bundesministeriums für Gesundheit, Nomos.

Zuckerman, B. (1994). Prenatal Cocaine Exposure - 9 Years Later. Mosby-Year Book Inc.

Zuckerman, B. & Bresnahan, K. (1991). Developmental and behavioral consequences of prenatal drug and alcohol exposure. Pediatric Clinics of North America, 38, 1387-1405.

Zuckerman, B., & Brown, E.R. (1993). Maternal substance abuse and infant development. In Zeanah C.H. (Ed.), Handbook of infant mental health (pp. 143–158). New York: Guilford Press.

Zuckerman, B., Frank, D. A., Hingson, R., Amaro, H., Levenson, S. M., Kayne, H., Parker, S., Vinci, R., Aboagye, K., Fried, L. E., Cabral, H., Timperi, R., & Bauchner, H. (1989). Effects of maternal marijuana and cocaine use on fetal growth. New England Journal of Medicine, 320, 762-768.

6

The Interactional Approach in the Treatment of Cocaine Addicts

Andrea Leonardi, Sonia Scavelli and Gianluca Ciuffardi

Fondazione Franceschi Onlus,
Italy

"A living system, due to its circular organization, is an inductive system and functions always in a predictive manner; what occurred once will occur again. Its organization (both genetic and otherwise) is conservative and repeats only that which works."
Humberto Maturana

1. Introduction

Over the last few years cocaine use has spread considerably to all social levels. According to statistical data currently available, cocaine is the psychoactive substance most frequently used in Europe, after cannabis (European Monitoring Centre for Drugs and Drug Addiction [EMDDA], 2011). Italy is one of the European countries where such consumption is more frequent: about 7% of the population report to have used cocaine at least once in their lifetime (Presidenza del Consiglio dei Ministri, 2007).

Cocaine is an alkaloid substance obtained from coca leaves, which acts on the central nervous system, especially on the dopamine system, compromising its functions. Cocaine use contributes to increased concentration of dopamine, a neurotransmitter that is present in different brain areas that governs cognition, emotional processes, motivation and associative processes related to feelings of pleasure. Normally, this neurotransmitter is released by neurons in response to a salient, pleasant stimuli, and then it is absorbed by the same cells that have produced it. Cocaine acts on these cells by blocking the recovery of dopamine, resulting in an accumulation of the neurotransmitter between synapses.

Repeated cocaine use damages the normal communication between neurons, leading to alterations in brain circuits for pleasure that is thought to contribute to the development of dependence. In addition, the brain needs progressively higher doses of the psychoactive substance to achieve the same effects and it needs increasing use in order to achieve the same levels of pleasure originally experienced (National Institute on Drug Abuse [NIDA], 2008).

The psychological effects of cocaine depend both on the amount consumed and on the route and modality of administration (Braglia et al., 2004): these effects consist mainly of sensations of euphoria, increased libido, reduction of hunger and thirst, and in the impression of increased perceptual abilities, but they may also generate panic attacks, mood disorders, paranoid ideation and induction of psychotic states with auditory, visual and tactile hallucinations (Braglia et al., 2004). Among the various routes of administration, the intravenous injection and the cocaine smoke are those causing a more rapid and intense action, while sniffing cocaine determines longer lasting effects, up to 30 minutes versus the 10 minutes of the smoke (NIDA, 2008).

Based on currently available data, cocaine addiction is a complex phenomenon in which various factors interact; there are those that are dependent on the central nervous system and therefore biological and those that are related to a certain lifestyle that from the point of view of the cocaine addict would encourage new opportunities for social meetings, sexual gratification and friendship (Rigliano, 2004).

2. Main therapeutic intervention protocols

Despite the considerable and ever increasing spread of cocaine, therapeutic intervention protocols that exist today in Europe are unfortunately still being tested and often result from treatment of other forms of addiction, such as heroin (EMCDDA, 2007a).

The pharmacological approach intervenes with the neurobiological systems involved in reinforcement and the long-term effects of drugs, thereby reducing the symptoms of abstinence. Most recently, some vaccines have also been developed based on the principle of using the properties of the immune system to counteract cocaine effects, preventing it from reaching the brain (Pirona & Hendrich, 2009).

The pharmacological approach, although representing a significant step forward in the care and treatment of cocaine dependence, has not proven sufficient to effectively treat cocaine addiction. The reason for this is that cocaine addicts continue to remember the pleasurable effects and states of arousal produced by the substance, and the attempt to reduce any pre-existing states of discomfort through the use of the psychoactive substance. Therefore, it is essential to integrate the pharmacological approach into a psychosocial and psychological treatment.

Among the various psychological orientations that have been proposed, those which have demonstrated a good level of effectiveness are as follows:

2.1 Cognitive Behavioural Therapy

Cognitive Behavioural Therapy (CBT) (Carroll, 1998) that treats cocaine addiction as a problematic behaviour depending on cognitive and environmental factors. Treatment is usually delivered on an outpatient basis and it lasts from 12 to 16 sessions, usually over 12 weeks. An individual format is preferred, because it makes possible to fit the treatment to the needs of each patient.

According to CBT, the learning processes are important factors for the development and the maintenance of cocaine use, but the same processes may be useful for helping the patient stop his drug use. So, CBT tries to assist the patient to recognize the situations in which he most probably takes cocaine, to avoid these circumstances if it is possible and to manage the difficulties and the problematic behaviours related to the cocaine use. CBT has two important components:

- *functional analysis*, that is, the identification of the patient's thoughts, feelings and circumstances before and after cocaine use. The functional analysis is helpful to assess the factors, or high-risk situations, that are likely to lead to cocaine consumption and it can gives insights into some of the causes of this use;

- *skills training*, aimed at unlearning the patient's habits associated with cocaine use and learning healthier skills and habits. At the beginning the skill training focuses on the practical and mental abilities which are useful to stop cocaine use. Then, the training is extended to other possible problems with which the patient may have difficulty facing (Carroll, 1998).

So, CBT encourages subjects to assume alternative behaviours than those associated with substance use (EMCDDA, 2007a).

2.2 Contingency Management Therapy

Contingency Management Therapy (Petry, 2002), based upon the principles of behaviour modification. This consists of providing positive reinforcement (in the form of clinic privileges, vouchers or payment) when the patient achieves given behaviours or treatment goals. In particular, for cocaine users this reinforcement is related to the urine tests carried out periodically (Higgins et al., 2000).

This therapy has four main values:

- *defining a target behaviour*, that is, what outcome the patient has to achieve. For example, drug abstinence and undertaking clinic and social activities related to a drug-free lifestyle;
- *regular monitoring of target behaviour* that has to be unequivocally assessed (for example, regular urine analysis would be undertaken to verify the patient's abstinence);
- *reward contingent on achievement of target behaviour*: at pre-established levels and frequencies, rewards are given to or retained by the patient depending on whether or not the target behaviours are achieved;
- *reinforcement* by brief counselling to reinforce the positive effects of the rewards (Weaver et al., 2007).

2.3 The Motivational Interview

The Motivational Interview (MI) (Miller & Rollnick, 2002) approach is a client-centred, directive method aimed at understanding the motives the patients have for addressing their substance use problems, to gather the clinical information needed to plan their care and to build and reinforce their readiness for change. The MI approach consists of short-term intervention to help the person in the changing process towards a healthier lifestyle through the resolution of ambivalence, that is, the tendency to provide opposite emotional responses to cocaine.

According to the MI, the patient can be in one of the following four stages of change:

- *pre-contemplation stage*, in which the patient does not want to change his behaviour;
- *contemplation stage*, when the patient would like to change, but he does not know how to do it;
- *preparation stage*, in which the person shows explicitly the intention to change;
- *action stage*, in which the patient realizes practical changes to feel better (Di Clemente & Velasquez, 2002).

2.4 Modified Dynamic Group Therapy

Modified Dynamic Group Therapy (MDGT) (Khantzian et al., 1990) aims to solve the problems of low self-esteem that lead the subjects to consume the substance. According to this theory, low self-esteem produces a "psychological vulnerability" which can predispose a person to drug use and decrease impulse control. The purpose of MDGT consists of helping patients become aware of their psychological vulnerability. This approach has four main therapeutic focuses:

- developing a better affective tolerance;
- improving self-esteem;
- improve interpersonal relationships;
- development of appropriate strategies of "self-care".

MDGT lasts about 6 months and has 3 main stages:

- during the first stage therapy consists of encouraging patients to address their vulnerability through better confidence resulting from the support of other members of the therapy and mutual listening;
- in the middle stage the attention is on members' attachment to the group, taken as a whole;
- in the last stage the older members take on the role of "co-therapists" and explain aspects of MDGT to new members.

So, the MDGT intervenes not only on drug use, but also in the self and on the relationship between some personality aspects and problems that can lead to relapse (Khantzian et al., 1990).

3. The interactional approach

The Interactional Approach (IA) is a type of psychological intervention that includes specific therapeutic techniques and procedures for the treatment of cocaine addiction.

Attempting to solve the problem of cocaine addiction, our research group has developed a short-term psychotherapeutic model, directed to increase the patient's interpersonal and communicative skills, to improve emotional control and the use of meta-cognitive resources, to adopt a healthy lifestyle, leading eventually to reduced risk of relapse. The proposed outpatient treatment has led to good results both in terms of effectiveness and efficiency (Leonardi et al., 2006, 2009; Leonardi & Velicogna, 2009).

At the basis of the psychological intervention there are studies on the processes of persuasive communication (Erickson et al., 1976; Erickson & Rossi, 1981), as well as theoretical models derived from constructivism (von Foerster, 1982; von Glasersfeld, 1984), the interactional approach (Jackson, 1961, 1965; Fisch et al., 1982; Watzlawick et al. 1967, 1974, 1984, 1997) and those derived from action research (Lewin, 1946).

Constructivism is a theoretical approach that challenges the idea that knowledge can be "objective", arguing that each man builds his own reality through cognition, sensory perception and communication processes. What the person sees and knows is a construction based on his own experiences. Therefore, from a psychological point of view it becomes essential to try to understand the meaning that individuals attribute to their experiences, how they organize their knowledge and the expectations they have about what will happen to them. Other authors who have contributed to develop this approach were Maturana and Varela (1980), who studied the way in which living systems are regulated and organized in their environment.

The interactional model is applied to relational aspects and it is based on the concept that psychological disorders depend on the interaction between the subject and his own perception of reality: the aim of the therapy is to facilitate the change through appropriate strategies, so that individuals can look at their problems in a different way and take the best solutions.

It often happens that just the *attempted solutions*[1], implemented by the person, contribute to complicate the problem inadvertently, while with appropriate strategies it becomes possible to change the patient's *perceptive-reactive system*, as well as his perspectives which are too rigid. The perceptive-reactive system is defined as the way a person constructs the three fundamental relationships: with himself, the others and the world. Thus, by intervening it is possible to change the processes of attribution of meaning to things over the perception of the problem (Nardone & Watzlawick, 1990).

In accordance with Franz Alexander (Alexander & French, 1946), the change is due to the *corrective emotional experience* that helps to modify initially set perceptions and in doing so engaging a virtuous process of learning new skills and competencies in the social sphere. Therefore, the scope of the interactional and constructivist therapy is to get the patient to change his perceptive-reactive system, through the experimentation with new and different strategies.

With regard to the interactional aspects, *injunctive and evocative language* is also really important: its aim is not to describe the surrounding reality, but to prescribe certain behaviours within a therapeutic relationship full of suggestion. Such injunctions can be very useful to interrupt the patient's dysfunctional patterns. The *injunctive and evocative language* is used to persuade the other to engage in specific tasks. Through the execution of such tasks the patient may perceive reality in a different way (Watzlawick, 1978).

Finally, our methodology of psychological treatment takes into consideration some aspects such as the neurological functional difference between the two hemispheres of the human brain. The left hemisphere uses a logical-analytical coding system and it specializes in the perception and in language, while the right one is involved in non-linguistic tasks such as recognition of their own and others' emotions or in activities that involve analogical processing such as the perception of images, configurations and contexts in their overview (Gazzaniga, 1972). The study of different functional specializations has been possible thanks to research on patients suffering from epilepsy and who had the corpus callosum surgically sectioned, a brain structure that represents the most important area linking the two hemispheres. Those studies revealed that the two hemispheres work in close synergy with each other, although responding to specific stimuli to their functional area, and that they are also highly integrated and complementary (Sperry, 1968).

According to Watzlawick (1978), a specific language is able to communicate and influence each of the two hemispheres, in order to activate one at the expense of the other: for example, evocative language and *hypnosis without trance*[2] (Erickson et al., 1976) are communicative modalities that can influence the right hemisphere. The purpose of these

---

[1] The *attempted solutions* are actions that a person does to try to solve his problem. If they do not lead to the resolution of the problem and if repeated, these solutions further complicate the situation preventing the change (Watzlawick et al., 1974). From the perspective of the therapist, the attempted solutions function as reducing complexity in the assessment of the clinical case examined.

[2] Without using formal hypnosis, Milton Erickson (Erickson et al., 1976) states that it is possible to realize a communicative exchange characterized by persuasion, control of attention and suggestion, which is able to bypass resistance to change.

communicative approaches consists of evoking certain images in the patient, as with the storytelling of metaphors, aphorisms and anecdotes. As a point of fact, these communicative modalities serve to bypass the normal resistance to change and provide easier access to unconscious psychological resources (Erickson et al., 1976).

In the therapeutic relationship, the use of suggestion, as well as the evocation of images, allows patients to gradually change their behaviours.

The experience "on their skin" of such behaviours allows the persons to realize that new ways of handling their problems are possible. The cognitive restructuring of these new experiences contributes to maintaining over time the modifications that have progressively occurred.

4. The five phases of the interactional model for the treatment of cocaine addiction

Our model is applied to both individual and group therapy. It can be divided into five phases of intervention that are interconnected with many levels of communication: each of these five phases is characterized by specific objectives and the achievement of each one allows access to the next level (Leonardi et al. 2006, 2009; Leonardi & Velicogna, 2009).

4.1 Evaluation-intervention

The purpose of the first phase is to collect useful information to explain how cocaine addiction has been established, to evaluate the level of motivation and to begin simultaneously the intervention aimed at changing.

Unlike what happens with other therapeutic approaches, such as Cognitive Behavioural Therapy (CBT) (Carroll, 1998), which uses more linear intervention strategies, our model consists of a sequence of self-corrective operations aimed at progressively increasing the effectiveness of care, which is accompanied by a circular type system of interaction with the patient. This happens from the first stage, in which there is no distinction between diagnosis and intervention. This distinction characterizes the traditional approach to the problem of cocaine addiction, where the time of diagnosis is considered free from possible communication influences.

During this initial phase, the therapist:

- investigates and assesses the overall situation;
- recalls situations associated with cocaine use;
- plans the most effective communication strategies to change the way the patient relates to the substance.

After collecting information on a person's life, the therapist identifies those elements that may have influenced the development of cocaine dependence (anamnesis). In parallel, he also seeks to assess the patient's level of motivation to change, which generally falls into one of the following categories:

- the person is motivated to seek help;
- the person is slightly motivated to seek help and forced into treatment by the family;

- the person is not motivated to change at all.

The elements of this scheme are additional to the already described usual resistance to change of the dysfunctional systems (Haley, 1963; Nardone, & Watzlawick, 1990).

The start time of problematic cocaine use and whether it coincided with a traumatic event should be assessed carefully (Leonardi & Velicogna, 2009).

It often happens that people who have occasionally used cocaine for fun or curiosity, increase their use considerably as a result of difficult situations that need to be addressed (such as bereavements, emotional loss, work problems, etc.), until the onset of a real physical and psychological dependence. Therefore, the therapist has to not only take care of the drug addiction behaviour, but he must attend also to the potential event that made things worse. Finding the possible reason that has contributed to the subsequent loss of control by the cocaine addict allows him to address the "real" problem that caused the suffering that he has tried to quell using cocaine (Leonardi & Velicogna, 2009).

Another important factor to take into consideration concerns modes of taking cocaine (which can be sniffed, smoked or injected into veins), because the therapeutic intervention must be calibrated depending on the method of intake of the substance. For example, in the case of cocaine injected into veins, in our experience we are often in the presence of a former heroin consumer that, maybe after years of abstinence, has decided to switch to cocaine and this must be taken into account in the psychological intervention. In the case of smoked and sniffed cocaine the sensory, perceptive and imagination techniques change, although the process of therapeutic intervention is similar.

During this first phase (see Table 1), the therapist adopts a style of communication aimed at increasing the level of the patient's motivation to overcome his natural resistance to change: through questions that explore the problem, we aim to change both the perceptions and reactions to the substance.

First phase of treatment	First level of therapeutic communication
• History and evaluation of general areas • Motivational levels • Outset • Intensity • Modality • Frequency	• Persuasive communication • Hypnosis without trance

Table 1. The evaluation-intervention.

For example, if a patient has just conjured up feelings of isolation and loneliness in relation to cocaine use, the therapist could explain this perception by means of a metaphor, comparing the patient to a person who is locked in by himself inside a cold and dark cell. This image evokes a painful sensation, but, at the same time, it produces a very refined restructuring because if a person has been able to enclose himself within a cell, he is also able to open it and to get out. As stated above, according to constructivist theory, the person may know and interact with the world around him through his own actions. Thus, an "objective" knowledge of reality is not possible, it depends upon the observer's point of view. But often the person is not aware of that building process. Rather, for that person knowledge has the value of "objective" truth and strongly influences his thoughts and actions (Nardone & Watzlawick, 1990).

On the one hand the interactional intervention works on the problem, on the other it has the aim of helping the patient to gradually build a different reality (De Shazer, 1985).

4.1.1 First clinical interviews

The first clinical interviews with cocaine users are crucial in order to explore the ways to develop the treatment. They serve to gather a preliminary knowledge of the individual and to lay the groundwork for increasing motivation to change: the patient describes in detail his problematic situation, which is compounded by drug-induced automatisms and compulsions.

Generally, people who seek psychological help for a problem of abuse and cocaine addiction have three levels of complexity that prevent the change:

- at the first level there is the inevitable resistance that occurs in this clinical setting, (Mascetti & Strepparola, 2006);
- at the second level lie the neurobiological modifications induced by cocaine use that render the brain less susceptible to changes (Shaham & Hope, 2005a; Edwards & Koob, 2010);
- finally, at the third level there is a lack of motivation of those who have been forced by family to undergo treatment.

Because of these difficulties, which are added to by the specific problems due to cocaine use, in this preliminary stage the use of the persuasive communication mode reaches noteworthy levels. In fact, by only "capturing" the attention of the patient it is possible to change his behaviour first and then, subsequently, also his perceptive-reactive system.

At this stage, the first question should be: "What is the problem?". According to our model, this simple question already contains an initial restructuring message, since the patient is not considered as a chronically ill patient, but he is treated as an individual who has a problem which can still be given a solution.

This is also the time to try to understand how the perceptive-reactive system works in relation to the problem of drug addiction. On the basis of our clinical experience gained over the years, we have found that cocaine users usually act like *sensation seekers* (Zuckerman, 1979), that is as people who actively and constantly seek strong pleasurable experiences.

Often, the first cocaine consumption happens randomly in a fun and entertaining context, such as in a club with friends. After a number of takings, which may vary from individual to individual, there is the loss of control leading to the emergence of a vicious circle which tends only to worsen (Serpelloni & Bertoncelli, 2006; Pavarin & Dionigi, 2009).

It is of the utmost importance to ask the patient to relive those first experiences of use: this re-enactment aims to make the patient conscious of the act of taking cocaine so that it ceases to be a mainly automatic process.

Generally, at the first interview the individual states that, after an initial phase characterized by extremely pleasurable sensations, side and opposite effects occurred (*paradox effect*). At this stage the therapist adopts a communication style characterized by suggestion and persuasion, emphasizing that cocaine has caused unpleasant effects which are opposite to those originally experienced and it is now those unpleasant effects that the patient wants to stop as soon as possible (Leonardi & Velicogna, 2009). To do that the therapist may use an analogy such as that of the cage, already mentioned above, to get the best view of the situation and to evoke the unpleasant feelings associated with cocaine use. The therapist ends the sentence with a post-hypnotic message: "The more you use it, the more you feel sick and the more you feel sick, the more you would like to free yourself of it."

The next step is to survey the attempted solutions that the patient uses to address cocaine addiction. Generally, there are three:

- appeal to the patient's willpower to resist the temptation to give in to drug use;
- avoid risk situations;
- try to not think about the substance.

In order to achieve the goal of getting out of vicious circles established by the failed attempts to solve problems, the questions asked by the therapist act as keys that unlock the ability to change. For example, at this stage a question feature is: "Now that you have decided to change your ways by coming here, what would you do to implement this?". This question prompts the person to feel *as if* he is actually changing and he is trying hard to do it, thus creating a prophecy that has a sensible hope of self-fulfilment[3].

Another category of questions is the one that puts the illusion of creating alternatives between two opposing choices. An example of this sequence of funnel-shaped questions could be the following: "Do you take more cocaine when you are with other persons or when you are alone?" If the answer is "alone", the therapist continues asking if this taking is usually done at home or outside. In this way we proceed with other questions of the same type, until the therapist summarizes all the collected information into a single sentence which aims to make the patient relive the intense feeling of loneliness that the drug causes every time, thus using the patient's arguments.

Change can be induced by other tools, such as metaphors, analogies and citations, because they have the advantage over the hedges of the analytical processes (Watzlawick, 1980), as well as having a strong educational and evocative component.

Towards[4] the end of the first session, the therapist applies a *therapeutic double bind*[4] (Bateson et al., 1956), thus constraining the individual to be even more motivated to change. An example of a double bind is when the therapist at the end of the interview states that "usually the treatment works, but I don't know if it is so in your case. We'll see...". If the patient wants treatment to work, here he must commit to belonging to that category of people for whom the treatment was successful.

---

[3] The *self-fulfilling prophecy* is a prediction that, because it has been formulated, sooner or later it will be fulfilled. People who are convinced that a certain event will happen in the future, in the short or medium-term, tend to alter their behaviour in a way that ends in causing the events that they had expected (Watlawick et al., 1967).

[4] The concept of the *therapeutic double bind* was formulated by Bateson to describe a contradiction at the level of communication, both verbal and non-verbal.

Finally, we give the *prescriptions*[5], which can be direct or indirect behavioural injunctions formulated by means of a strongly suggestive language, so that the patient performs the task assigned between sessions. The behavioural prescriptions are intended to unhinge the attempted solutions used until then.

4.1.2 Psychological assessment

Although the interactional model is not planned to frame people by the diagnosis, however, our team has used a series of psychological assessment instruments to obtain statistically valid measures for research purposes.

The assessment procedure aims to evaluate personality elements and those related to self-esteem, cognitive processes and social skills. Therefore, diagnostic tools used in the research project investigate the relationship between behaviour, personality factors and attitudes.

The survey instruments are:

- the Eysenck Personality Questionnaire Revised Short Form (EPQ-RS) (Eysenck et al., 1985), which measures some personality traits like introversion and extroversion;
- the Parental Bonding Instrument (PBI) (Parker et al., 1979), which provides a reliable and valid evaluation about the relationship with both parents, especially with regard to the level of care received and the feelings of security;
- the Basic Self-Esteem Scale (SE-BASIC) (Forsman et al., 2003), which consists of a rating scale of self-esteem in adulthood, seen as a stable personality trait over time and whose score is independent of the skills and feedback received from others.
- other indices of cognitive and behavioural assessment that have been extrapolated during the psychological observation of patients, with particular reference to verbal and non-verbal communication factors.

4.2 Motivational intervention

In the second phase we address the problem of dependence, encouraging the patient to speak freely about the difficulties encountered in the relational and family field, which may have favoured the use of cocaine. This work is important not only because it allows defining the possible critical areas for the person, but also because it helps to shift attention from the main problem, cocaine, and it helps to decrease obsessive ideation about the dependence on the substance.

In fact, two seemingly contradictory phenomena can be detected in the problem of cocaine addiction: obsessive ideation about the substance and mental dissociation that occurs during the use. To counter these two aspects of the problem, patients should be stimulated in sensory, perceptual and cognitive awareness (Main, 1991; Bara et al., 2005; Leonardi & Velicogna, 2009; Belin et al., 2011) of the occurrence of the abuse of cocaine.

---

[5] *Direct prescriptions* are clear instructions to carry out specific actions. They are aimed at the resolution of the problem or at reaching one of a series of goals on the road to change. *Indirect prescriptions* are behavioural injunctions whose real objectives are hidden. The therapist prescribes an action that will produce a different result from the one that was seemingly being specified (Nardone & Watzlawick, 1990).

To effectively achieve the treatment objectives, it is necessary to establish a relationship with the patient geared to the understanding of the problem and to mutual cooperation. The therapist must try to convey the message to the patient that he is not judging him by the fact of being dependent on a substance. In addition, rather than commiserate or treat him as an incompetent, the therapist encourages the patient to take responsibility and develop better decision-making capacity. Depending on different situations, the relationship with the patient can take directive or non-directive aspects.

At this stage (see Table 2), we use specific intervention techniques to re-enact sensations and perceptions induced by cocaine on the imaginative level, thus increasing the patient's capacity to recall the context in which the drug abuse developed and to prevent a possible relapse.

Second phase of treatment	Second level of therapeutic communication
• Further evaluation-intervention	• Therapeutic capture
• Intervention on the use of cocaine	• Sensory and perceptual intervention

Table 2. The motivational intervention.

A special technique was developed called the transformational re-enactment technique (Leonardi & Velicogna, 2009). This re-enactment is much more intense than just simple memory recalling, because it becomes possible to highlight the unpleasant moments connected with the use of the substance.

Here now we provide an example of a case study to explain how this technique is structured, based on our previous publication (Leonardi & Velicogna, 2009, p. 48):

(…) Gaetano, 35 years, has had a problem of cocaine addiction for about five years. He is a building contractor by profession, married and childless. In the past, he had abused heroin from the age of fifteen, but he was able to solve this problem after a period of one year in a drug rehabilitation centre. Abstinent for a long time, then he begins to take cocaine underestimating the risks and he loses control very quickly.

During the motivational phase, the therapist applies the transformational re-enactment technique, asking the patient to recall a typical situation of cocaine abuse. Despite encountering some difficulties in the initial stage, the patient gradually achieves very satisfactory results: in fact, Gaetano claims to perceive a certain aversion in reviewing that situation, underlining that he had never thought previously about the specific moment of cocaine use.

Continuing with the treatment, the therapist puts a new element in, representative configuration of use, which takes advantage of the discomfort the patient feels in "seeing" himself during the action of using cocaine (principle of use, Erickson et al., 1976). In fact, the patient tries to live again the moments immediately preceding the situation of abuse, during cocaine use and then after, as if he was reviewing them in front of a mirror. The effect obtained is very strong, because it completely changes the perception that the person had so far: whereas before the use was associated only with pleasure, now painful and negative feelings appear. Taking advantage of the difficulty of see himself, the therapist assists in leading to a greater fear in the patient, through the dual action to see the scene and to be able to review his actions.

The next step was to create an alternative sequence in which Gaetano was able to avoid the situation of abuse, reviewing with satisfaction: him reducing the use until complete cessation and then focusing his attention on relationship problems and the lack of self-esteem that had led him to cocaine addiction.

Using the transformational re-enactment technique, the therapist achieves three different objectives:

- to avoid automatisms. This technique allows the patient to review, at sensory and perceptual level, three fundamental aspects of cocaine consumption: what happens before, during and after use. It has, also, the *prescription of the symptom*[6] function, because it forces the patient to re-think in detail something that until now escaped control: the dependence;
- to insert in the patient's memory of cocaine use minimal elements with an aversive content against the substance. Thus, the patient lives painful and unpleasant sensations at perceptual level, every time he thinks about the substance;
- the modification of the patient's mental patterns into more adaptive ones, so that he can imagine himself doing affirmative actions for his mental and physical health.

Patients treated with this technique have gradually reduced cocaine use, often eventually complete cessation of using the drug, so that in a short time they were able to focus on their relationship problems and lack of self-esteem (Leonardi & Velicogna, 2009).

4.3 Development and consolidation.

The third stage is used to consolidate the results achieved in the previous two phases, proceeding in this way to restructure the cognitive level, in terms of less rigid alternatives in the perception of the reality.

In this phase, which may occur during group or in individual sessions, we try to ensure that the patient thinks of new skills acquired through the therapeutic treatment. The course within a group has some advantages in terms of learning, because the person interacts with other individuals who share similar problems. Many circular exchanges occur in a group and they can improve the patient's capacity to communicate with himself, the others and the world. So, the thought moves from the main problem: cocaine. In this way the mobilization of meta-cognitive resources helps to control the impulsivity that is typical of drug addicts and has been shown to contribute to compulsivity (Belin et al., 2008; Dalley et al., 2011). The ability of meta-communication (Sluzki, 1966; Watzlawick et al., 1967; Bateson, 1972; Belin et al., 2011) about cocaine addiction also helps the individual to reflect on interactions with his social environment.

The development and consolidation phase (see Table 3) serves also to decrease the risk of relapse that may occur after several months or even years after cessation of use. Indeed, the prolonged use of cocaine produces changes at the neurobiological level (Huang et al., 2009; Dobi et al., 2011, for review see Belin et al., 2009), which likely involves the formation of a

---

[6] The prescription of the symptom is a type of paradoxical prescription. The patient has to perform voluntarily actions that were previously involuntary and uncontrollable, and that he had always tried to avoid. The voluntary performance of the symptom eliminates it, as it is no longer spontaneous and uncontrollable (Nardone & Watzlawick, 1990).

long-term memory trace (Lee & Dong, 2011) about the pleasurable effects caused by cocaine, even after a single exposure (Ungless et al., 2001). Thus, working on meta-cognition it becomes possible to act on the mechanisms of impulsivity that may promote relapse in cocaine addiction.

Third phase of treatment	Third level of therapeutic communication
• Therapy admission	• Increased collaboration
• The seven therapeutic topics	• Decrease in the evocative language

Table 3. Development and consolidation.

4.3.1 The seven learning topics

The intervention we propose acts on the specific problem of addiction and on the possible situations that led to its appearance. For this reason, we use seven learning topics that are connected to each other and relate to many psychological areas. Considering and confronting each other about these topics we invite the patients to act in a more constructive way (O'Connell & Palmer, 2003).

4.3.1.1 Choosing a healthy lifestyle

The difficulties that a person normally encounters in the management of his lifestyle can be exacerbated by cocaine addiction (Serpelloni & Bertoncelli, 2006). At this phase, the focus of the therapy is on the possible choices which the patient can make to improve his own life. The purpose of this topic is to increase the ability to organize and direct daily activities towards healthier life choices. Adherence to more balanced rules of life, such as living by time schedules, eating a healthy diet and doing sport, allows individuals to build a healthier lifestyle.

4.3.1.2 Avoidance of relapses

Through group discussion assisted by the facilitator, we focus on the reasons that led to the patient using cocaine in the past. These may be different, such as difficulties in managing specific emotional states, the problems related to significant emotional relationships or risk underestimation in certain circumstances.

Awareness of the factors that can lead to relapse may be increased through reflection on the choices made, on automatic thoughts[7] and on emotional experiences occurring in certain circumstances. In accordance with the principle of use, we try to exploit even possible relapses in a positive way: instead of judging them as failures, they are redefined as opportunities to move on with greater and renewed commitment. According to Milton Erickson (Erickson et al., 1976), the principle of use is based on identifying the patient's available resources, on the understanding of his belief system, on connecting the resources to deal with the problem and on conveying confidence to the patient about the fact that the present problems will soon be overcome.

---

[7] *Automatic thoughts* are ideas and unexpected images that the patient has when their beliefs related to addiction are activated. These thoughts may act to trigger and increase drug withdrawal (Newman & Ratto, 1999). Through repeated observations, the patient is able to consider objectively their automatic thoughts and recognize their possible unreliable and non-adaptive features. Beck (1975) calls this process *distancing*.

4.3.1.3 Increasing social skills

Cocaine tends to alter the state of consciousness, distorting the perception and, therefore, it worsens the person's ability to significantly relate to others. The experience of being part of a group is a powerful tool by which he constructs a network of shared meanings with other members. The facilitator helps group members to focus on the present moment, inviting them to feel the emotions that they are experiencing during the dialogue with others.

4.3.1.4 Development of communication and meta-communication skills

The communication can never be separated from the interactional aspects: the person learns to communicate through the discussions that take place in the group, drawing on the resources of the verbal and non-verbal sphere. The development of communication skills helps to contrast feelings of isolation that often accompany the experience of cocaine addiction.

4.3.1.5 Increasing meta-cognitive resources

Meta-cognition is the ability to reflect on your thought processes, because it is assumed that an increase of this ability may encourage the person to make global changes in his lifestyle and in the management of feelings evoked by the use of cocaine. The group facilitator invites the members to meta-communicate and reflect on their and others' thinking, in order to stimulate greater awareness in emotion management.

4.3.1.6 A more balanced emotion management

Group members are instructed to recognize their own emotions and those of others: in other words, everyone is invited to wonder what he feels and what the others feel. To do this, the group members are invited to observe their sensations here and now and to realize the emotions of others. The same process can be referred also to remember particular events, such as the cocaine use situation. Observation and acceptance of their emotional states play important roles in the recognition of unpleasant emotions associated with the use of the substance.

4.3.1.7 Increasing problem solving skills

Increasing the capacity to solve problems effectively is obtained by assigning to the group members problem solving exercises to stimulate learning more appropriate strategies. This capacity can also improve the perceived sense of self-efficacy and thus the level of self-esteem of the person.

The self-efficacy refers to all the beliefs the person has about their ability to organize and execute the necessary actions to achieve their goals (Bandura, 1997).

4.4 Gradual release

Once you have completed the phase of development and consolidation, the next step requires the patient to acquire greater autonomy and self-confidence. The therapeutic session takes place during this phase with a collaborative attitude, in order to monitor any signs which could have anticipated the risk of relapse in cocaine addiction. At this stage, the patient has gained a greater autonomy and confidence in his ability to continue alone down the road of change. In this regard, it is interesting to focus on the concept of deutero-learning, introduced by Bateson (1972), to indicate the learning level higher than that of the basic stimulus-response scheme: briefly, it describes the process by which an individual "learns to learn".

This step is essential to encourage the patient to develop a greater degree of autonomy (see Table 4), as well as a greater sense of security, such as he becomes able to deal with various difficult situations.

Fourth phase of treatment	Fourth level of therapeutic communication
• Increasing autonomy • Increased complexity of the arguments of the group • Deutero-learning	• Demonstration-rational language • Perceptual and sensory forms of intervention

Table 4. Gradual release.

During this phase, the therapist also aims to improve the quality of inner dialogue, for example, through a specific training technique called inner conversation (Leonardi & Velicogna, 2009), whereby the patient imagines himself thinking as speaking aloud, focusing so that his linguistic performance is as correct as possible. This exercise leads to a progressive increase in reflective ability (self-regulation of thought) with a corresponding decrease in impulsivity, which is one of the reasons of possible relapse in cocaine use, as demonstrated by preclinical studies (Economidou et al., 2009).

4.5 Follow-up

After treatment, the phase of periodic review of results begins and it is realized by monitoring urine tests and follow-up interviews. This is the time (see Table 5) to understand whether or not the therapy has reached its objectives: the patient should become more cooperative towards the therapist, as well as more inclined to discuss any other issues that have occurred in other areas of his life.

In order to avoid possible relapses, at this stage the therapist also uses training techniques and imaginative simulation procedures, similar to the transformational re-enactment technique described above.

Fifth phase of treatment	Fifth level of therapeutic communication
• Verification, development and consolidation of achievements	• Increased collaboration • Collaborative language

Table 5. Follow-up.

5. Evaluation of the effectiveness and efficiency of treatment

Cocaine addiction is a highly complex field of study, in which communicative, interpersonal and neurobiological processes act. In order to collect data about the *effectiveness* (that means to cease cocaine use) and *efficiency* (to reach this goal as soon as possible) of the interactional approach, our research group has used both quantitative tools, such as urinary tests, and qualitative tools, such as self-evaluation questionnaires completed by the patients directly.

Through these evaluations indexes, given before, during and after treatment, we think it is possible to obtain a reliable evaluation of the treatment outcome.

Data collected are used:

- to assess whether treatment produces concrete results and if it responds adequately to the initial expectations;
- to identify which aspects of the treatment are valid and which ones are ineffective and, therefore, modifiable;
- to improve further those treatment components that have shown to be effective.

One of the rules of scientific method is to never be satisfied with the results achieved, because in another context or with other patients the same results achieved in the past may not be obtained. So we need a constant monitoring of these activities, in order to modify certain aspects of the psychological intervention, if necessary.

In a previous article (Leonardi et al., 2006), we underlined the importance of this *circular deepening principle* which derives from Lewin's Action Research model (1946). According to this model, the research and intervention phases are interconnected and constantly changing thanks to a feedback mechanism. After theoretically defining the working hypotheses, the real finding phase, during which data are collected, follows. Through the analysis of these data it becomes possible to effectively coordinate the intervention. The evaluation of achievements generates new working hypotheses, thus determining the beginning of a circular process whereby it becomes possible to make corrections and changes to the treatment itself.

This cycle also allows us to adjust the treatment to very different realities compared to the initial sample which has been processed. As Trombetta and Rosiello (2000) claimed, the circularity of this process is characterized by a collection of new material to be analysed, which is then used in constructing and implementing new strategies and action plans.

The principle of circularity just described is consistent with systemic theory (von Bertanlaffy, 1971), which underlines the importance of feedback mechanisms that act through the different phases: in our case, these feedback processes concern the continuous analysis of clinical individual and group interviews, as well as observation of results achieved (urinary tests, remission of symptoms and change in behavioural style).

Over the years, this circular process has meant continuous improvements to the treatment protocol, thus increasing the final effectiveness.

The research process can be divided into three macro areas:

- observation of individual and group interviews;
- quantitative and qualitative monitoring of the results obtained, and the administration of cognitive and personality tests;
- theoretical study in the field of general psychology and drug addiction.

The evaluation of therapeutic work mainly consists of studying the interviews or the group meetings carried out, with particular reference to the interactional aspects which occur between the therapist and the patient.

As noted elsewhere (Leonardi et al., 2006), monitoring of the clinical situation through periodic urine tests represents an element of fundamental importance and is the primary tool to verify the abstinence from cocaine and thus, indirectly, to obtain an *objective evaluation index* on the effectiveness of treatment.

According to our intervention protocol, urine tests should be carried out twice a week during treatment. These data provide an objective parameter for achieving and maintaining abstinence from cocaine, and they are also used to detect the possible occurrence of relapses. The statistical analysis of urine test results also allows the detection of the presence of some critical periods during the course of treatment, when abstinence from the drug is relatively more likely to be established (see Leonardi et al., 2006, for more details).

To monitor the validity of the therapy we also use some *subjective evaluation indices* that refer to how the patients views the therapeutic activity, the skills that they believe they have acquired during the treatment and the personal areas where they would require further therapeutic intervention. These evaluations are obtained through semi-structured interviews.

Finally, the study of general psychology and drug addiction literature has allowed expanding the existing knowledge, implementing it with new ways to observe and act on the person. The updating of bibliographic material is designed to deepen knowledge about the neurological, cognitive and social aspects related to the phenomenon of cocaine addiction.

6. Conclusions

Solving the problem of cocaine addiction presents considerable difficulties because of frequent relapses in the use of the substance. For this reason, a gradual change of subjective models for the construction of reality should also be combined with the psychological change, which begins to develop from the first session.

The interactional model has allowed us to reach good levels of effectiveness and efficiency of treatment. For example, as reported in Leonardi et al. (2006), in a group of 22 subjects who finished the treatment successfully, 73% resulted in abstinence from cocaine after 12 weeks. A 12 week outpatient study of Carroll et al. (1991), comparing the effectiveness of CBT with Interpersonal Psychotherapy or IPT (Klerman et al., 1984), reported that in a group of 42 subjects, 57% of the patients assigned to CBT and 33% of those assigned to IPT attained three or more continuous weeks of abstinence.

Our results (see Leonardi et al., 2009, for more details) were achieved by continuous research and correction of what was not fully satisfactory for the purpose of the therapy. On the basis of the results and data collected over time, we have developed a specific protocol for dealing with the problem of cocaine addiction, characterized by the following principle: try constantly to adapt the treatment to changes occurring during the therapeutic work.

7. References

Alexander, F. & French, T.M. (1946). Psychoanalytic Therapy: Principles and Applications, Ronald Press Company, New York.

Bandura, A. (1997). Self-Efficacy: the exercise of control, W.H. Freeman & Company, ISBN 978-0716726265, New York.

Bara, G.B., Colle, L., Bosco & F.M. (2005). Metacognizione: aspetti rilevanti per la clinica, In: Bara, B.G. (Ed.), Nuovo manuale di Psicoterapia Cognitiva, Vol. I, Bollati Boringhieri, ISBN 978-8833957685, Torino.

Bateson, G. (1972). Steps to an Ecology of Mind: Collected Essays in Anthropology, Psychiatry, Evolution, and Epistemology, University Of Chicago Press, ISBN 0226039056, Chicago.

Bateson, G., Jackson, D.D., Haley, J. & Weakland, J. (1956). Toward a Theory of Schizophrenia, *Behavioural Science*, 1(4): 251-264.

Belin, D., Daniel, M.L., Lacoste, J., Belin-Rauscent, A., Bacconnier, M. & Jaafari, N. (2011). Insight: perspectives étiologiques et phénoménologiques dans la psychopathologie des désordres obsessionnels compulsifs. *Annales Médico-psychologiques, revue psychiatrique*, 169(7): 420-425.

Belin, D., Mar, A., Dalley, J., Robbins, T. & Everitt, B. (2008). High Impulsivity Predicts the Switch to Compulsive Cocaine-Taking. *Science*, 320(5881):1352–1355.

Belin, D., Jonkman, S., Dickinson, A., Robbins, T.W. & Everitt, B.J. (2009). Parallel and interactive learning processes within the basal ganglia: Relevance for the understanding of addiction, *Behavioural Brain Research*, 199(1):89–102.

Bertalanffy, Von, L. (1969). General System Theory. Foundations, development, applications, George Braziller, ISBN 978-0807604533, New York.

Beck, A.T. (1975). Cognitive Therapy and the Emotional Disorders, International Universities Press, ISBN 978-0823609901, New York.

Braglia, D., Gerra, G., Mezzelani, P., Quaglio, G., Timpano, M.E., Zaimovic, A. & Zambelli., U. (2004). Cocaina: Farmacocinetica, abuso, dipendenza, detossificazione e trattamento. In: Trattato completo degli abusi e delle dipendenze, Nizzoli, U. & Pissacroia, M. (Eds.), Piccin, ISBN 978-8829916481, Padova.

Carroll, K.M., Rounsaville, B.J. & Gawin F.H. (1991). A comparative trial of psychotherapies for ambulatory cocaine abusers: relapse prevention and interpersonal psychotherapy, *The American Journal of Drug and Alcohol Abuse*, 17(3):229-247.

Carroll, K.M. (1998). A Cognitive-Behavioural Approach: Treating cocaine addiction, NIH Publication 98-4308, National Institute on Drug Abuse, Rockville, Retrieved from archives.drugabuse.gov/TXManuals/CBT/CBT1.htm

Childress, A.R., Mozley, P.D., McElgin, W., Fitzgerald, J., Reivich, M. & O'Brien, C.P. (1999). Limbic activation during cue-induced cocaine craving, *American Journal of Psychiatry*, 156: 11-18.

Dalley, J.W., Everitt, B.J., Robbins, T.W. (2011) Impulsivity, compulsivity, and top-down cognitive control, *Neuron*, 69(4):680–694.

De Shazer, S. (1985), Keys to Solutions in Brief Therapy, W.W. Norton & Company, ISBN 978-0393700046, New York.

Di Clemente, C.C., & Velasquez, M. (2002). Motivational Interviewing and the Stages of Change, In: Miller, W.R. & Rollnick, S. (Eds.), Motivational Interviewing: Preparing People to Change, The Guilford Press, ISBN 978-1572305632, New York.

Dobi, A., Seabold, G.K., Christensen, C.H., Bock, R. & Alvarez, V.A. (2011). Cocaine-induced plasticity in the nucleus accumbens is cell-specific and develops without prolonged withdrawal, *The Journal of Neuroscience*, 31(5): 1895–1904.

Economidou, D., Pelloux, Y., Robbin, T.W., Dalley, J.W. & Everitt, B.J. (2009). High impulsivity predicts relapse to cocaine-seeking after punishment-induced abstinence, *Biological Psychiatry*, 65(10): 851-856.

Edwards, S. & Koob, G.F. (2010). Neurobiology of dysregulated motivational systems in drug addiction, *Future Neurology*, 5(3): 393-401.

Erickson, M.H. & Rossi, E. (1981). Experiencing Hypnosis. Therapeutic Approaches to Altered States, Irvington Publishers, ISBN 0829002464, New York.

Erickson, M.H., Rossi E. & Rossi S. (1976), Hypnotic Realities: The Induction of Clinical Hypnosis and Forms of Indirect Suggestion, Irvington Publishers, ISBN 978-0829001129, New York.

European Monitoring Centre for Drugs and Drug Addiction, (2007a), EMCDDA Literature reviews - Treatment of problem cocaine use: a review of the literature, European Monitoring Centre for Drugs and Drug Addiction, ISBN 9291682748, Lisbon, Retrieved from http://www.emcdda.europa.eu/attachements.cfm/att_44787_EN_cocainetreatment_literature_review.pdf

European Monitoring Centre for Drugs and Drug Addiction, (2011), 2011 Annual report on the state of the drugs problem in Europe, European Monitoring Centre for Drugs and Drug Addiction, ISBN 978-9291684700, Lisbon, Retrieved from http://www.emcdda.europa.eu/attachements.cfm/att_143743_EN_EMCDDA_AR2011_EN.pdf

Eysenck, S.B.G., Eysenck, H.J. & Paul Barrett, P. (1985) A revised version of the psychoticism scale, *Personality and Individual Differences*, 6(1):21-29.

Forsman, L., Johnson, M., Ugolini, V., Bruzzi, D. & Raboni, D., (2003), Basic SE. Basic self-esteem scale. Valutazione dell'autostima di base negli adulti, Edizioni Erickson. ISBN 978-8879465304, Trento.

Fisch, R., Weakland, J. & Segal, L. (1982). The Tactics of Change. Doing Therapy Briefly, Jossey-Bass, ISBN 978-0875895215, San Francisco.

Foerster, Von, H. (1982). Observing systems, Intersystems Publications, ISBN 978-0914105190 Seaside.

Gazzaniga, M.S. (1972). One brain - two minds?, *American Scientist*, 60(3): 311-317.

Glasersfeld, Von, E. (1984). An Introduction to Radical Constructivism, In: The invented reality: How do we know what we believe we know? (Contributions to Constructivism), Watzlawick, P. (ed.), pp. 17-40, W.W. Norton & Company, ISBN 978-0393017311, New York.

Haley, J. (1963). Strategies of psychotherapy, Grune & Stratton, ISBN 0808901680, New York.

Higgins, S.T., Wong, C.J., Badger, G.J., Odgen, D.E. & Dantona, R.L. (2000). Contingent reinforcement increases cocaine abstinence during outpatient treatment and 1 year of follow-up, *Journal of Consulting and Clinical Psychology*, 68(1): 64-72.

Huang, Y.H., Lin, Y., Mu, P., Lee B.R., Brown T.E., Wayman, G., Marie, H., Liu, W., Yan, Z., Sorg, B.A., Schlüter, O.M., Zukin, R.S., & Dong, Y. (2009). In vivo cocaine experience generates silent synapses, *Neuron*, 63(1): 40–47.

Jackson, D. (1961). Interactional psychotherapy, In: Contemporary Psychotherapies, Stein, M. (Ed.), pp. 256-271, The Free Press of Glencoe, New York.

Jackson, D. (1965). The study of the family, Family Process, 4(1): 1-20.

Khantzian, E.J., Halliday, K.S. & McAuliffe, W.E. (1990). Addiction and the vulnerable self: Modified Dynamic Group Therapy for drug abusers, Guilford Press, ISBN 978-0898621723, New York.

Klerman, G.L., Weissman, M.M., Rounsaville, B.J., & Chevron, E.S. (1984). Interpersonal Therapy of Depression, Basic Books, New York.

Lee, B.R. & Dong, Y. (2011). Cocaine-induced metaplasticity in the nucleus accumbens: silent synapse and beyond, Neuropharmacology, 61(7): 1060–1069.

Leonardi, A., Fioravanti, P., Scavelli, S. & Velicogna, F. (2006). Programma Conoscenza: trattamento psicoeducativo integrato ed evoluto per problemi di cocaina. In: Cocaina. Manuale di aggiornamento tecnico scientifico, Serpelloni G., Macchia T., Gerra G. (Eds.), Progetto "START" del Dipartimento Nazionale per le Politiche Antidroga, ISBN 978-8895149004, Retrieved from http://iport.dronet.org/com/filedownloadlink/allegatoA.php?key=116&lingua=1

Leonardi, A., Fioravanti, P., Scavelli, S. & Velicogna, F. (2009). Programma Conoscenza. Psycho-educational, integrated and evolved treatment for cocaine addiction. International Journal of Mental Health and Addiction, 7(4):513–529.

Leonardi, A. & Velicogna, F. (2009). Cocaina: dipendenza e trattamento. Un modello di intervento psicologico, Franco Angeli, ISBN 987-8856812848, Milano.

Lewin, K. (1946), Action Research and minority problems, Journal of Social Issues, 2(4):34-46.

Main, M. (1991). Metacognitive knowledge, metacognitive monitoring and singular (coherent) vs. multiple (incoherent) models of attachment: findings and directions for future research, In: Parkes, C., Stevenson-Hinde, C.M & Marris, P. (Eds.), Attachment across the life cycle, Tavistock & Routledge, ISBN 0415056519, London.

Mascetti, W. & Strepparola, G. (2006). I disturbi da uso di sostanze, In: Bara, B.G. (Ed.), Nuovo manuale di Psicoterapia Cognitiva, Vol. III, Bollati Boringhieri, ISBN 978-8833957708, Torino.

Maturana, H.R. & Varela, F.J. (1980). Autopoiesis and Cognition: the realization of the living, D. Reidel Publishing Company, ISBN 978-9027710161, Boston.

Miller, W.R. & Rollnick, S. (2002), Motivational Interview: Preparing people to change, Guilford Press, ISBN 978-1572305632, New York.

Nardone, G. & Watzlawick, P. (1990). L'arte del cambiamento, Ponte alle Grazie, ISBN 978-8879284653, Firenze.

National Institute on Drug Abuse, (2008). Cocaine, NIDA InfoFacts, Retrieved from http://www.nida.nih.gov/pdf/infofacts/Cocaine08.pdf

Newman, C.F. & Ratto, C.L. (1999). Cognitive therapy of substance abuse. In: Comparative treatments of substance abuse, Dowd, E.T., Rugle, L. (Eds.), Springer Publishing Company, ISBN 0826112765, New York.

O'Connell, B. & Palmer, S. (2003). Handbook of Solution-Focused Therapy, Sage Publications, ISBN 978-0761967842, London.

Parker, G., Tupling, H., & Brown, L.B. (1979). A Parental Bonding Instrument, British Journal of Medical Psychology, 52(1):1-10.

Pavarin, R.M. & Dionigi, A., (Eds.), (2009). Cocaina. Percezione del danno, comportamenti a rischio e significati, CLUEB , ISBN 978-8849133325, Bologna.

Petry, N.M. (2002). Contingency management in addiction treatment, *Psychiatric Times*, 19(2): 52-56.

Pirona, A. & Hedrich, D. (2009). Treatment of cocaine use – a short update, European Monitoring Centre for Drugs and Drug Addiction, Retrieved from http://www.emcdda.europa.cu/attachements.cfm/att_76877_EN_EMCDDA cocaine%20treatment-update.pdf

Presidenza del Consiglio dei Ministri (Eds.). (2007). Relazione sullo stato delle tossicodipendenze in Italia anno 2007, Retrieved from http://www.governo.it/GovernoInforma/Dossier/relazione_droga_2007/Relazio ne_2007.pdf

Rigliano, P. (2004). Piaceri drogati. Psicologia del consumo di droghe, Feltrinelli, ISBN 978-8807817908, Milano.

Serpelloni, G. & Bertoncelli, S. (2006). Cocaina: profili dei soggetti in base alle modalità d'uso, agli aspetti comportamentali e sociali, In: Cocaina. Manuale di aggiornamento tecnico scientifico, Serpelloni G., Macchia T., Gerra G. (Eds.), pp. 637-653, Progetto "START" del Dipartimento Nazionale per le Politiche Antidroga, ISBN 978-8895149004, Retrieved from http://iport.dronet.org/com/filedownloadlink/allegatoA.php?key=141&lingua=1

Shaham, Y. & Hope, B.T. (2005a). The role of neuroadaptations in relapse in drug seeking, *Nature Neuroscience*, 8(11): 1437-1439.

Sluzki, C. (1966). Seminario sobre metacomunicacion: nota, *Acta Psiquiatrica y Psicologica de América Latina*, 12:119.

Sperry, R.W. (1968). Hemisphere deconnection and unity in conscious awareness, *American Psychologist*, 23(10): 723-733.

Ungless, M.A., Whistler, J.L., Malenka, R.C. & Bonci, A. (2001). Single cocaine exposure in vivo induces long-term potentiation in dopamine neurons, *Nature*, 411(6837): 583-587.

Watzlawick, P. (1978). The Language of Change: elements of therapeutic communication, Basic Books, ISBN 978-0465037926, New York.

Watlawick, P. (Ed.)(1984). The invented reality. How do we know what we believe we know? (Contributions to Constructivism), W. W. Norton & Company, ISBN 978-0393017311, New York.

Watzlawick, P., Beavin, J. & Jackson, D. (1967). Pragmatics of human communication. A study of interactional patterns, pathologies and paradoxes, W. W. Norton & Company, ISBN 978-0393010091, New York.

Watlawick, P. & Nardone, G. (1997). Terapia Breve Strategica, Raffaello Cortina Editore, ISBN 978-8870784718, Milano.

Watlawick, P., Weakland, J., & Fisch, J. (1974). Change. Principles of problem resolution. W. W. Norton & Company, ISBN 978-0393011043, New York.

Weaver, T., Hart, J., Fehler, J., Metrebian, N., D'Agostino, T. & Benn, P. (2007), Are contingency management principles being implemented in drug treatment in England?, National Treatment Agency for Substance Misuse, Retrieved from

http://www.drugsandalcohol.ie/11939/1/NTASM_rb33_contingency_manageme
nt_summary.pdf

Zuckerman, M. (1979). Sensation seeking: beyond the optimal level of arousal, L. Erlbaum, ISBN 978-0470268513, Hillsdale.

7

HCV and Drug Use – What Can Be Learned from the Failure to Control This Epidemic?

Philippe Chossegros
UHSI Lyon, Hospives Civils de Lyon,
French National Coordination of Healthcare Networks,
France

1. Introduction

Around 10 million intravenous drug addicts (IDUs) have been infected by the virus of hepatitis C (HCV) and around 1.2 million are HBsAg positive. Clear geographical differences exist in prevalence ranging in Western Europe between 37 and 98 % (1). At WHO's 63rd World Health Assembly in May, 2010, a resolution was passed to establish "goals and strategies for disease control, increasing education and promoting screening and treatment of people infected with HBV and HCV". In 2011, the WHO argued that injecting drug users (IDUs) are a key group that needs to be specifically targeted for prevention and treatment of viral hepatitis. At a time when a worldwide significant reduction in the HIV epidemic among drug users (DU) is observed, the spread of HCV infections is not controlled. If large variations are observed between countries and regions, prevalence of HCV infection of more than 70 % has been reported among recent-onset DUs (2) and, in 2009, in a city, Vancouver, with one of the most diversified and publicized panel of care services for substance users, Grebely et al. could make the statement that "overall, the rate of new HCV seroconversions in this cohort in the study period was about 25 times the rate of HCV treatment uptake. There are extremely low rates of HCV treatment initiation and very limited effectiveness, despite a high prevalence of HCV infection in this large community-based cohort of inner city residents with access to universal healthcare". It underlines the limits of the risk reduction policy which has been advocated and promoted for the last 20 years (3).

This quasi universal observation may be explained by differences between the viral epidemics of HIV, HBV, HCV and HDV and between their local management. I will confront my own experience and what I have understood of this epidemic in France to a selection of the international literature to propose what, I believe, could improve the care not only of hepatitis but of DUs themselves.

2. A scientific look at the HCV epidemic among DUs

An attempt at understanding the HCV epidemic can be considered as an object of science and discussed as such.

2.1 What is known of HCV hepatitis?

Our knowledge of HCV has grown tremendously since its discovery in 1988. However, gray areas persist. To develop effective control strategies, it is crucially important to determine how epidemiological significant organisms infect us, what is their natural history and what efficacy for its treatment. In most cases these evaluations are not easy.

2.1.1 HCV transmission among DUs: A reappraisal

In 2008, Rhodes et al. observed that "there was much confusion and uncertainty concerning HCV knowledge, including its medical and transmission risks" among drug injectors. Most IDUs viewed HCV prevalence as high and HCV transmission as an inevitable consequence of injecting, HCV risk was perceived as ubiquitous and unavoidable" (4). Is this confusion and uncertainty to be assigned to the messages they receive or our limited understanding of this disease and of its communication?

2.1.1.1 Drug use and HCV: the mystery of the contamination of non injecting drug users (NIDU)

The discovery of HCV followed a search for a viral cause of the remaining post-transfusion hepatitis after HBV had been excluded. Injections make a difference:

- Blood borne transmission through syringe and needle sharing (NSS) has never been questioned and the evidence linking drug injection and NSS to HCV infections are overwhelming. However the level of infectivity of the HCV containing blood remaining in a needle or a syringe after injecting is not known. It is likely that the viral load will be a limiting factor and it is obvious that HCV is able to survive in the environment but we do not for how long? HCV infection is robustly associated with the duration of injections, the number of receptive injecting episodes and of needles and syringes exchanges (NSS), but despite these associations, IDUs may remain hepatitis free after years of risks and others may be contaminated after a unique exchange The observation of Smyth and al. that accidental and unnoticed sharing of injecting equipment may be an important contributor to an IDU's increasing risk of infection over time (5) tallies with my own experience.
- The incidence of contamination through other drug paraphernalia is still debated. Cross-sectional studies have given conflicting results, but cohort studies were able to show significant relations between HCV contamination and sharing drug cookers and filtration cottons among IDUs who did not share syringes (6,7).
- Despite a much higher HCV prevalence (35.3 %) in non injecting drug users (NIDUs) than in non-drug users in some studies (8), the role of equipment (straws, bills, pipes,…) in HCV transmission remains unclear since statistical correlation has never been consistently found, since some misclassification of previous injectors could have occurred and since other possible modes of contamination such as tattooing or sexual transmission were often present (8). However, in some other studies, this prevalence was in the low range observed in individuals living in the same household as HCV carriers. Since it is obvious that every contact is not infectious, a comparison relating their number, the state of the nasal and buccal mucosa (cocaine, heroin) and the lips (crack) (9,10) at the time of sharing , as well as the HCV status of the DUS with whom the equipment was shared could help to understand the cause of these staggering discrepancies.

2.1.1.2 Possible modes of HCV contamination: blood but what else?

An early assimilation to HBV and to HIV, led to the hypothesis that HCV was a sexually transmitted disease. In 1990, a study conducted in Barcelona, in an AIDS clinic, found that 11 % of the partners of infected drug users and 16 % of the partners of infected homosexuals were seropositive for HCV (11). In 1999, using HCV genotypes, Neumayr et al., exploring heterosexual transmission of hepatitis C, finding no other cause of contamination concluded that sexual intercourse could be the cause of contamination in half of the cases (2,3 %) despite any significant relationship with any sexual practice (12). The same year, a metaanalysis computed an order of 1-3 % probability of being found infected among sexual partners of HCV carriers with no other known risk of contamination. The authors had no clue to counsel on their sexual practice viremic HCV carriers with a long term relationship who had not transmitted their infection (13). Overall, since the allocation of these contaminations to sexual intercourse was not significantly related with any history of particular sexual practice, room is left for other possible but never proven modes of contamination such as sharing razor or toothbrushes or, once every other suspected modes of contamination have been excluded, the mysterious "household" transmission (14).

Recent studies rediscovered the risk of sexual transmission among men who have sex with men (MSM) with high-risk sexual behavior (15–17). The HIV epidemic with its mortality and its transient behavioral changes may have hidden its existence for a while, but a Canadian cohort study of HIV positive MSM was able to trace their first contaminations to 1996, with an increase in the incidence of HCV contamination from 0.9 to 2.2 per 1000 person-year to 23.4 and 51.1 % in 2007 which could be related to an increase in the HCV prevalence among MSM as well as an increased level of risks taken during sexual intercourse (18).

Needles are used to perform tattoos and piercings. They are an obvious risk of transmission of HCV and they have been involved in small epidemics. Today, sterile material is used in professional parlors. Thus it is not surprising that non professional tattooing may be associated with a significant risk of HCV transmission among high-risk groups (19). However, like snorting drug, these contaminations, if possible, remain epidemiologically marginal when compared with NSS (20).

2.1.1.3 New insights and new tools could change our understanding of the HCV epidemic

- A consensual belief that HCV antibodies can always be detected years after a contamination has been recently contradicted. If a previous contamination with HCV gives usually rise to antibody production (humoral response) 45–68 days after HCV infection, the presence of a cellular immunity in absence of antibodies has been known for more than 10 years but its epidemiological implication has been ignored until recently (21,22). The discovery that some acute HCV hepatitis could occur and be spontaneously cured without any detection of anti HCV through sequential studies of new expositions has confirmed this hypothesis. It was observed in as many as 33 % of RNA positive cases (23). HCV has also been found in the liver or lymphoid tissue despite the absence of detectable HCV RNA and, even, of HCV antibodies. These occult infections could be the cause of some cases of persistently elevated transaminases (24). However, the clinical meaning of these silent forms which include persistence of HCV in the tissue after clearance of HCV viremia is still a subject of debate (24,25). There was no difference in the prevalence of HCV markers between family members of patients with occult HCV infection and family members of patients with a chronic hepatitis C (26).

Among IDUS different profiles have been described: but existing data are too scarce and sometimes contradictory to decide what is the real occurence of these evolutions:

- In IDUs engaging in risky behaviors for years without being infected by HCV, the prevalence of HCV-specific T cell response was significantly higher than that of healthy controls in an English study (58/19 %, p=.004) (27). In another study, this response reached 62 % of at risk IDUs lacking antibodies (28). The authors report a 100 % positive response for subjects who indicated that they had shared syringes during the previous 6 months as compared to 50 % who had not, implying a possible disappearance of cellular immunity with time.
- The studies of reinfections occurring in IDUs followed up with repeated blood testing added a new understanding to the clearance of HCV infections: When the rate of NSS remains high and if the tests are repeated at short intervals, a significant incidence of reinfections is observed with a new clearance of HCV RNA observed in more than 40 % of the cases (29,30). It confirms the well known notion of an absence of a total protection by a previous immunization against HCV, as well as the possible immunity in some cases (31,32), but points out a high prevalence of repeated HCV clearance which was not known.
- At last, genotyping HCV core sequences may identify phylogenic clusters and help to better understand HCV transmissions among IDUs and NIDUs (33).

These notions could be of use to explain some of the confusing observation of dissimilar serological status among couples and IDUs with the same risky behaviors in the same neighborhood.

2.1.2 The evolution of HCV chronic hepatitis: A lottery governed by genes?

Currently, HCV, a positive-strand RNA virus distantly related to the Flaviviriadae family, is classified in 6 major genotypes and multiple subtypes. An excellent description of the disease can be found online in the 2004 EMCDDA monography (34).

2.1.2.1 What prognosis for the HCV infections of IDUs?

If some chronic HCV infections progress to cirrhosis, liver cancer and death, this evolution is still unpredictable:

- It is assumed that, after an acute infection, 20 % of the subjects will clear spontaneously the virus. Using antibody screening followed by RNA amplification, 20 % of the cases occurring among IDUs following an acute infection resolve spontaneously (35,36) with a lower clearance rate in HIV infected and African-Americans (37). This prevalence of viral clearance is not significantly different from the general population.
- Progression toward cirrhosis of HCV hepatitis has been studied by two meta-analysis, the second selecting DUs (38,39). The first concluded that cirrhotic progression was comprised between 7 and 18 % after an evolution of 20 years, the second was more precise with a progression rate of 14,8 % with a confidence interval of 7.5 to 25.5 %. Male sex and alcohol consumption added an additional 5 % each. However, when the original studies were independently considered the progression rate could vary from

0.3 to 34.9 %, and the computation was performed using the data of 47 papers selected out of 764 potentially relevant articles and 6 679 abstracts. Significant bias could explain these ranges such as a selection of symptomatic patients or the different proposal to perform liver biopsies and their acceptance. In my own series of 650 DUs recruited through my addiction network and in prison with liver biopsies proposed and performed (acceptance 98 %) whenever HCV RNA was present independently of the level of transaminases, after 20 years, the prevalence of cirrhosis was 10.5 % (alcoholics non alcoholics 3.6 %; alcoholics 12.5 %). In a study conducted in the general population in Italy, HCV infection was associated with a severe liver disease in less than 50 % of the cases (40). In these studies as well as in a study of DUs, a high daily intake of alcohol (3 or more drinks) explained most early progression to cirrhosis in DUs (36).

- The prognosis of post-transfusional hepatitis mortality has been the first to be studied. They are characterized by their high rate of early death, their old age at contamination and the one-shot infection. It is believed that infections occurring at a younger age have a more benign evolution. Nurses infected by contaminated gammaglobulins had a 1 % prevalence of cirrhosis with no death after 25 years (41). This benign evolution has been confirmed by others (42). In 5 transfusion retrospective studies, 25 years after exposure all-cause mortality was not different between cases with an history of acute hepatitis and controls and the liver-related death significantly higher than controls was lower than 3 % (42). 16 years after contamination, a national cohort had no excess mortality compared to controls, but the risk of death directly from liver diseases was higher (Hazard ratio: 2.71, 95% CI 1.09-6.75). An excessive alcoholic consumption was present in 30 % of those deaths (43) Progression after 20 years is "less" known but the overall mortality of HCV liver diseases is usually considered to be in a range of 20 to 30 %. The higher rate of death observed among veterans. infected by HCV by Butt et al in 2009 could be related to the presence of other comorbidities such as alcohol, tobacco, violence... since the cause of death was not recorded (44). However, modelisation of the impact of C hepatitis treatment on patients' survival should consider the high rate of other causes of death among IDUs. They represent a significant proportion of infected people (44) : In a cohort of acute HCV hepatitis followed 25 years, if 8 % were cirrhotic, the death rate by overdose was eight times higher than the risk of dying of a liver disease (45) suicide, violence are common and, in older DUs, cardiovascular or pulmonary diseases compete with HIV and HCV (46-4).. In a more recent study conducted in of long-term heroin addicts in California, premature mortality was high, but "only" 14 % of the deaths were related to liver diseases (50).

A search of prognosis markers of progression in hepatitis C has led to the identification of modifiable and non-modifiable factors which influence its evolution. An older age at infection, a longer evolution, being male or African-American (cancer), viral genotype 3 are non-modifiableOn the contrary, an alcohol consumption greater than 30-50 g/day, smoking (cancer), iron overload, coinfection in HBV and/or immunocompromised HIV positive patients, presence of a metabolic syndrome (obesity, steatosis, insulin resistance) can be acted upon to improve individual prognosis (51). More recently, a search for more accurate predictors of progression to cirrhosis led to genome wide association studies (GWAS), screening the entire human genome. They identified single nucleotide polymorphisms (SNP) which are not often responsible for functional effects but serve as tag for the causal variant that is not genotyped:

- The study of patients resistant to HCV infection has shown that multiple independent protective genetic factors could explain their diverse evolution: clearance of HCV remaining anti HCV positive (52,53) and "protection" against HCV without production of antibodies (53).

- A link between fibrosis progression and genetic predisposition has been considered after the observation of familial clusters of HCV-related cirrhosis (54). An independent GWAS identified a genetic variant, already associated with alcoholic and non-alcoholic fatty liver disease (55), associated with steatosis and fibrosis severity in HCV related hepatitis (56). The screening of host genetic factors has led to a selection of seven single-nucleotide polymorphisms used to compute a Cirrhosis Risk Score (CRS) which could be able to stratify patients' cirrhosis risk prior to liver biopsy (57). This CRS was able to predict progression to cirrhosis in male patients at a F0 stage of fibrosis, result which could lead to treat them early without having to wait for the development of a significant liver disease. The prognosis value of the CRS held true even in patients who abused alcohol (58).

2.1.2.2 Coinfections of HCV hepatitis with other viruses have worse disease progression and outcome

Since high risk practices are common among IDUs, concomitant or successive contaminations by HBV, HCV and HDV, as well as HIV may be observed:

- HBV is a partially double stranded, enveloped DNA virus of the Hepadna family and HDV is a defective RNA virus which requires the presence of an active HBV infection for its multiplication. The evolution of coinfections is dependent of the innate and adaptative immune host response. The results of their interactions are unforeseeable, but it seems that the newcomer will act as a dominant virus which can lead to the clearance of preexisting infections. Acute HBV, HDV or HCV coinfections or superinfection of HBV or HCV may be the cause of fulminant or subfulminant hepatitis. These interactions may also lead to occult, serologically silent HBV or HCV infections. Coinfections are believed to result in worse disease progression with a higher risk of cirrhosis and hepatocellular carcinoma when compared to HBV or HCV alone (46,59,60).

- Up to one-third of HIV-infected patients are infected with hepatitis C virus. The advent of Highly Active Antiviral treatment (HAART) has transformed the prognosis of HIV infected patients with the occurrence of significant liver related death related to the prolongation of their life expectancy. A meta-analysis of 17 studies including 3567 individuals confirmed that chronic hepatitis C outcomes are worse among coinfected individuals with a prevalence of cirrhosis of 49 % (40 to 59 %), twice the rate observed in monoinfected patients (21 %; 16-28 %). This acceleration is mainly observed in immunocompomised patients and could be acccentuated by an immune reactivation occurring after the introduction of HAART. On the other hand, HAART might lessen progression of chronic liver disease and improve response to anti-HCV therapy without fully correcting the adverse effect of HIV infection on HCV prognosis (61-63) . If hepatic side effects of antiretroviral treatments are common, they do not seem to have a significant effect on the progression of liver fibrosis (64).

2.1.3 Hepatitis C management: Toward a potential Copernician revolution (at a price)

2.1.3.1 Less invasive diagnosis tools

Medical tools have also evolved with less invasive tests for the diagnosis and the follow-up of HCV hepatitis:

- Individuals who perform a test are eager to know its result without waiting for days. Blood access of IDUs is often problematic. Rapid tests answer these problems. After HIV, they have become available for HCV diagnosis. They can be performed using saliva, whole blood, serum or plasma. The frame of their use is controversial. In France, they can only be used by healthcare professionals with a complementary traditional test as confirmation. In the United-states where HIV auto-tests are available, in a DTP 24 % of preferred to remain anonymous, preference which reached 38 % if the test was free (65).
- To detect an ongoing infection, an amplification of the viral RNA is performed which is prone to contamination and false positive results. HCV core antigen detection, easily automated, and requiring less technical skill, has been advocated. Its limitations are noted in some HBV/HCV coinfections (66–68).
- Liver biopsy is often believed to be dangerous and painful by some patients and most general practitioners becoming a barrier to the care of hepatitis C patients. Non invasive tests are proposed: either scores computed from the results of different blood tests or a measure of the elastance (fibroscan) of the liver. Diverse algorithms have been proposed to improve their results but they are today an indisputable alternative to liver biopsy even in HIV/HCV coinfected patients (69,70). The fibroscan does not need a blood sample and gives immediate results (71).

2.1.3.2 Treat all, cure all?

- For 10 years, the treatment of HCV hepatitis has been an association of a long lasting form of alpha interferon with ribavirine. It is able to reduce significantly HCV related mortality (71) Today, there is a clear-cut difference of the response rate to treatment between the types of HCV viruses. Among the 6 genotypes, 2 and 3 need only 6 months of treatment with 80 to 90 % sustained viral response (SVR) whereas, genotype 1 and 4 usually need 12 months for a SVR of 50 %. Response rate of DUs are in the same range as the general population (72). Our finding of a significantly better SVR of genotype 1 infected DUs treated by buprenorphine as compared to methadone remains to be explored in a prospective study exploring that difference (73). An "à la carte" adaptation of the duration of treatment has been proposed for genotype 1 following the time of RNA clearance at 4, 12 or 32 weeks followed by respective treatment duration of 24, 48 or 72 weeks which has been confirmed for HIV/HCV coinfections (74,75). For patients with advanced diseases, treatment has been completed thanks to the use of growth factors which improved their tolerance (76)).
- This individual response could be predicted before treatment prescription: A better knowledge of the immune response against hepatitis C gives a central role to regulatory T lymphocytes which are present in the necroinflammatory infiltrate of the liver. By studying a single nucleotide polymorphisms (SNPs) linked to the IFN-lambda 3 (IL28B) gene it is now possible to predict a better prognosis for patients infected with genotype 1 with the CC genotype. They are more than twice as likely to respond to 48 weeks of treatment than non-CC genotypes (CT,TT) (77,78). This association has also been found in hepatitis C virus genotype 2 or 3 patients (79) and in HIV coinfected patients (80), but not in genotype 5 (81).

- However, new drugs which have been specifically tailored to HCV will improve these results. The first antiproteases on the market, Telaprevir and boceprevir improved the SVR for genotype 1 from 50 to 70 % for naïve patients and improved significantly SVRs of previous relapsers or non-responders (82,83). Since these drugs are added to interferon/ribavirine side–effects are more frequent and severe with serious cutaneous reactions (telaprevir) or a need for more growth factors (boceprevir). Early responder could benefit of shorter treatments. Other drugs are in the pipeline which could still have better results. The combination of two antivirals to the association of interferon/ribavirine led to a 100 % viral response, 12 weeks after the completion of treatment in previous non responders of a classical bitherapy. In a near future, association of 2 antivirals tailored for HCV should be able to cure almost every infected patient. This improvement has a cost: A full treatment course of telaprevir (12 weeks fixed-duration) will cost £30 000, whereas a full treatment course of boceprevir will range from to €22 000 to €40 000 (84) which should be added to the €16 000 of 48 weeks of bitheray by interferon and vidarabine for a genotype 1 (for a genotype 2 or 3, 24 weeks of a classic bitherapy are usually sufficient) and to the €1 000, annual cost of the care. The latest communications in international hepatology meetings promise a second generation of antivirals more effective with less side-effects which could be used in association without interferon and, in some cases, ribavriine in a near future. They should be able to cure almost all the hepatitis whatever their genotype. We do not know yet what will be their cost.

- Among HCV/HIV coinfected DUS at risk for liver disease progression a combination of interferon and ribavirin, is not highly effective; it has lower rates of SVR than monoinfected patients, especially for coinfected patients with HCV genotype 1 and those of African descent. Direct-acting antivirals might overcome factors such as immunodeficiency that can reduce the efficacy of IFN with the additional problem of interaction with antiretrovirals which should lead to early treatment independent of the stage of the liver disease, before the introduction of an HIV antiviral treatment (85).

- Most of the infectious epidemics observed in humans have been controlled by vaccination campaign. Novel vaccine candidates have been studied based on molecular technology such as recombinant proteins (E1 and/or E2 glycoprotein), poly peptides, virus-like particles, plasmid DNA and recombinant viral vectors which can be combined with novel adjuvants. Some of them have reached Phase I/II human clinical trials with, in some cases, production of robust antiviral immunity but the challenge is to move to test their efficacy in at-risk of infected population to prevent new infections. Their cost has led to preferential studies of their efficacy as adjuvant for existing treatment (86,87).

2.1.4 Conclusion: DUs confusion and uncertainty are founded (they are not alone in that situation)

We may know for certain that HCV infection follows conditions or practices causing blood transmission whether through contaminated needles or through mucosal traumatism and/or bleeding during hetero or homosexual intercourse. However, the studies of HCV transmission explore only the expected associations the researchers believe to be relevant. One must be cautious not to mix up low statistical significant association with causal relationship and remember that our inability to explain some HCV contamination may be related to, until now, unknown or overlooked modes of contamination: Animal bites were found significantly related to HCV infections (88) and a model of transmission of HCV by biting arthropods could explain the maintenance of long-term endemic transmission of HCV in Africa and South-East Asia (89). The route of contamination of patients on hemodialysis has not yet been understood leading to a debate on the interest of their isolation (90).

Today, our prevention messages are "simple"!!!:

- Do not inject and if you do, never share syringes, needles or any injecting paraphernalia.
- Never share bills and straws you use for sniffing or pipes you use to smoke cocaine.
- Use condoms for every sexual intercourse.
- Choose a reliable professional to perform your tattoos or piercings
- Never share your toothbrush and your razor.
- If, despite these counsels, you have taken some risks make a blood test.
- If positive for HCV, ask to be treated.

But, even if a DU could follow these very restricting recommendations, it is not possible to guarantee an absence of contamination. Confusion and indetermination are not gone. We are not on the eve of a simple training course for professionals as well as for the public at large which would explain hepatitis C and give coherent and always effective recommendations for prevention. We have to wait for effective vaccines.

2.2 The epidemic of HCV hepatitis among DUs is not controlled

More than 20 years after the discovery of the hepatitis C virus, much of the ongoing epidemic is attributable to unsafe drug injections. An evaluation of the drug consuming population and of the DUs infected with HCV is recognized as an arduous exercise. One can consider snapshots taken at one time or can study a trend in a cohort. Both approaches must consider the evolution of:

- The population of DUs and the nature of drug consumption. Younger addicts cannot be treated as the older ones minus ten or twenty years. The French OFDT study "le matos" (the works), interviewing a panel of injectors, has been documenting these changes since the nineteen seventies. These different attitudes may coexist in different age groups (91). Despite globalization, each country and, even, each region, has its own history and market. I have described its course in France in a short overview in 2007 (92). A series of publications relevant to the French drug consumption can be downloaded from the site of the Observatoire Français des Drogues et des Toxicomanies (OFDT) in free acess (http://www.ofdt.fr/ofdtdev/live/publi.html).
- Illegal drugs' use has cycles. Cocaine will succeed heroin, designer drugs will find a new public. A new drug is detected each week in the European market (93). Recently, high levels of amphetamine injection have been reported around the Baltic, as well as Slovakia and Hungary…. A tremendous growth of the drug business occurred since the beginning of a war on drugs and the repressive laws of the 1970s. It is related to the huge profitability of the trafficking and the increasing demand of new consumers for psychoactive drugs, licit or illicit.

2.2.1 How many (intravenous) drug users and what proportion is infected by HCV?

Despite these recognized problems, figures are none the less produced: in counties of Western Europe, HCV prevalence among IDUs fall in a range comprised between 47.1 % (Austria) and Netherland (86.2 %) (94). The number of infected DUs in Western Europe could reach 727 500 (95% CI 497 000 – 1018 000).

France is the only country were different approaches have been used at different times to estimate the number of DUs and of people infected by HCV. A comparison of their results gives an idea of the accuracy of these estimations:

* The OFDT recently produced and discussed an estimation of the prevalence of problem drug users in France following a methodology shared by all the European countries: 5,4 to 6,4 /1 000 hab 15-64 years old. This estimate is almost twice that of Germany but lower than Italy, Spain and UK which had the highest prevalence. It has certain limits which are listed in the publication with a rare honesty (95):
  * First, the changing definition of the subject of the estimate. In 1993, "heroin addicts" were, at least, 160 000. In 1995, the estimate was of 142-172 000 "opiate problem users". In 2006, a new definition, taking into account the change in the drug market, considered "intravenous drug users or regular users of opiates, cocaine or amphetamines", led to an increase of 44 %. The change in these estimates may be more related to a difference in definition than to a real change in the size of the population.
  * Second, the proposed estimate of 230 000 problem users (210 to 250 000) cannot hide the fact that the real range computed through the four different methods before its narrowing by the experts to a definite number, without convincing arguments explaining their choice, was 147 000 to 367 000.
  * Third, these approaches ignored the users who have not been and will not be in contact with one of the information sources used (arrest, treatment, health problems, death, etc.)". For cocaine which is considered to be one of the most "addictive" drugs, no more than 20 % of users become addicted after 20 years of use, 80 % may not be accounted for by these evaluation (Wagner 2002). This statement is of importance, since this population is not negligible and can influence the evaluation of the number of patients infected by HCV through their drug use (96,97). In the nineties, most patients 30 to 40 years old, carriers of HCV, who came in our unit without any history of a possible contamination, confessed that 10 years before, on one or two "festive" occasions, they had injected drugs with friends and shared their syringes. They were not "addicts" and they did not consider themselves as such.
* The Veille Sanitaire (VS), the French organization studying public health, conducted 4 different surveys leading to four different results:,
  * Starting from HCV prevalence in the general population, two successive studies were conducted ten years apart (1994-2004) (98,99). Both addressed people covered by the French public welfare system (only 9 % of the recruited population agreed to make a test). They differed only by their scope. The second being much larger than the first. The interval of the first estimate was 500 000 to 600 000. Among IDUs, HCV prevalence was 78 %. Ten years later, what was presented as a more accurate

estimation of 367 000 was given with 65 % of viremic patients. The only explanation given to this spectacular decrease was the better methodology of the second study. Among the 0,38 % who recognized a previous history of injecting drugs, HCV prevalence was 55,5 % which would lead to a total of 150 000 French people with an history of at least one drug injectors in 2004, 82 500 of whom would be infected by HCV.

- In 2003, the number of DUs infected by HCV and of the incidence of new contaminations started with an hypothesis of a number of active injectors ranging from 80 to 100 000, given, at the time, by the OFDT and a prevalence of 60 to 70 %. The proposed number of infected IDUs was 48 000 to 70 000 and the number of new infections ranged from 2 700 to 4 400 for an estimated yearly new contaminations of 11 % (100).

- The fourth study was a cross-sectional multicenter survey of DUs having injected or snorted drugs at least once in their life conducted in 2004, the same year as the second population prevalence study (101). It was a two stage random survey of DUs selected to represent the diversity of drug use. Fingerprick blood samples were collected on blotting paper in 75 % of the screened population. The overall prevalence of HIV and HCV were respectively 10.8 (0.3 % under 30 years of age) and 59.8 % (NIDUs 27.9 %; IDUs 73,8 %; under 30 years 28%). In multivariate analysis, factors independently associated with HCV seropositivity were age over 30, HIV seropositivity, having ever injected drugs, opiate substitution treatment (OST), crack use, and precarious housing. HIV seroprevalence was not related to an history of injecting, but increased with age with a geographic difference of prevalence.

Contrary to the OFDT, no explanation was given of these discrepancies: a decrease of one third of the number of people infected by HCV between 1994 and 2004, and, the same year, 2004, a discrepancy of 18.3 % between two estimations using different methodologies to assess HCV prevalence among IDUs.

2.2.2 Is it possible to know HCV prevalence and incidence among DUs and what is the efficacy of harm reduction programmes?

2.2.2.1 Cohorts the incidence and risk factors of new infections can only be studied in cohorts of IDUs initially seronegative

Ideally, these cohorts should begin when IDUs start to inject and no drop out should occur or, at least, the drop outs should not differ from the rest of the cohort. Of course, these requirements are almost impossible to fulfill. In some cases, infection incidence rate was even computed from a retrospective selection of patients who had at least two serum samples available and found initially seronegative (102–104). In a prospective study in the north and east of France, 28.6 % were lost to follow-up and differed significantly from the others who remained in the study (6). These studies can inform on the modes of contamination. They can never accurately predict the true HCV incidence among all the DUs. However, the incidence rate of new HCV contaminations among NIDUs remained low in the few cohort studies which included them: 1/422 (0.4/100 PY (95 % CI 0.0-1.2) (105), none in those who did not start injection (106).

The four randomized studies of the impact of interventions to prevent hepatitis C infection among IDUs were not able to show significant differences (106–108). Despite an exclusion of severe psychiatric or somatic illnesses, which represent a significant bias, the drop-out rates were high. For example, Abou-Saleh et al. explored behavioral interventions among DUs already followed by drug treatment services. Among the 206 IDUS (initially 1354) who remained after exclusion of HCV positivity, of severe mental or physical illnesses or serious legal problems, 54 % refused or dropped out during the inclusion process, 95 were randomized, 82 % and 65 % were followed at six months and 12 months. In a per-protocol approach, the rate of contamination was higher at the end of six months (18 %) than after 12 months (12 %) and there was no significant difference between the two interventions even if the trend was "in the anticipated direction" (108). In an intention to treat, drop-outs would have been considered as possible contaminations raising the contamination rate over 50 %.

Hagan et al. (109), mixed up these studies with different other interventions from bleach disinfection of syringes to behavioral interventions, in a report with strong methodological bias. First, the majority of the 26 studies were not intended to assess the efficacy of an intervention but to measure the rate of new infections among a cohort of IDUs. Then, they included the univariate odds-ratios of seroconversion even if they were not retained in multivariate analysis. For example, in the French study, a 60 % reduction in HCV incidence was observed between the patients treated with oral substitution treatment (OST) and the others. However, once the level of cotton and syringe sharing were included, this difference disappeared because these levels were not equally distributed between the two groups.

These observations explain why the quality of evidence of intervention impacts is found to be lacking and why it is so difficult to prove the efficacy of any harm reduction procedures. At best they can show that DUs retained in a programme fare better than those who stay outside or who quit. But they cannot prove that the decision to take part in the programmes does not select less risky behaviors and, most of all, that the proposal of these programmes to every DU would result in a significant decrease of new contaminations, which, of course, should be their aim.

2.2.2.2 Cross sectional studies

The results of repeated cross-sectional studies have the advantage of not being dependent of the retention rate in a programme. However, the population recruitment must be representative of the population studied and its modalities must not change from one period to the next. An incidence survey has been added to the cross-sectional approach in some cases. The community based study by Mehta et al. in Baltimore (110) and the study of IDUs attending Needle and Syringe Programs (NSP) in Autsralia by Falster et al. (111) can be considered as models:

- Mehta et al. studied a cohort of IDUs initially recruited in 1988-1989 and then added new IDUs in 1994-1995, 1998 and 2005-2008. They followed those who were seronegative for HCV and HIV and compared the new recruits. They observed a significant decrease in HIV infection from 5.5 cases/100 patient/year in 1988-1989 to 0/100 py in 2005-2008, whereas there was no significant change in HCV incidence. The prevalence study observed a decline in HCV prevalence among the youngest (39 years) and those who had a shorter injection history (<15 years). An increase in the duration of injection to reach a 80 % prevalence was observed between 1988-1989 (5-9 years) and

2005-2008 (15-19 years). After adjustment for demographic and time since injection, significant differences were observed between HCV prevalence in 1988-1989 and 1994-1995 on one hand and 2005-2008 on the other. A small proportion of this decline was explained by changes in drug-related risk behavior over time. It could be the consequence of a decrease of HCV prevalence.

- In Australia all IDUs attending a NSP site participating in the study were invited to complete an anonymous questionnaire and to provide a capillary blood sample (participation rate: 41 to 61 %) every year between 1995 and 2004 (Falster 2009). After adjustment for covariates, HCV antibody seropositivity remained associated with a longer duration of injecting, older age, participation in the state of New South Wales, opiates as the last drug injected, imprisonment in the last year, female sex, daily or more frequent injection, sharing needles and syringes in the last month, sex work, and survey participation in 2000–2004. An increase in HCV prevalence was found within injection initiation cohorts over time, with prevalence appearing to reach saturation around 90% in the older cohorts. An increase from 1895-1996 to 2003-2004 in the prevalence of HCV infection among IDUs who had injected less than 7 years could reflect an increase in the prevalence of HCV in that population.

2.2.2.3 France and Lyon: the course of an epidemic

Knowing the methodological limits of any evaluation of an HCV epidemic among DUs and of the effectiveness of harm reduction programs, I will present the results of the studies I conducted in Lyon and in France and, taking into account the other French evaluation on the subject and my experience of thirty years of care to DUs, I will give a tentative interpretation of the course of the epidemic in France.

2.2.2.3.1 Prison

I conducted studies in Lyon's prison because it was the only place, outside of complex snowball enquiries, were no bias was met, in the recruitment of IDUs, which could be related to a care demand. Every IDU entering Lyon's prisons between 19987-1989, 1997-1999 and 2009-2011 were asked to answer a questionnaire and to provide a blood sample. Acceptance was high (>90 %).

- Among DUs entering prison, before 1990, injection was the rule (90 %) and heroin was the main product. This study showed a sharp decrease of "indiscriminate" sharing from 65 % for those who had begun their drug use before 1980, to 15 % for those whose first use began after 1987. This change was related to the occurrence of the AIDS epidemic in 1984-1985 and predated the free access to sterile needles and syringes of 1987 which, nevertheless, had an additional impact. After 1985, an increasing number of pharmacists agreed to sell syringes answering an increasing demand of IDUs. Follow-up studies conducted in the same environment among injectors confirmed this trend in the change of behavior and of viral prevalence with a quasi disappearance of indiscriminate syringe sharing after 1992. Conversely, the absence of any sharing reported by less than 5 % of IDUs who had begun to inject before 1980, reached 70 % after 1990.
- In 2009-2010, a radical change in drug consumption had occurred from heroin injection associated by less than 10 % of DUs to cocaine in speedballs in the eighties to an almost equal number of heroin and cocaine consumers (cocaine 82 %; heroin 70 %; 52,6 % used

both drugs). Only one fourth had injected. These results underline the change in drug use observed at a national level (95). The prevalence of injection was higher (29.5 %) among heroin addicts than among cocaine abusers (18.3 %) but, among injectors syringe and needle sharing was not different. There was no difference in HCV prevalence between non drug users (2.4 %) and NIDU (3.9 %, OR 1.7 95 % CI=0.7-4.2). This prevalence rose to 48.6 % for IDUs who said they had never shared their needles (OR/NIDU 23.9 95 percent CI=8.0-65.8) and to 66.7 % for those who had (OR/NIDU 44.7 95 percent CI=13.6-167.4). HCV detection was also related to an older age and a longer drug use but had no relation, among injectors, with the nature (heroin or cocaine) of the drug used. One fourth (24,4 %) were nationals of countries belonging to the exUSSR which is in accordance with a trend observed in most French hepatitis units for some years.

• In a comparison of IDUs entering prison in 1987-1989, 1997-1999 and 209-2011, the decrease of syphilis infections among that population as soon as 1986 (11 % before to 4.7 % after) and its disappearance after 1990 demonstrated the decrease of the trade of sex for drug. In a multivariate analysis controlling for date of first injection, duration of injection, place of injection (for HIV alone) and risk sharing the Odds ratio of viral infection in 1987-1988 compared to 1997-1998 were 15,4 for HIV, 7,8 for HBV and 3,3 for HCV, indicating a decrease (certain for HBV and HIV, possible for HCV) in the prevalence of these infections among injecting drug users. On the contrary, no difference was observed between 1978-199 and 2009-2011.

2.2.2.3.2 Multicenter cross-sectional studies

In 1996 a multicenter study, at that time the largest state funded study of DUs, recruited 1302 DUs in 3 French towns (Lille, Lyon, Paris) among GPs and their referral hospitals. 120 data were collected. It confirmed the trend observed in Lyon's prison with a decrease of the indiscriminate needle sharing. A consistent increase in age for first drug use since the end of the eighties was observed. Before 1981 and after 1991, the prevalence of syringe sharing without precaution was divided by 8 while that for spoons was only divided by 1.4, for cotton wool by 1.6 and that for back loading by 1.3. Needle sharing was more frequent at night (60% versus 30 %). The proportion of nightly exchanges increased during periods when patients were "high" (59%), during withdrawal (61 %) and at the time of a relapse (76 %). This sharing at the time of relapse was unpredictable and represented approximately 25% of cases. Shared material other than syringes were in decreasing order: spoons (46%), filtration cotton (39%) and 'back loading' (20%). 9 years after the legalization of the purchase of needles and syringes in pharmacies and 5 years after the opening of the first NSP in Paris, a very small proportion attended NSPs (7%) or vending machines (2%). Socio-economic variables were not associated with the extent of needle sharing (a continuous professional activity was only found in 20% of cases but only 3% of drug addicts in this study did not benefit from any kind of social assistance). Gender, living with a partner and housing were not significant. Only the level of education and, to a lesser degree, professional situation was of importance. The prevalence of needle exchanges without precautions decreased from 29% in users who had primary level of education compared to 12 % in those who had started high school. Prostitution was seldom reported by men (3 %), but 29 % of women recognized this practice which declined from 33 % before 1980 to 21 % after 1990, most frequently observed in occasional "hookers" (28 to 16 %). The prevalence of cutaneous abscesses (23 %) and of overdoses (29 %) had not changed with time.

2.2.2.3.3 Discussion

These studies confirmed the disappearance of the HIV epidemic and, on the contrary, a persistence of the HCV epidemic. This observation is concordant with the results of national surveys. In 2008, the estimated French total number of new HIV infections among IDUs was 70 (95 % CI 0-190) with, for the first time, a majority of DUs newly discovered being born abroad (112)(Levu 2011). A credible story can be told:

- Before the AIDS epidemic, if hepatitis were known to be present among DUs, they were ignored since their symptoms were few, no treatment was available and their death rates (fulminant or subfulminant hepatitis) were exceptional, much lower than those of deaths by overdoses, violence or suicides. With the sudden onset of the HIV epidemic, everything changed. DUs wasted and died and as soon as 1984-1985 everybody knew that AIDS was an infectious disease transmitted through sexual intercourse and blood transmission. The message had all the characteristics which make a message "stick": it was simple (HIV infection led to death), unexpected (people paid attention), concrete (it was understood and remembered), credible (people agreed and believed), emotional (people cared) and led people to act (a credible story was told with a solution: condoms and sterile works). Paraphernalia use (the impact was obvious on needle and syringes, filters were mostly ignored) as well as sexual practices changed significantly. I observed a decrease in NSS which begun well before the law of 1987 on the free access to needle and syringes, sex for drug and the prevalence of syphilis declined at the same time and, furthermore, DUs died (those who took the most risks). As a result, the HIV epidemic disappeared in regions like Lyon were its prevalence had been low when the epidemic was discovered. In others (Paris, Bordeaux, the south of France), a small pool of DUs infected with HIV survived. They were slow progressors and were able to access HIV infectious specialists and wait until HAART were available. They remained a reservoir for some occasional contaminations (the respective role of injection and homo or heterosexual transmission in these new infections is unknown). This is in accordance with our multicenter study of 1996 and explains the discrepancy between the high rate of HIV prevalence observed in Marseille and the national observation of a very low incidence of new infections (113). Contrary to Jauffret-Roustide (101), I believe that the difference in HIV prevalence between Lille and Marseille in 2004, is not mainly related to a prevalence of injection, which was not significantly related to HIV seroprevalence in their survey, but to a difference in the course in the epidemic shown by our 1996 study: Marseille had already one of the highest HIV prevalence in the early eighties and the explosion of drug use in Lille occurred in the late eighties, when people were aware of the HIV epidemic, explaining the constant low HIV prevalence. However, recent changes are observed with the occurrence of new cases coming form countries were HIV prevalence is high among IDUs (today countries from the ex-USSR, maybe Africa were drug use is expanding tomorrow). The impact of this new epidemic on native DUs is still unknown.
- The course of the HBV epidemic followed that of HIV. To be infected, one must encounter a infectious carrier: 90 % of adults newly infected will spontaneously clear the virus and only a fraction of them will be infectious through sexual contacts and through NSS. If in the eighties and most of the nineties, a diagnosis of infection through drug use could be made when HBV together with HCV markers were detected, it was not the case anymore after 2000, or earlier with younger addicts only infected with

HCV. HDV, which needs an HBV coinfection, had disappeared at the end of the eighties, but comes back, sporadically, with eastern migrants.

- For HCV, the course of the epidemic is radically different. It is obvious that in the early eighties, HCV, like HBV prevalence was high among IDUs, in the range of 80 to 90 %. There was no difference between French regions. Harm reduction did not exist. The 3 surveys I conducted before 2000 give a coherent picture of their evolution. Before the discovery of the AIDS epidemic, the majority of IDUs took no precaution with their "works" (even if they injected only once in a recreational setting). Since most IDUs were infected the first year of injection, HCV prevalence among IDUs with an history of only few injections did not differ significantly from that of those who had been indiscriminate. A decrease in NSS occurred in the eighties resulting in a delay when duration of injection was considered, but the influence of the level of NSS, when it had occurred, was not significant, reflecting the persisting high HCV prevalence. The 1996 survey emphasizes the low access to harm reduction programs such as NSP or vending machines at a time when most of the changes in the course of the HIV and HCV epidemic had occurred. NSS occurred at a time when pharmacies were closed, at a place where vending machines were absent and when a sudden craving was felt. Behavior reported by most of the few IDUs I followed who seroconverted. This situation was not exceptional in DUs receiving OST after 1996. A small but significant trend was noted toward a reduction in the epidemic when comparing IDUs who had begun injecting before 1990 and between 1990 and 1999. This decrease was sustained in 2009 but the size of the sample is too small to make final conclusions. However, differences may exist between French regions. In Alsace, in a GP network, HCV prevalence among DUs under 30 years of age was only 7 % (114). This dissociation in the evolution of HIV and HCV epidemic has been observed in Vancouver (115) and in most countries were drug injection was present before 1980 (116,117).

2.3 From an addition of successive layers of harm reduction to the recognition of the complexity of the control of risky behaviors

A thorough synthesis and evaluation of harm reduction effectiveness has been published in an EMCDDA monograph in 2010 (118) following others (119–121) with the same conclusions: the absence of high-quality review evidence leading to question this efficacy. I will try to consider the respective impact of past harm reduction programmes and the improvement which could be implemented to improve their efficiency in the French context.

2.3.1 Prevention

2.3.1.1 Oral substitution treatment

The massive introduction of OST in France in 1996 was followed by an instantaneous and tremendous change in the care for DUs. In 2002, it was assumed that one third of problematic opiate users (52 000) were engaged in long-term treatment with an additional 22 000 receiving prescriptions on an irregular basis (122). OST introduction occurred at a time when the HIV epidemic among DUs was already controlled. Its impact is, thus, difficult to assess. However, OST in community setting is considered to reduce HIV seroconversion and to have a possible role in reducing the number of HCV seroconversions among DUs who remain in the programmes. From my experience and from the results of a study of the migration of IDUs inside Lyon's healthcare and penal institutions I conducted in 1989, OSTs have delayed the time of transition to injection among heroin users. But since many other variables have changed during that period, and since we still do not know the evolution of the prevalence of injectors, this assumption remains speculative. The problem which remains is what to do with the non compliant DUs, most at risk of infection or with those who do not attend OSTs? The change in the nature of the drugs consumed by DUs observed in the last years with an increase in cocaine/crack use could limit the impact of OST on these consumers and should lead to an evolution of the DPs even if, recently a disaffection for cocaine and a come-back of heroin through micronetworks of users-sellers (123) has been reported in France.

2.3.1.2 Reduction of syringe and needle sharing (NSS)

The first harm reduction programme implemented in France occurred in 1987 with a law allowing free access to needles and syringes in French pharmacies. The motivation behind this decision, like the decision, in 1996, to offer an easy access to OST, was more a protection of the heterosexual community from HIV and hepatitis viruses than an improvement of DUs' care. For someone who lived that period, it is obvious that, this decision increased significantly a preexisting trend and was significantly associated to a quasi disappearance of indiscriminate NSS among IDUs. From my study in prison and the national survey of 1996 as well as my own experience with the IDUs I followed at that time when no OST, beside neocodion, was available, it is "obvious" that it answered a demand of IDUs and decreased significantly NSS after they had discovered and realized the risk inherent to that practice. Following this first move, steribox containing needles, syringes, filters and condoms have been sold to IDUs for a low price or have been available through NSP which have been opened in the early nineties. In 1998, with an estimation of 2.8 injections per IDU per day, Lurie and al. estimated that between 920 million and 1.7 billion injections by IDUs took place each year in the United States (estimated 12 million in San Francisco and >80 million in New York City) (124). Using the same level of daily injections, with a conservative estimation of 80-100 000 IDUs, 80 and 100 000 million of injections could take place in France. An annual estimation of syringes sold to IDUs in France between 1996 and 2003 made by the INVS increased from 1996 to 1999 (14.7 to 17.7 M) and then decreased dramatically from 1999 to 2003 (10.9 M) (125). This decrease was ascribed to an increase in OST during the same period. NSP accounted for only 1.5 M exchanges with large differences in the number of steribox exchanged yearly (253-10 000) between as many as 129 programmes or vending machines. The observation that a syringe can be reused 10 times is not a surprise. Pharmacies after they began to give free steribox have been shown to quadruple in the first 6 months the number they dispensed to the same number of IDUs (126). In a survey of 35 large metropolitan areas in the US, the range of the number of syringes distributed was 2 per 10 injection events to 3 per 10 000 injection events (127). Sterile syringes for each shoot may be desired, but can this goal be reached and would it be sufficient to prevent receptive exchanges? For cocaine users, distribution of glass stems, rubber mouthpieces, brass screens, chopsticks, lip balm and chewing gum, reducing the harms associated with smoking crack, may decrease the number of injections (128).

Considering what is unknown about the number of IDUs, their access to harm reduction programmes (HRPs), the efficacy of theses HRPs and the modes of viral contamination, one can be surprised that models fitting strategies to control the HCV epidemic can be proposed.

However, models exist even if they are oversimple and if some (many) of their initial assumptions on the rate of viral transmission or the efficacy of NSP and OST to prevent infection, may be problematic. The conclusion that high-risk DUs are infected early and that the rate of infection among low-risk groups will continue for years are truisms (34). Percolation-based approximations can be highly biased when one incorrectly assumes that infectious periods and when deterministic models assume that every contact is with a new individual. Thus, models should be significantly improved, for example, with the use of stochastic models which take into account lasting relationships and inclusion in groups, but they should also use additional data on specific populations (129,130). Despite these limits, Vickerman et al. suggest that, in the UK, NSP and OST have been able to limit 50 000 new infections in the UK, but even with their initial optimistic assumptions, they conclude that a reduction by half in chronic HCV prevalence would need OST and 100% NSP to be scaled up to 80 % coverage for at least 20 years (131).

French results do not support a significant impact of harm reduction programmes on the course of the HIV and HCV epidemic outside of the free access to sterile needles and syringes in pharmacies (112).

2.3.2 Hepatitis treatment

The treatment of DUs' viral infections has been considered since the occurrence of the AIDS epidemic. In the nineteen eighties, our diagnosis tools were limited and available treatments were experimental. In Lyon we used the first anti HBV antiviral in continuous perfusions of four weeks durations for severe HBV hepatitis as early as 1979, then with beta interferon for HBV/HDV coinfections and NonA NonB hepatitis in 1984 and alpha interferon for both since 1989 after the first randomized trials of 1987. This know-how encompassed also HIV infections and at every step we treated active IDUs years before OST could be prescribed (1996) in France. Our recruitment was biased, but we were able to screen and treat most of the DUs who asked for heroin detoxification or hepatitis and HIV treatment. On another level, a national consultation in 1991, concluded that HIV infected DUs did not differ from the other patients. Compliance was related to housing problems whatever the modalities of infection. Having treated DUs for their HIV infections since 1984 and for their hepatitis since 1986, we did not agree with the recommendations of the French consensus conferences which denied the treatment of HCV hepatitis to active DUs in 1997. This position, initially controversial, has become the norm with an emerging consensus that DUs can be treated for their hepatitis on a case by case basis. In a study of the perception of their disease in 2000, 60 IDUs successively entering Lyon's prisons were interviewed. At least one liver biopsy had been performed in 49 (90 % of those whose hepatitis had been discovered more than 5 years earlier). 80 % of viremic DUs who had a significant fibrosis (> F1) had been treated and 50 % of the others on account of fatigue or a desire to be treated. The multi-disciplinary management we developed with success in the early nineteen nineties is now proposed as a possible solution to improve access to treatment (132–134). The possible impact of treating HCV infected DUs on the course of the epidemic has even been studied by different models which are the subject of debates (135,136).

In France when we proposed to study the possibility of treating HCV hepatitis to decrease HCV prevalence in a nationally funded Clinical Hospital Research Programme in 2002, few hepatitis units received IDUs. In 2004, in a national observational study of 40 hepatitis units, only two hepatitis reference centers treated a significant number of HCV hepatitis of drug users. In 2011, after three successive national plans, the situation has changed. 90 % of the 31 hepatitis reference centers who treat two third of French HCV hepatitis declared that DUs' hepatitis care was a strategic decision. Differences in history and location, as well as the size of the HCV specialist team (range 0.8-10) made each centre a special case. Various innovative solutions have been implemented, in some cases before the allocation of resources. A partnership was present with drug treatment programs (DTP) (85.2 %) and GPs' network (25.9 %). 44.7 % found that care for DUs hepatitis did not need a specific competence. Perceived problems were reported by only 34.3 % of HCV specialists (absenteeism) and 48.3 % of nurses (absenteeism, blood access). Waiting times were similar for DUs and non-DUs. Our results support collaboration between services involved in DUs' care. However their complete and complex integration may only be needed for the most precarious such as homeless adolescents.

3. HCV, drug use, and the world complexity

Biomedical knowledge of the HCV epidemic among DUs is obviously not enough to be able to control its course. My practice taught me that if objectification of DUs as well as of their hepatitis was inescapable, an understanding of its limits implies an integration of other aspects of our "being-here" (Dasein) such as the brain, society, social systems and ethics.

- The "rationality" of one's decision includes his lifetime experience, "being-here". The human brain constructs the world from gestation onward in an interaction with its environment. This process governed by genes and their expression (epigenetic) (137) leads to more and more complex "logical" choices following statistical "Bayesian inferences" (138), the results of which may be forgotten but still predetermine future decisions by limiting the scope of one's expectations. Its integrated complexity is mainly unconscious and organizes a memory which is more concerned by one's future efficiency than by an accurate memorization of past events. It leaves a small place to what we consider as consciousness which has to decide among a limited number of preselections networked through sleep and "mind wandering" (139–142). Brain exercise like meditation could improve its efficiency. The development of the brain is crucially sensitive in its first months and years to its relations with its human environment which will make up the limits of its future "creativity" through the secure basis of its attachment (143–145). At adolescence, the brain restructuration will settle its adult functional frame (146) . Drug use and addiction represent only one dimension of this complex adaptative interaction which cannot be "revolutionized" by a single logical argumentation. The impact of the initial AIDS epidemic, with its massive death toll, observed in France in the nineteen eighties will not occur anymore. It was "one shot". Prevention messages, treatment proposals have to take into account these changing individual ecologies. One can be immediately convinced by the description of the risk of NSS but will nevertheless engage in NSS when its result is an instant improvement in well being compared with an improbable success of hepatitis prevention over the future years of addiction and the high probability of dying before the advent of an improbable liver cancer.
- Modern society, faced with the management of its growing complexity, has organized itself functionally around social systems which rationally objectify the world (147).

They follow an initial selection of their missions through binary codes (health/disease for medicine, presence or absence of an hepatitis for HCV specialists) which makes them "blind" to what has been excluded (the complexity of the world) and gives them a meaning which is the basis of their communication with their environment. These self-referential systems fight to survive and extend their territories responding to stimulations (irritations) of their environment through the limited structural couplings they themselves made possible. Hepatologists will use scientific medical mathematics to modelize the HCV epidemic from scarce and improbable data to convince politics and economics to maintain and, even, increase their funding. Publication of these computations will improve the academic status of biostatisticians. The pharmaceutical industry will fund these studies which secure the outlet of their products and so on. For an hepatitis specialist DU exists first as a carrier of an HCV infection for an hepatitis specialists This practical discovery explains the absence of specificity of DUs' hepatitis management reported by French HRCs: The only limit of HCV treatment was compliance, problem which was not restricted to DUs and, in our French study of HRCs, did not need a specific management for consulting DUs. The question of the control of the HCV epidemic was irrelevant. The global failure of society faced with the problem of drug use and of its management, the awareness of its social complexity are the source of the demand by the professionals of an association in the same place of diverse services addressing belonging to multiple social systems: they would "have to" manage the failures of one particular service which, once its limits recognized, would not be considered as such.

- This organization ignores the complexity of one's "being-here" and is the source of a modern reactivation of the ethical debate (148–151). A DU does not exist as such outside its representation by society's Other. The practical success of HCV care cure but also prevention) is related to the capacity of each individual to recognize and make recognized the inscrutable "otherness" present in every human being. Rational objectification, which is at the core of every scientific approach, is supported by the emptiness of universal concepts which deny this recognition. This otherness is the source of an infinite demand which founds inter human relations. The limited offer which one can propose in return, leaves to this "neighbour", who is to be "loved like oneself ", the freedom to make the right choice. In its absence, the quenching of the scientific rational solution (see Descartes's discourse of a method), when it is implemented, may be transformed into an unbearable violence which will force one to step out of the symbolic order to express one's freedom and say no to an impossible but irrefutable proposal (see paragraph II.1.3.): "death drive" for Freud, "radical negativity" for German Idealism. This "acting-out" has its own inescapable rationality: the immediacy of one's (emotional and conscious) survival in the "death struggle" of the Hegelian demand for recognition. Care and cure cannot be summed up as an accurate diagnosis and prescription. In my practice, this (not so) simple recognition of the other's freedom had a constant practical impact. One of society's responses is the development of a "third sector", non-profit organizations outside of organized social systems which answer its latencies such as individual and social complexity but whose precarious survival depends on their perceived immediate social utility.

4. Finally, let us try to be creative

At the end of this general survey, limiting their scope to the HCV epidemic, four options are possible.

- The first would keep the status quo, leaving the community with the belief that harm reduction is efficient, efficiency which could be boosted by additional funding of each of these actions and a better collaboration between services leading to integration in drug treatment programmes which would encompass them all. The sole aim of many papers published in journals dedicated to drug use and DUs is to convince their reader of its validity. This position is held by each subsystem which, to survive and even grow has to convince its environment of its performance. In my opinion, it may appear as the less costly in energy and financial involvement, but I believe, in the long term, it will be the less efficient.

- The second is more ambitious. It considers HCV hepatitis as an epidemic which should be controlled and DUs as users of services supplied by the healthcare system which may not be spontaneously desired by DUs but which use such as the treatment of HIV and hepatitis should be implemented to control these epidemics. From a DU's stand point HCV hepatitis cannot be considered alone. It is never more than a part of his "being-here" for which society's goals of harm reduction may not be relevant. To succeed society has to propose an environment "good-enough" to enable him to live without a continuous help of drugs. This option depends on the assumption that a better knowledge and a better management could control the HCV epidemic. Today, it remains a "wishful thinking" of existing social systems:

  - The initial assumption would be that the control of the HCV epidemic should associate prevention of new infections to the treatment of "all" (at least a large majority) the infected DUs (even not in DTP) to decrease viral prevalence to a level which would, by itself, limit the new contaminations, passing from an epidemic to sporadic cases, evolution observed for HIV in most countries where the initial prevalence remained low.

  - The first step would design and conduct an ethno-epidemiological study of a population in a geographical delimited area relevant for the proposed intervention. It would collect its socio-demographics, health status, social networks, drugs consumed and risks associated to that consumption, viral status and use of social and health care as well as its motivations, desires and plans (152).

  - From that collection, an analysis would define potentially different subgroups which would be targeted for different interventions which would try to build a "cultural" environment including a positive vision of HCV care and the conscience of the necessity of a global commitment needed to control the HCV epidemic. It would try to understand its course among these different subgroups including the possible viral reservoirs among DUs who do not attend healthcare services. The first goal of these programmes would be to win the trust of the concerned DUs by proposing services answering their need (desires). Beside proposing substitution treatments or social help to find work or housing, considering the cost of harm reduction and HCV treatment, one could propose conditional cash transfer or vouchers which have been used successfully in many countries to improve access to school or healthcare programmes and which is one of the few incentives proven to be efficient in cocaine addiction (153,154). Heroin treatment should be considered. It has been shown to be significantly more effective than methadone for difficult to maintain patients (155,156). This efficacy was also present in DUs without previous maintenance treatments (157). It can be delivered intranasally or orally (158). It has been shown to be cost-effective (159).

HCV prevention and treatment would only come second, tailored to the course of the epidemic, targeting opinion leaders through peers' interventions explaining the ethical goal of the project which would not be limited to the individual gain of the cure of one's hepatitis but would want to control the HCV epidemic in the area, control which would benefit not only DUs but also their family, friends and neighbors. Their success would be conditioned by a complete appropriateness between the discourse and the means: To improve the impact of NSP, a significant rise would be mandatory to decrease significantly the occurrence of receptive exchanges. It could mean a tenfold increase in the number of syringes exchanged, but it would not be enough. NSP should shift from exchange to distribution (160) allowing IDUs to store sterile syringes for future use and "providers" to distribute syringes to other IDUs who are in need of sterile syringes and cannot access a NSP or a pharmacy (161) This would help to cover unexpected "craving" episodes in former IDUs at times when pharmacies and NSP are closed which represent, at least in my experience, a significant cause of new contaminations. Home self-test for the diagnosis of HIV and HCV infection should be an option (65). As long as the HCV prevalence remains high, to be efficient, NSP as well as potential consumption rooms should be located in the neighborhood of every drug scene (162-164) embedded within existing spatial and social relations of DUs (165). Outreach, bringing services to the DUs with the lowest social functioning can also decrease NSS). Open scenes, where users could come to buy their drugs, find NSP and meet harm reduction services, could reduce the level of NSSHCV screening could only be considered if a treatment could be proposed to every infected DU. Interventions should be adapted to the evolution of each case. Building trust takes time, even more when every partner (from customers to professionals) are concerned.

- The simplistic idea that one would only need to bring potential actors together to carry out a community project is long overdue [166]. Understanding the implications of the affiliation of professionals to social sub-systems could help them as well as those responsible for leading and managing programs to consider the limits of their individual scope, the need for an evolution of their missions and for new cooperative programs. The evolution of the French care of DUs' hepatitis C bears witness of its feasibility. To reach these goals, time and specific resources must be allocated and a common will and trust between the different actors is mandatory to overcome the existing barriers to an effective integration of prevention and treatment of hepatitis C (167-169). The proposed approach makes the control of the HCV epidemic an example of a new health policy paradigm: efficient integrated services (medical and social) based on the knowledge of the health of a population in a designated area as advocated by most groups working on the improvement of clinical effectiveness. This multilevel approach to change should include the individual, group/team, organization, and larger environment/system level (170).

- The third alternative would be the legalization (not a simple depenalization) of drug consumption. Of course this proposal may appear heretic when one considers drug related deaths and comorbidities. However, the rational behind the "war on drugs" was its possible success. 40 year after its implementation, one is forced to observe its failure,

failure which has a precedent with alcohol prohibition in the United States (171-181). The belief that this legalization would result in a huge increase in drug consumption can be compared to the fantasy of an increase in sexual promiscuity induced by sexual education in the eighties, which was proven to be false. The obvious benefit would be the huge amount of taxes which escapes today every government. The drug market is still one of the most perfect examples of a free market economy adapting its products to its customers and one of the most profitable. Of course, it would mean a negative impact on many social sub-systems devoted to this war like justice, police, customs or, even, medicine with a significant reduction of state spending. They would not able to "understand" a proposal which would negate the mission which justifies their existence and reduce their "power". A global vision would be mandatory. One must also not forget drug dealers who have an interest in keeping their trade illegal and can spend large sums of money to bribe people who are able prevent that evolution. An initial transfer of marijuana market from organized crime to state management could assess the risks and benefits of this change of policy. Of course, its impact on the HCV epidemic would wait heroin and cocaine legalization which would only reduce the number of new contaminations.

- The fourth and last solution would be the development of a vaccine comparable to the HBV vaccine and which could be implemented on a population basis at least at adolescence. Of course this solution, when available, could improve each one of the previous solutions.

5. References

[1] Matheï C, Buntinx F, van Damme P. Seroprevalence of hepatitis C markers among intravenous drug users in western European countries: a systematic review. J.Viral. Hepat. 2002 May;9(3):157-73.

[2] Hagan H, Des Jarlais DC, Stern R, Lelutiu-Weinberger C, Scheinmann R, Strauss S, et al. HCV synthesis project: preliminary analyses of HCV prevalence in relation to age and duration of injection. Int. J. Drug Policy. 2007 oct;18(5):341-51.

[3] Grebely J, Raffa JD, Lai C, Krajden M, Kerr T, Fischer B, et al. Low uptake of treatment for hepatitis C virus infection in a large community-based study of inner city residents. J. Viral Hepat. 2009 mai;16(5):352-8.

[4] Rhodes T, Treloar C. The social production of hepatitis C risk among injecting drug users: a qualitative synthesis. Addiction. 2008 oct;103(10):1593-603.

[5] Smyth BP, Barry J, Keenan E. Irish injecting drug users and hepatitis C: the importance of the social context of injecting. Int. J. Epidemiol. 2005 feb;34(1):166-72.

[6] Maher L, Jalaludin B, Chant KG, Jayasuriya R, Sladden T, Kaldor JM, et al. Incidence and risk factors for hepatitis C seroconversion in injecting drug users in Australia. Addiction. 2006 oct;101(10):1499-508.

[7] Lucidarme D, Bruandet A, Ilef D, Harbonnier J, Jacob C, Decoster A, et al. Incidence and risk factors of HCV and HIV infections in a cohort of intravenous drug users in the North and East of France. Epidemiol. Infect. 2004 août;132(4):699-708.

[8] Scheinmann R, Hagan H, Lelutiu-Weinberger C, Stern R, Des Jarlais DC, Flom PL, et al. Non-injection drug use and Hepatitis C Virus: a systematic review. Drug Alcohol Depend. 2007 juin 15;89(1):1-12.

[9] Macías J, Palacios RB, Claro E, Vargas J, Vergara S, Mira JA, et al. High prevalence of hepatitis C virus infection among noninjecting drug users: association with sharing the inhalation implements of crack. Liver Int. 2008 juill;28(6):781-6.

[10] Nurutdinova D, Abdallah AB, Bradford S, O'Leary CC, Cottler LB. Risk factors associated with Hepatitis C among female substance users enrolled in community-based HIV prevention studies. BMC Res Notes. 2011;4:126.

[11] Tor J, Llibre JM, Carbonell M, Muga R, Ribera A, Soriano V, et al. Sexual transmission of hepatitis C virus and its relation with hepatitis B virus and HIV. BMJ. 1990 nov 17;301(6761):1130-3.

[12] Neumayr G, Propst A, Schwaighofer H, Judmaier G, Vogel W. Lack of evidence for the heterosexual transmission of hepatitis C. QJM. 1999 sept;92(9):505-8.

[13] G Rooney, Gilson RJ. Sexual transmission of hepatitis C virus infection. Sex Transm Infect. 1998 déc;74(6):399-404.

[14] Tsai P-S, Chang C-J, Chen K-T, Chang K-C, Hung S-F, Wang J-H, et al. Acquirement and disappearance of HBsAg and anti-HCV in an aged population: a follow-up study in an endemic township. Liver Int. 2011 août;31(7):971-9.

[15] Ghosn J, Thibault V, Delaugerre C, Fontaine H, Lortholary O, Rouzioux C, et al. Sexually transmitted hepatitis C virus superinfection in HIV/hepatitis C virus co-infected men who have sex with men. AIDS. 2008 mars 12;22(5):658-61.

[16] Urbanus AT, van de Laar TJ, Stolte IG, Schinkel J, Heijman T, Coutinho RA, et al. Hepatitis C virus infections among HIV-infected men who have sex with men: an expanding epidemic. AIDS. 2009 juill 31;23(12):F1-7.

[17] van de Laar T, Pybus O, Bruisten S, Brown D, Nelson M, Bhagani S, et al. Evidence of a large, international network of HCV transmission in HIV-positive men who have sex with men. Gastroenterology. 2009 mai;136(5):1609-17.

[18] van der Helm JJ, Prins M, del Amo J, Bucher HC, Chêne G, Dorrucci M, et al. The hepatitis C epidemic among HIV-positive MSM: incidence estimates from 1990 to 2007. AIDS. 2011 mai 15;25(8):1083-91.

[19] Tohme RA, Holmberg SD. Transmission of hepatitis C virus infection through tattooing and piercing: a critical review. Clin. Infect. Dis. 2012 avr;54(8):1167-78.

[20] Hwang L-Y, Kramer JR, Troisi C, Bull L, Grimes CZ, Lyerla R, et al. Relationship of cosmetic procedures and drug use to hepatitis C and hepatitis B virus infections in a low-risk population. Hepatology. 2006 août;44(2):341-51.

[21] Koziel MJ, Wong DK, Dudley D, Houghton M, Walker BD. Hepatitis C virus-specific cytolytic T lymphocyte and T helper cell responses in seronegative persons. J. Infect. Dis. 1997 oct;176(4):859-66.

[22] Bronowicki JP, Vetter D, Uhl G, Hudziak H, Uhrlacher A, Vetter JM, et al. Lymphocyte reactivity to hepatitis C virus (HCV) antigens shows evidence for exposure to HCV in HCV-seronegative spouses of HCV-infected patients. J. Infect. Dis. 1997 août;176(2):518-22.

[23] Kim JY, Won JE, Jeong S-H, Park SJ, Hwang SG, Kang S-K, et al. Acute hepatitis C in Korea: different modes of infection, high rate of spontaneous recovery, and low rate of seroconversion. J. Med. Virol. 2011 juill;83(7):1195-202.

[24] Pham TNQ, Coffin CS, Michalak TI. Occult hepatitis C virus infection: what does it mean? Liver Int. 2010 avr;30(4):502-11.

[25] MacParland SA, Pham TNQ, Guy CS, Michalak TI. Hepatitis C virus persisting after clinically apparent sustained virological response to antiviral therapy retains infectivity in vitro. Hepatology. 2009 mai;49(5):1431-41.

[26] Castillo I, Bartolomé J, Quiroga JA, Barril G, Carreño V. Hepatitis C virus infection in the family setting of patients with occult hepatitis C. J Med Virol 2009 juill;81(7):1198-203.

[27] Thurairajah PH, Hegazy D, Chokshi S, Shaw S, Demaine A, Kaminski ER, et al. Hepatitis C virus (HCV)--specific T cell responses in injection drug users with apparent resistance to HCV infection. J. Infect. Dis. 2008 déc 15;198(12):1749-55.

[28] Mizukoshi E, Eisenbach C, Edlin BR, Newton KP, Raghuraman S, Weiler-Normann C, et al. Hepatitis C virus (HCV)-specific immune responses of long-term injection drug users frequently exposed to HCV. J. Infect. Dis. 2008 juill 15;198(2):203-12.

[29] Aitken CK, Lewis J, Tracy SL, Spelman T, Bowden DS, Bharadwaj M, et al. High incidence of hepatitis C virus reinfection in a cohort of injecting drug users. Hepatology. 2008 déc;48(6):1746-52.

[30] Osburn WO, Fisher BE, Dowd KA, Urban G, Liu L, Ray SC, et al. Spontaneous control of primary hepatitis C virus infection and immunity against persistent reinfection. Gastroenterology. 2010 janv;138(1):315-24.

[31] Mehta SH, Cox A, Hoover DR, Wang X-H, Mao Q, Ray S, et al. Protection against persistence of hepatitis C. Lancet. 2002 avr 27;359(9316):1478-83.

[32] Grebely J, Conway B, Raffa JD, Lai C, Krajden M, Tyndall MW. Hepatitis C virus reinfection in injection drug users. Hepatology. 2006 nov;44(5):1139-45.

[33] Sacks-Davis R, Daraganava G, Altken C, Higgs P, Jenkinson R, Tracy SI, Bawden S, Robins G, Pattison P, Grebely J, Barry AE, Helard M. Molecular epidemiolgical evidence that social network research can identify hepatitis C transmission pathways in people who inject drugs. Hepatology. 2011;54(S1):1164A.

[34] Jager JC, European Monitoring Centre for Drugs and Drug Addiction. Hepatits C and injecting drug use: impact, costs and policy options. Luxembourg: European Monitoring Centre for Drugs and Drug Addiction; 2004.

[35] Loomba R, Rivera MM, McBurney R, Park Y, Haynes-Williams V, Rehermann B, et al. The natural history of acute hepatitis C: clinical presentation, laboratory findings and treatment outcomes. Aliment. Pharmacol. Ther. 2011 mars;33(5):559-65.

[36] Page K, Hahn JA, Evans J, Shiboski S, Lum P, Delwart E, et al. Acute hepatitis C virus infection in young adult injection drug users: a prospective study of incident infection, resolution, and reinfection. J. Infect. Dis. 2009 oct 15;200(8):1216-26.

[37] Thomas DL, Astemborski J, Rai RM, Anania FA, Schaeffer M, Galai N, et al. The natural history of hepatitis C virus infection: host, viral, and environmental factors. JAMA. 2000 juill 26;284(4):450-6.

[38] Thein H-H, Yi Q, Dore GJ, Krahn MD. Natural history of hepatitis C virus infection in HIV-infected individuals and the impact of HIV in the era of highly active antiretroviral therapy: a meta-analysis. AIDS. 2008 oct 1;22(15):1979-91.

[39] John-Baptiste A, Krahn M, Heathcote J, Laporte A, Tomlinson G. The natural history of hepatitis C infection acquired through injection drug use: meta-analysis and meta-regression. J. Hepatol. 2010 août;53(2):245-51.

[40] Bellentani S, Tiribelli C. The spectrum of liver disease in the general population: lesson from the Dionysos study. J. Hepatol. 2001 oct;35(4):531-7.

[41] Kenny-Walsh E. The natural history of hepatitis C virus infection. Clin Liver Dis. 2001 nov;5(4):969-77.

[42] Seeff LB, Hollinger FB, Alter HJ, Wright EC, Cain CM, Buskell ZJ, et al. Long-term mortality and morbidity of transfusion-associated non-A, non-B, and type C hepatitis: A National Heart, Lung, and Blood Institute collaborative study. Hepatology. 2001 févr;33(2):455-63.

[43] Harris HE, Ramsay ME, Andrews NJ. Survival of a national cohort of hepatitis C virus infected patients, 16 years after exposure. Epidemiol. Infect. 2006 juin;134(3):472-7.

[44] Butt AA, Wang X, Moore CG. Effect of hepatitis C virus and its treatment on survival. Hepatology. 2009 août;50(2):387-92.

[45] Grønbaek K, Krarup HB, Møller H, Krogsgaard K, Franzmann M, Sonne J, et al. Natural history and etiology of liver disease in patients with previous community-acquired acute non-A, non-B hepatitis. A follow-up study of 178 Danish patients consecutively enrolled in The Copenhagen Hepatitis Acuta Programme in the period 1969-1987. J. Hepatol. 1999 nov;31(5):800-7.

[46] Amin J, Law MG, Bartlett M, Kaldor JM, Dore GJ. Causes of death after diagnosis of hepatitis B or hepatitis C infection: a large community-based linkage study. Lancet. 2006 sept 9;368(9539):938-45.

[47] Neal KR, Ramsay S, Thomson BJ, Irving WL. Excess mortality rates in a cohort of patients infected with the hepatitis C virus: a prospective study. Gut. 2007 août;56(8):1098-104.

[48] Guiltinan AM, Kaidarova Z, Custer B, Orland J, Strollo A, Cyrus S, et al. Increased all-cause, liver, and cardiac mortality among hepatitis C virus-seropositive blood donors. Am. J. Epidemiol. 2008 mars 15;167(6):743-50.

[49] Omland LH, Krarup H, Jepsen P, Georgsen J, Harritshøj LH, Riisom K, et al. Mortality in patients with chronic and cleared hepatitis C viral infection: a nationwide cohort study. J. Hepatol. 2010 juill;53(1):36-42.

[50] Smyth B, Hoffman V, Fan J, Hser Y-I. Years of potential life lost among heroin addicts 33 years after treatment. Prev Med. 2007 avr;44(4):369-74.

[51] Missiha SB, Ostrowski M, Heathcote EJ. Disease progression in chronic hepatitis C: modifiable and nonmodifiable factors. Gastroenterology. 2008 mai;134(6):1699-714.

[52] Dring MM, Morrison MH, McSharry BP, Guinan KJ, Hagan R, O'Farrelly C, et al. Innate immune genes synergize to predict increased risk of chronic disease in hepatitis C virus infection. Proc. Natl. Acad. Sci. U.S.A. 2011 avr 5;108(14):5736-41.

[53] Knapp S, Warshow U, Ho KMA, Hegazy D, Little A-M, Fowell A, et al. A polymorphism in IL28B distinguishes exposed, uninfected individuals from spontaneous resolvers of HCV infection. Gastroenterology. 2011 juill;141(1):320-325, 325.e1-2.

[54] Pagliaro L, Pasta L, D'Amico G, Madonia S, Pietrosi G. Familial clustering of (mostly) HCV-related cirrhosis. A case-control study. J. Hepatol. 2002 déc;37(6):762-6.

[55] Sookoian S, Pirola CJ. Meta-analysis of the influence of I148M variant of patatin-like phospholipase domain containing 3 gene (PNPLA3) on the susceptibility and histological severity of nonalcoholic fatty liver disease. Hepatology. 2011 juin;53(6):1883-94.

[56] Trépo E, Gustot T, Degré D, Lemmers A, Verset L, Demetter P, et al. Common polymorphism in the PNPLA3/adiponutrin gene confers higher risk of cirrhosis and liver damage in alcoholic liver disease. J. Hepatol. 2011 oct;55(4):906-12.

[57] Huang H, Shiffman ML, Friedman S, Venkatesh R, Bzowej N, Abar OT, et al. A 7 gene signature identifies the risk of developing cirrhosis in patients with chronic hepatitis C. Hepatology. 2007 août;46(2):297-306.

[58] Marcolongo M, Young B, Dal Pero F, Fattovich G, Peraro L, Guido M, et al. A seven-gene signature (cirrhosis risk score) predicts liver fibrosis progression in patients with initially mild chronic hepatitis C. Hepatology. 2009 oct;50(4):1038-44.

[59] Riaz M, Idrees M, Kanwal H, Kabir F. An overview of triple infection with hepatitis B, C and D viruses. Virol. J. 2011;8:368.

[60] Jamma S, Hussain G, Lau DT-Y. Current Concepts of HBV/HCV Coinfection: Coexistence, but Not Necessarily in Harmony. Curr Hepat Rep. 2010;9(4):260-9.

[61] Greub G, Ledergerber B, Battegay M, Grob P, Perrin L, Furrer H, et al. Clinical progression, survival, and immune recovery during antiretroviral therapy in patients with HIV-1 and hepatitis C virus coinfection: the Swiss HIV Cohort Study. Lancet. 2000 nov 25;356(9244):1800-5.

[62] Vallet-Pichard A, Pol S. Natural history and predictors of severity of chronic hepatitis C virus (HCV) and human immunodeficiency virus (HIV) co-infection. J. Hepatol. 2006;44(1 Suppl):S28-34.

[63] Weis N, Lindhardt BO, Kronborg G, Hansen A-BE, Laursen AL, Christensen PB, et al. Impact of hepatitis C virus coinfection on response to highly active antiretroviral therapy and outcome in HIV-infected individuals: a nationwide cohort study. Clin. Infect. Dis. 2006 mai 15;42(10):1481-7.

[64] Mehta SH, Thomas DL, Torbenson M, Brinkley S, Mirel L, Chaisson RE, et al. The effect of antiretroviral therapy on liver disease among adults with HIV and hepatitis C coinfection. Hepatology. 2005 janv;41(1):123-31.

[65] Skolnik HS, Phillips KA, Binson D, Dilley JW. Deciding where and how to be tested for HIV: what matters most? J. Acquir. Immune Defic. Syndr. 2001 juill 1;27(3):292-300.

[66] Morota K, Fujinami R, Kinukawa H, Machida T, Ohno K, Saegusa H, et al. A new sensitive and automated chemiluminescent microparticle immunoassay for quantitative determination of hepatitis C virus core antigen. J. Virol. Methods. 2009 avr;157(1):8-14.

[67] Mederacke I, Potthoff A, Meyer-Olson D, Meier M, Raupach R, Manns MP, et al. HCV core antigen testing in HIV- and HBV-coinfected patients, and in HCV-infected patients on hemodialysis. J. Clin. Virol. 2012 févr;53(2):110-5.

[68] Hosseini-Moghaddam S, Iran-Pour E, Rotstein C, Husain S, Lilly L, Renner E, et al. Hepatitis C core Ag and its clinical applicability: Potential advantages and disadvantages for diagnosis and follow-up? Rev. Med. Virol. 2012 mai;22(3):156-65.

[69] Ahmad W, Ijaz B, Gull S, Asad S, Khaliq S, Jahan S, et al. A brief review on molecular, genetic and imaging techniques for HCV fibrosis evaluation. Virol. J. 2011;8(1):53.

[70] Cacoub P, Carrat F, Bédossa P, Lambert J, Pénaranda G, Perronne C, et al. Comparison of non-invasive liver fibrosis biomarkers in HIV/HCV co-infected patients: the fibrovic study--ANRS HC02. J. Hepatol. 2008 mai;48(5):765-73.

[71] Lucidarme D, Foucher J, Le Bail B, Vergniol J, Castera L, Duburque C, et al. Factors of accuracy of transient elastography (fibroscan) for the diagnosis of liver fibrosis in chronic hepatitis C. Hepatology. 2009 avr;49(4):1083-9.

[72] Huckans MS, Loftis JM, Blackwell AD, Linke A, Hauser P. Interferon alpha therapy for hepatitis C: treatment completion and response rates among patients with substance use disorders. Subst Abuse Treat Prev Policy. 2007;2:4.

[73] Chossegros P, Mélin P, Hézode C, Bourlière M, Pol S, Fhima A, et al. A French prospective observational study of the treatment of chronic hepatitis C in drug abusers. Gastroenterol. Clin. Biol. 2008 oct;32(10):850-7.

[74] Moreno C, Deltenre P, Pawlotsky J-M, Henrion J, Adler M, Mathurin P. Shortened treatment duration in treatment-naive genotype 1 HCV patients with rapid virological response: a meta-analysis. J. Hepatol. 2010 janv;52(1):25-31.

[75] Martin-Carbonero L, Nuñez M, Mariño A, Alcocer F, Bonet L, García-Samaniego J, et al. Undetectable hepatitis C virus RNA at week 4 as predictor of sustained virological response in HIV patients with chronic hepatitis C. AIDS. 2008 janv 2;22(1):15-21.

[76] Falasca K, Ucciferri C, Mancino P, Gorgoretti V, Pizzigallo E, Vecchiet J. Use of epoetin beta during combination therapy of infection with hepatitis c virus with ribavirin improves a sustained viral response. J. Med. Virol. 2010 janv;82(1):49-56.

[77] Rauch A, Kutalik Z, Descombes P, Cai T, Di Iulio J, Mueller T, et al. Genetic variation in IL28B is associated with chronic hepatitis C and treatment failure: a genome-wide association study. Gastroenterology. 2010 avr;138(4):1338-1345, 1345.e1-7.

[78] Suppiah V, Gaudieri S, Armstrong NJ, O'Connor KS, Berg T, Weltman M, et al. IL28B, HLA-C, and KIR variants additively predict response to therapy in chronic hepatitis C virus infection in a European Cohort: a cross-sectional study. PLoS Med. 2011 sept;8(9):e1001092.

[79] Mangia A, Thompson AJ, Santoro R, Piazzolla V, Tillmann HL, Patel K, et al. An IL28B polymorphism determines treatment response of hepatitis C virus genotype 2 or 3 patients who do not achieve a rapid virologic response. Gastroenterology. 2010 sept;139(3):821-827, 827.e1.

[80] Neukam K, Nattermann J, Rallón N, Rivero A, Caruz A, Macías J, et al. Different distributions of hepatitis C virus genotypes among HIV-infected patients with acute and chronic hepatitis C according to interleukin-28B genotype. HIV Med. 2011 sept;12(8):487-93.

[81] Antaki N, Bibert S, Kebbewar K, Asaad F, Baroudi O, Alideeb S, et al. IL28B polymorphisms do not predict response to therapy in chronic hepatitis C with HCV genotype 5. Gut [Internet]. 2012 févr 16 [cité 2012 avr 23]; Available de: http://www.ncbi.nlm.nih.gov/pubmed/22345656

[82] Kwo PY, Lawitz EJ, McCone J, Schiff ER, Vierling JM, Pound D, et al. Efficacy of boceprevir, an NS3 protease inhibitor, in combination with peginterferon alfa-2b and ribavirin in treatment-naive patients with genotype 1 hepatitis C infection (SPRINT-1): an open-label, randomised, multicentre phase 2 trial. Lancet. 2010 août 28;376(9742):705-16.

[83] Sherman KE, Flamm SL, Afdhal NH, Nelson DR, Sulkowski MS, Everson GT, et al. Response-guided telaprevir combination treatment for hepatitis C virus infection. N. Engl. J. Med. 2011 sept 15;365(11):1014-24.

[84] Ramachandran P, Fraser A, Agarwal K, Austin A, Brown A, Foster GR, et al. UK consensus guidelines for the use of the protease inhibitors boceprevir and telaprevir in genotype 1 chronic hepatitis C infected patients. Aliment. Pharmacol. Ther. 2012 mars;35(6):647-62.

[85] Sulkowski MS, Benhamou Y. Therapeutic issues in HIV/HCV-coinfected patients. J. Viral Hepat. 2007 juin;14(6):371-86.

[86] Halliday J, Klenerman P, Barnes E. Vaccination for hepatitis C virus: closing in on an evasive target. Expert Rev Vaccines. 2011 mai;10(5):659-72.

[87] Habersetzer F, Honnet G, Bain C, Maynard-Muet M, Leroy V, Zarski J-P, et al. A poxvirus vaccine is safe, induces T-cell responses, and decreases viral load in patients with chronic hepatitis C. Gastroenterology. 2011 sept;141(3):890-899.e1-4.

[88] Bellentani S, Pozzato G, Saccoccio G, Crovatto M, Crocè LS, Mazzoran L, et al. Clinical course and risk factors of hepatitis C virus related liver disease in the general population: report from the Dionysos study. Gut. 1999 juin;44(6):874-80.

[89] Pybus OG, Markov PV, Wu A, Tatem AJ. Investigating the endemic transmission of the hepatitis C virus. Int. J. Parasitol. 2007 juill;37(8-9):839-49.

[90] Agarwal SK. Hemodialysis of patients with HCV infection: isolation has a definite role. Nephron Clin Pract. 2011;117(4):c328-332.

[91] Sous le signe du «MATOS» Contextes, trajectoires, risques et sensations liés à l'injection de produits psychoactifs.

[92] Chossegros P. [Management of drug addiction in France (a short history)]. Gastroenterol. Clin. Biol. 2007 sept;31(8-9 Pt 3):4S44-50.

[93] EMCDDA–Europol 2011 Annual Report on the implementation of Council Decision 2005/387/JHA.

[94] Nelson PK, Mathers BM, Cowie B, Hagan H, Des Jarlais D, Horyniak D, et al. Global epidemiology of hepatitis B and hepatitis C in people who inject drugs: results of systematic reviews. Lancet. 2011 août 13;378(9791):571-83.

[95] Prévalence de l'usage problématique de drogues en France - estimations 2006. Saint-Denis, OFDT, 2009,. OFDT;

[96] Kuebler D, Hausser D, Gervasoni JP. The characteristics of « new users » of cocaine and heroin unknown to treatment agencies: results from the Swiss Hidden Population Study. Addiction. 2000 oct;95(10):1561-71.

[97] Fontaine A, Fontana C. Drogues, activité professionnelle et vie privée. OFDT. 2003;

[98] Dubois F, Desenclos JC, Mariotte N, Goudeau A. Hepatitis C in a French population-based survey, 1994: seroprevalence, frequency of viremia, genotype distribution, and risk factors. The Collaborative Study Group. Hepatology. 1997 juin;25(6):1490-6.

[99] INVS. Estimation des taux de prévalence des anticorps anti-VHC et des marqueurs du virus de l'hépatite B chez les assurés sociaux du régime général de France métropolitaine, 2003-2004. Analyse descriptive [Internet]. 2005. Available on: http://www.invs.sante.fr/publications/2005/analyse_descriptive_140205/index.html

[100] Emmanuelli J, Jauffret-Roustide M, Barin F. Epidémiologie du VHC chez les usagers de drogues, France, 1993-2002. BEH. 2003;97-9.

[101] Jauffret-Roustide M, Le Strat Y, Couturier E, Thierry D, Rondy M, Quaglia M, et al. A national cross-sectional study among drug-users in France: epidemiology of HCV

and highlight on practical and statistical aspects of the design. BMC Infect. Dis. 2009;9:113.

[102] Villano SA, Vlahov D, Nelson KE, Lyles CM, Cohn S, Thomas DL. Incidence and risk factors for hepatitis C among injection drug users in Baltimore, Maryland. J. Clin. Microbiol. 1997 dec;35(12):3274-7.

[103] van Beek I, Dwyer R, Dore GJ, Luo K, Kaldor JM. Infection with HIV and hepatitis C virus among injecting drug users in a prevention setting: retrospective cohort study. BMJ. 1998 aug 15;317(7156):433-7.

[104] Smyth BP, O'Connor JJ, Barry J, Keenan E. Retrospective cohort study examining incidence of HIV and hepatitis C infection among injecting drug users in Dublin. J Epidemiol Community Health. 2003 avr;57(4):310-1.

[105] Fuller CM, Ompad DC, Galea S, Wu Y, Koblin B, Vlahov D. Hepatitis C incidence--a comparison between injection and noninjection drug users in New York City. J Urban Health. 2004 mars;81(1):20-4.

[106] Stein MD, Herman DS, Anderson BJ. A trial to reduce hepatitis C seroincidence in drug users. J Addict Dis. 2009 oct;28(4):389-98.

[107] Garfein RS, Golub ET, Greenberg AE, Hagan H, Hanson DL, Hudson SM, et al. A peer-education intervention to reduce injection risk behaviors for HIV and hepatitis C virus infection in young injection drug users. AIDS. 2007 sept 12;21(14):1923-32.

[108] Abou-Saleh M, Davis P, Rice P, Checinski K, Drummond C, Maxwell D, et al. The effectiveness of behavioural interventions in the primary prevention of hepatitis C amongst injecting drug users: a randomised controlled trial and lessons learned. Harm Reduct J. 2008;5:25.

[109] Hagan H, Pouget ER, Des Jarlais DC. A systematic review and meta-analysis of interventions to prevent hepatitis C virus infection in people who inject drugs. J. Infect. Dis. 2011 juill 1;204(1):74-83.

[110] Mehta SH, Astemborski J, Kirk GD, Strathdee SA, Nelson KE, Vlahov D, et al. Changes in blood-borne infection risk among injection drug users. J. Infect. Dis. 2011 mars 1;203(5):587-94.

[111] Falster K, Kaldor JM, Maher L. Hepatitis C virus acquisition among injecting drug users: a cohort analysis of a national repeated cross-sectional survey of needle and syringe program attendees in Australia, 1995-2004. J Urban Health. 2009 janv; 86(1):106-18.

[112] Jauffret-Roustide M, Emmanuelli J, Desenclos JC. [Limited impact of the harm-reduction policy on HCV among drug-users. The ANRS-Coquelicot survey example]. Rev Epidemiol Sante Publique. 2006 juill;54 Spec No 1:1S53-51S59.

[113] Cazein F, Le Strat Y, Pillonel J, Lot F, Bousquet V, Pinget R, Le Vu S, Brand D, Brunet S, Thierry D, Leclerc M, Benyelles L, Couturier S, Da Costa C, Barin F, Semaille C. Dépistage du VIH et découvertes de séropositivité, France, 2003-2010. BEH. 2011;(43/44):446-54.

[114] Di Nino F, Imbs JL, Melenotte GH, le réseau RMS3, Doffoel M. Dépistage et traitement des hépatites C par le réseau des microstructures médicales chez les usagers de drogues en Alsace, France, 2006-2007. BEH. 2009;

[115] Patrick DM, Tyndall MW, Cornelisse PG, Li K, Sherlock CH, Rekart ML, et al. Incidence of hepatitis C virus infection among injection drug users during an outbreak of HIV infection. CMAJ. 2001 oct 2;165(7):889-95.

[116] Skidmore CA, Robertson JR, Robertson AA, Elton RA. After the epidemic: follow up study of HIV seroprevalence and changing patterns of drug use. BMJ. 1990 janv 27;300(6719):219-23.

[117] Tempalski B, Lieb S, Cleland CM, Cooper H, Brady JE, Friedman SR. HIV prevalence rates among injection drug users in 96 large US metropolitan areas, 1992-2002. J Urban Health. 2009 janv;86(1):132-54.

[118] Harm reduction: evidence, impacts and challenges. EMCDDA, Lisbon, April 2010:

[119] Institute of Medicine (U.S.). Committee on HIV Screening and Access to Care. HIV screening and access to care exploring the impact of policies on access to and provision of HIV Care. Washington, D.C.: National Academies Press; 2011.

[120] Colvin HM, Mitchell AE, Institute of Medicine (U.S.). Committee on the Prevention and Control of Viral Hepatitis Infections, Institute of Medicine (U.S.). Board on Population Health and Public Health Practice. Hepatitis and liver cancer a national strategy for prevention and control of hepatitis B and C [Internet]. Washington, DC: National Academies Press; 2010 [cité 2012 juin 8]. Available on: http://site.ebrary.com/id/10395833

[121] Expertise collective. Réduction des risques infectieux chez les usagers de drogues. INSERM; 2010.

[122] Costes JM, Cadet-Tairo A. Drug maintenance treatments in France: recent results 2004. OFDT; 2004.

[123] Phénomènes marquants et émergents en matière de drogues illicites (2010-2011). OFDT; 2012.

[124] Lurie P, Jones TS, Foley J. A sterile syringe for every drug user injection: how many injections take place annually, and how might pharmacists contribute to syringe distribution? J. Acquir. Immune Defic. Syndr. Hum. Retrovirol. 1998;18 Suppl 1:S45-51.

[125] Emmanuelli J, Desenclos J-C. Harm reduction interventions, behaviours and associated health outcomes in France, 1996-2003. Addiction. 2005 nov;100(11):1690-700.

[126] Bonnet N. [Pharmacy syringe exchange program for injection drug users]. Presse Med. 2006 déc;35(12 Pt 1):1811-8.

[127] Tempalski B, Cooper HL, Friedman SR, Des Jarlais DC, Brady J, Gostnell K. Correlates of syringe coverage for heroin injection in 35 large metropolitan areas in the US in which heroin is the dominant injected drug. Int. J. Drug Policy. 2008 avr;19 Suppl 1:S47-58.

[128] Leonard L, DeRubeis E, Pelude L, Medd E, Birkett N, Seto J. « I inject less as I have easier access to pipes »: injecting, and sharing of crack-smoking materials, decline as safer crack-smoking resources are distributed. Int. J. Drug Policy. 2008 juin;19(3):255-64.

[129] Volz E, Miller JC, Galvani A, Ancel Meyers L. Effects of heterogeneous and clustered contact patterns on infectious disease dynamics. PLoS Comput. Biol. 2011 juin;7(6):e1002042.

[130] Kretzschmar M, Mangen M-JJ, Pinheiro P, Jahn B, Fèvre EM, Longhi S, et al. New Methodology for Estimating the Burden of Infectious Diseases in Europe. PLoS Med. 2012 avr;9(4).

[131] Vickerman P, Martin N, Turner K, Hickman M. Can needle and syringe programmes and opiate substitution therapy achieve substantial reductions in HCV prevalence? Model projections for different epidemic settings. Addiction (Abingdon, England) [Internet]. 2012 mai 7 [cité 2012 mai 11]; Available de: http://www.ncbi.nlm.nih.gov/pubmed/22564041

[132] Birkhead GS, Klein SJ, Candelas AR, O'Connell DA, Rothman JR, Feldman IS, et al. Integrating multiple programme and policy approaches to hepatitis C prevention and care for injection drug users: a comprehensive approach. Int. J. Drug Policy. 2007 oct;18(5):417-25.

[133] Sylvestre DL, Zweben JE. Integrating HCV services for drug users: a model to improve engagement and outcomes. Int. J. Drug Policy. 2007 oct;18(5):406-10.

[134] Wilkinson M, Crawford V, Tippet A, Jolly F, Turton J, Sims E, et al. Community-based treatment for chronic hepatitis C in drug users: high rates of compliance with therapy despite ongoing drug use. Aliment. Pharmacol. Ther. 2009 janv;29(1):29-37.

[135] Vickerman P, Martin N, Hickman M. Can Hepatitis C virus treatment be used as a prevention strategy? Additional model projections for Australia and elsewhere. Drug Alcohol Depend. 2011 janv 15;113(2-3):83-85; discussion 86-87.

[136] Zeiler I, Langlands T, Murray JM, Ritter A. Optimal targeting of Hepatitis C virus treatment among injecting drug users to those not enrolled in methadone maintenance programs. Drug Alcohol Depend. 2010 août 1;110(3):228-33.

[137] Keverne EB, Curley JP. Epigenetics, brain evolution and behaviour. Front Neuroendocrinol. 2008 mai;29(3):398-412.

[138] Perfors A, Tenenbaum JB, Griffiths TL, Xu F. A tutorial introduction to Bayesian models of cognitive development. Cognition. 2011 sept;120(3):302-21.

[139] Cichy RM, Chen Y, Haynes J-D. Encoding the identity and location of objects in human LOC. Neuroimage. 2011 févr 1;54(3):2297-307.

[140] Dijksterhuis A, Aarts H. Goals, attention, and (un)consciousness. Annu Rev Psychol. 2010;61:467-90.

[141] Kompus K. Default mode network gates the retrieval of task-irrelevant incidental memories. Neurosci. Lett. 2011 janv 10;487(3):318-21.

[142] Holyoak KJ, Cheng PW. Causal learning and inference as a rational process: the new synthesis. Annu Rev Psychol. 2011;62:135-63.

[143] Winnicott DW. Playing and Reality. 2e éd. Routledge; 2005.

[144] Bowlby J. Attachment and Loss: Separation - Anxiety and Anger v. 2. New Ed. Penguin Books Ltd; 1975.

[145] Wallin DJ. Attachment in Psychotherapy. 1er éd. Guilford Press; 2007.

[146] Schmithorst VJ, Yuan W. White matter development during adolescence as shown by diffusion MRI. Brain Cogn. 2010 janv;72(1):16-25.

[147] Luhmann N. Social Systems. 1er éd. Stanford University Press; 1996.

[148] Lacan J. Les psychoses, 1955-1956. Editions du Seuil; 1981.

[149] Critchley S. Infinitely Demanding: Ethics of Commitment, Politics of Resistance. Verso Books; 2008.

[150] Zizek S, Santner EL, Reinhard K. The Neighbor: Three Inquiries in Political Theology. New edition. University of Chicago Press; 2006.

[151] Dahlstrom DO. Heidegger's Concept of Truth. 1er éd. Cambridge University Press; 2009.

[152] Moore D, Dray A, Green R, Hudson SL, Jenkinson JL, Siokou C, Perez P, Bammer G, Maher L, Dietze P. Extending drug ethno-epidemiology using agent-based modeling. Addiction. 2009. 104(12):1991-7.

[153] Festinger DS, Marlowe DB, Dugosh KL, Croft JR, Arabia PL. Higher magnitude cash payments improve research follow-up rates without increasing drug use or perceived coercion. Drug Alcohol Depend. 2008 juill 1;96(1-2):128-35.

[154] García-Fernández G, Secades-Villa R, García-Rodríguez O, Sánchez-Hervás E, Fernández-Hermida JR, Higgins ST. Adding voucher-based incentives to community reinforcement approach improves outcomes during treatment for cocaine dependence. Am J Addict. 2011 oct;20(5):456-61.

[155] Schulte B, Schütt S, Brack J, Isernhagen K, Deibler P, Dilg C, et al. Successful treatment of chronic hepatitis C virus infection in severely opioid-dependent patients under heroin maintenance. Drug Alcohol Depend. 2010 juin 1;109(1-3):248-51.

[156] Rehm J, Frick U, Hartwig C, Gutzwiller F, Gschwend P, Uchtenhagen A. Mortality in heroin-assisted treatment in Switzerland 1994-2000. Drug Alcohol Depend. 2005 août 1;79(2):137-43.

[157] Haasen C, Vertheim U, Eiroa-Orosa FJ, Schäfer I, Reimer J Is heroin-assisted treatment effective for patients with no previous maintenance treatment? Results form the German randomized controlled trial Eur. Addict. Res 2010

[158] Dijkgraaf MGW, van der Zanden BP, de Borgie CAJM, Blanken P, van Ree JM, van den Brink W. Cost utility analysis of co-prescribed heroin compared with methadone maintenance treatment in heroin addicts in two randomised trials. BMJ. 2005 juin 4;330(7503):1297.

[159] Frick U, Rehm J, Zullino D, Fernando M, Wiesbeck G, Ammann J, et al. Long-term follow-up of orally administered diacetylmorphine substitution treatment. Eur Addict Res. 2010;16(3):131-8.

[160] Small D, Glickman A, Rigter G, Walter T. The Washington Needle Depot: fitting healthcare to injection drug users rather than injection drug users to healthcare: moving from a syringe exchange to syringe distribution model. Harm Reduction J. 2010 january;7(1): 10.1186/1477-7517-7-1

[161] Snead J, Downing M, Lorvick J, Garcia B, Thawley R, Kegeles S, et al. Secondary syringe exchange among injection drug users. J Urban Health. 2003 juin;80(2):330-48.

[162] Hutchinson SJ, Taylor A, Goldberg DJ, Gruer L. Factors associated with injecting risk behaviour among serial community-wide samples of injecting drug users in Glasgow 1990-94: implications for control and prevention of blood-borne viruses. Addiction. 2000 juin;95(6):931-40.

[163] Cooper HLF, Des Jarlais DC, Ross Z, Tempalski B, Bossak B, Friedman SR. Spatial access to syringe exchange programs and pharmacies selling over-the-counter syringes as predictors of drug injectors' use of sterile syringes. Am J Public Health. 2011 juin;101(6):1118-25.

[164] Parkin S, Coomber R. Injecting drug user views (and experiences) of drug-related litter bins in public places: a comparative study of qualitative research findings obtained from UK settings. Health Place. 2011 nov;17(6):1218-27.

[165] Rhodes T, Kimber J, Small W, Fitzgerald J, Kerr T, Hickman M, et al. Public injecting and the need for « safer environment interventions » in the reduction of drug-related harm. Addiction. 2006 oct;101(10):1384-93.

[166] Building knowledge about community change : moving beyond evaluation. The Aspen Institute; Roundtable on community change 2004.

[167] Sobeck J, Agius E. Organizational capacity building: Addressing a research and practice gap. Evaluation and Program Planning 2007;30:237–246.

[168] Baser H. and Morgan P. 2008. Capacity, Change and Performance Study Report. (ECDPM Discussion Paper 59B). Maastricht: ECDPM.

[169] Owen J., Cook T., Jones E. Evaluating the early excellence initiative: the relationship between evaluation, performance management and practitioner participation Evaluation 2005;11:331-349.

[170] Tooke J. 283028/Report of the High Level Group on Clinical Effectiveness A report to Sir Liam Donaldson Chief Medical Officer Department of Health 2007

[171] Wodak A. Drug prohibition: it's broke, now go and fix it. Int. J. Drug Policy. 2012 janv;23(1):22-3.

[172] Room R, Reuter P. How well do international drug conventions protect public health? Lancet. 2012 janv 7;379(9810):84-91.

[173] Bewley-Taylor D, Jelsma M. Regime change: re-visiting the 1961 Single Convention on Narcotic Drugs. Int. J. Drug Policy. 2012 janv;23(1):72-81.

[174] Okrent D. Last call: The rise and fall of prohibition. Scribner 2011.

[175] Drug war facts. Ed; McVay A. 2007. www.drugwarfacts.org.

[176] Marez C. Drug wars: the political economy of narcotics. Univ Of Minnesota Press 2004.

[177] Wyler LS, Cook N. Illegal drug trade in Africa: Trends and U.S. policy. CRS Report for Congress 2009.

[178] World drug reports –Global illicit drug trends UNODC 1999-2012. http://www.unodc.org/unodc/en/data-and-analysis/WDR.html

[179] MacCourt RJ. Reuter P. Drug war heresies: learning from other vices, times, and places (RAND studies in Policy Analysis). Cambridge University Press 2001.

[180] McCoy. The politics of heroin: CIA complicity in the global drug trade 1991

[181] Scott PD, American war machine: deep politics, the CIA global drug connection and the road to Afghanistan. Rowman & Littlefield Publishers 2010.

Permissions

The contributors of this book come from diverse backgrounds, making this book a truly international effort. This book will bring forth new frontiers with its revolutionizing research information and detailed analysis of the nascent developments around the world.

We would like to thank David Belin, PhD, for lending his expertise to make the book truly unique. He has played a crucial role in the development of this book. Without his invaluable contribution this book wouldn't have been possible. He has made vital efforts to compile up to date information on the varied aspects of this subject to make this book a valuable addition to the collection of many professionals and students.

This book was conceptualized with the vision of imparting up-to-date information and advanced data in this field. To ensure the same, a matchless editorial board was set up. Every individual on the board went through rigorous rounds of assessment to prove their worth. After which they invested a large part of their time researching and compiling the most relevant data for our readers. Conferences and sessions were held from time to time between the editorial board and the contributing authors to present the data in the most comprehensible form. The editorial team has worked tirelessly to provide valuable and valid information to help people across the globe.

Every chapter published in this book has been scrutinized by our experts. Their significance has been extensively debated. The topics covered herein carry significant findings which will fuel the growth of the discipline. They may even be implemented as practical applications or may be referred to as a beginning point for another development. Chapters in this book were first published by InTech; hereby published with permission under the Creative Commons Attribution License or equivalent.

The editorial board has been involved in producing this book since its inception. They have spent rigorous hours researching and exploring the diverse topics which have resulted in the successful publishing of this book. They have passed on their knowledge of decades through this book. To expedite this challenging task, the publisher supported the team at every step. A small team of assistant editors was also appointed to further simplify the editing procedure and attain best results for the readers.

Our editorial team has been hand-picked from every corner of the world. Their multi-ethnicity adds dynamic inputs to the discussions which result in innovative outcomes. These outcomes are then further discussed with the researchers and contributors who give their valuable feedback and opinion regarding the same. The feedback is then collaborated with the researches and they are edited in a comprehensive manner to aid the understanding of the subject.

Apart from the editorial board, the designing team has also invested a significant amount of their time in understanding the subject and creating the most relevant covers. They scrutinized every image to scout for the most suitable representation of the subject and create an appropriate cover for the book.

The publishing team has been involved in this book since its early stages. They were actively engaged in every process, be it collecting the data, connecting with the contributors or procuring relevant information. The team has been an ardent support to the editorial, designing and production team. Their endless efforts to recruit the best for this project, has resulted in the accomplishment of this book. They are a veteran in the field of academics and their pool of knowledge is as vast as their experience in printing. Their expertise and guidance has proved useful at every step. Their uncompromising quality standards have made this book an exceptional effort. Their encouragement from time to time has been an inspiration for everyone.

The publisher and the editorial board hope that this book will prove to be a valuable piece of knowledge for researchers, students, practitioners and scholars across the globe.

List of Contributors

David Belin
INSERM European Associated Laboratory, Psychobiology of Compulsive Habits, UK
INSERM U1084 - LNEC & Université de Poitiers, AVENIR Team Psychobiology of Compulsive Disorders, Poitiers, France

Jérôme Lacoste
Unité de Recherche Clinique Intersectorielle, Centre Hospitalier Henri-Laborit, Poitiers, France

Jennifer E. Murray
Department of Experimental Psychology, University of Cambridge, Cambridge, UK
INSERM European Associated Laboratory, Psychobiology of Compulsive Habits, UK

Zheng-Xiong Xi
National Institute on Drug Abuse, Intramural Research Program, National Institutes of Health, Baltimore, MD, USA

Marta Rodríguez-Arias and María Asunción Aguilar
University of Valencia, Spain

Cynara Teixeira Ribeiro
Pontifícia Universidade Católica de São Paulo (PUC/SP), Brazil
Universidade Federal da Bahia (UFBA), Brazil
Universidade Federal Rural do Semi-Arido (UFERSA), Brazil

Andréa Hortélio Fernandes
Université de Paris VII, France
Universidade Federal da Bahia, Brazil

Paolo Stocco
Therapeutic Community "Villa Renata", Venice, Italy

Nicoletta Capra
Mother-Child Therapeutic Community "Casa Aurora e Villa Emma," Venice, Italy

Alessandra Simonelli and Francesca De Palo
Department of Developmental and Social Psychology, Padua University, Italy

Andrea Leonardi, Sonia Scavelli and Gianluca Ciuffardi
Fondazione Franceschi Onlus, Italy

Philippe Chossegros
UHSI Lyon, Hospives Civils de Lyon, French National Coordination of Healthcare Networks, France

Printed in the USA
CPSIA information can be obtained
at www.ICGtesting.com
JSHW011411221024
72173JS00003B/504

9 781632 424099